# LPN *to* RN
# TRANSITIONS

# LPN *to* RN TRANSITIONS

## ACHIEVING SUCCESS IN YOUR NEW ROLE

Second Edition

**Nicki Harrington, RN, MAEd, MSN, EdD**
Superintendent / President
Yuba Community College District
Marysville, California

**Cynthia Lee Terry, RN, MSN, CCRN**
Associate Professor
Health Sciences Division
Lehigh Carbon Community College
Schnecksville, Pennsylvania

Staff Nurse per Diem
Warren Hospital
Phillipsburg, New Jersey

Outdoor Emergency Care Instructor
National Ski Patrol
Blue Mountain Ski Area
Palmerton, Pennsylvania

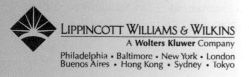
LIPPINCOTT WILLIAMS & WILKINS
A **Wolters Kluwer** Company
Philadelphia • Baltimore • New York • London
Buenos Aires • Hong Kong • Sydney • Tokyo

Acquisitions Editor: Lisa Stead
Assistant Editor: Susan Rainey
Senior Production Editor: Rosanne Hallowell
Senior Production Manager: Helen Ewan
Managing Editor / Production: Erika Kors
Design Coordinator: Brett MacNaughton

Interior Design: Joan Wendt
Cover Design: Melissa Walter
Manufacturing Manager: William Alberti
Indexer: Alexandra Nickerson
Compositor: Lippincott Williams & Wilkins
Printer: R. R. Donnelley

Second Edition

9 8 7 6 5 4 3 2 1

**Library of Congress Cataloging-in-Publication Data**
Harrington, Nicki.
  LPN to RN transitions : achieving success in your new role / Nicki harrington, Cynthia Lee Terry.-- 2nd ed.
    p. ; cm.
Includes bibliographical references and index.
ISBN 0-7817-3693-5 (pbk. : alk. paper)
  1. Nursing--Vocational guidance. 2. practical nurses. I. Terry, Cynthia Lee. II. Title.
[DNLM: 1. Nursing—Examination Questions. 2. Career Mobility--Examination
Questions. 3. Nurses--psychology--Examination Questions. 4. Nursing,
Practical--Examination Questions. WY 18.2 H311L2003]
RT82.H37 2003
610.73'06'9--dc21                                        2002043365

Care has been taken to confirm the accuracy of the information presented and to describe generally accepted practices. However, the authors, editors, and publisher are not responsible for errors or omissions or for any consequences from application of the information in this book and make no warranty, express or implied, with respect to the content of the publication.

The authors, editors, and publisher have exerted every effort to ensure that drug selection and dosage set forth in this text are in accordance with the current recommendations and practice at the time of publication. However, in view of ongoing research, changes in government regulations, and the constant flow of information relating to drug therapy and drug reactions, the reader is urged to check the package insert for each drug for any change in indications and dosage and for added warnings and precautions This is particularly important when the recommended agent is a new or infrequently employed drug.

Some drugs and medical devices presented in this publication have Food and Drug Administration (FDA) clearance for limited use in restricted research settings. It is the responsibility of the health care provider to ascertain the FDA status of each drug or device planned for use in his or her clinical practice.

LWW.com

*To all the LPN/LVN students and their families and significant others who gave up so much of their personal lives to nurture and grow another professional registered nurse for the good of humankind*

*—Nicki Harrington*

*To my father and mothers: To Don Shoop, my father, who has been an excellent mentor and role model—you have led by example and showed me that it is tough but rewarding to "stay the course" and "climb the ladder" of life. To Shirley Shoop, my birth mother—I thank you for your friendship, counsel, and loyalty through good and troubled times. To my newest mother, Nancy Shoop—you are kind, gentle, caring and supportive, which is more welcomed than you know.*

*—Cindy Terry*

# Reviewers

**Carol Ann Alexander, MSN, RN**
Associate Professor
Nursing Department
Palm Beach Community College
Lake Worth, Florida

**Fran Hammerly, RN, MSN, CNS**
Associate Professor
Associate Degree in Nursing Department
Stark State College of Technology
Canton, Ohio

**Eileen Klein, EdD, MSN, RN**
Task Force Chair Health Sciences
Austin Community College
Austin, Texas

**Roselena Thorpe**
Professor and Department Chairperson
Nursing Department
Community College of Allegheny County, Allegheny Campus
Pittsburgh, Pennsylvania

**Lisa Wehner**
Associate Professor
Nursing and Allied Health Department
State University of New York at Delhi
Delhi, New York

# Preface

The huge leap into the rigors of academic life is a monumental decision for the LPN/LVN. The process is a personal and financial risk, fraught with extreme highs and frustrating lows. In keeping with the ever-changing health care arena and with the practice of nursing, the revisers and editors of *LPN to RN Transitions: Achieving Success in Your New Role*, second edition, have attempted to take constructive criticism from our student and faculty users. Our hope is that we have simplified some of the complexities that existed in the first edition and added some exciting new features to help ensure a successful transition to the RN role.

We have added vignettes involving real student experiences at the beginning of each chapter. This is our attempt to assist the reader in realizing that the adventure of associate degree nursing is not an isolated one, but is shared by other students making the same journey. We have also rearranged chapters in the first section so students will not have to wade through theory (Chapters 2 through 4) before obtaining practical information (Chapter 1) that will be immediately useful in their transition process. Also, the chapter on communication (Chapter 10) now comes before the chapter on teaching (Chapter 11). The Legal and Ethical Issues chapter in the first edition was split into two separate chapters in this edition: Chapter 15, Legal Accountability, and Chapter 16, Ethical Issues.

NCLEX-RN style questions have been added to most chapters to help the student adjust to this testing style. The new National League for Nursing Core Competencies for Associate Degree Nurses have also been added. The Thinking Critically feature and the Student Exercises have been retained and can be useful when explored by the student independently, in class, or during on-line discussions. Updated resources and websites have been added at the end of chapters; it is our hope that students will use these for further individual exploration or as a beginning point for future projects. All of these features should provide the student with useful tools to successfully balance career, school, and personal lives while pursuing their goals.

*Nicki Harrington, RN, MAEd, MSN, EdD*
*Cynthia Lee Terry, RN, MSN, CCRN*

# Acknowledgments

I would like to thank my LPN students, who have challenged and shifted my vision of nursing and nursing education. I would also like to thank the 7P-7A shift staff in the ICU at Warren Hospital, Phillipsburg, New Jersey. You keep me grounded—thank you. A thanks goes out to Acquisitions Editor Lisa Stead who has edited this project from the get-go, and to Assistant Editor Susan Rainey. Your consistent patience, wisdom, and faithfulness to Nicki and me made this project happen. Thanks to Nicki Harrington who has been the historian for this project and who gave us all a "West Coast" perspective.

*— Cindy Terry*

I would like to thank the many individuals who supported me in the writing of this book. To the many LVN-to-RN students in the past with whom I shared learning experiences in the classroom as their teacher, I thank you for your inspiration which continues with me today. It was the memory of your struggles that kept me focused on your needs throughout my writing.

To my co-author, Cindy Terry, thank you for your hard work, patience, and perseverance, and your contributions to the profession of nursing.

To my father, whose spirit is still with me, and to my mother, who continues to believe in me and support me, I thank you for the values you have modeled and instilled in me throughout my life.

Finally, and with greatest appreciation, I want to thank Jim, my husband, partner, and best friend in life, for his enduring love and support, and Cayden Chance, our beautiful son, who always keeps me focused on the most important things in life—God's gifts of love and life.

*— Nicki Harrington*

# Contents

**UNIT II**
# Core Competencies for Professional Nursing Practice

# UNIT   III
# Role Concepts Essential for RN Practice

## PART A:  Provider of Care

## PART B:  Manager of Care

# The Transition Process

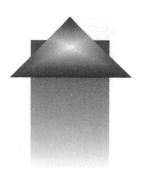

# C H A P T E R 1

# Lifelong Learning: Returning to School

*By the end of this chapter, the student will be able to:*

1. Describe the importance of lifelong learning in nursing.
2. Describe the process of re-entry into the role of student.
3. Outline the stages of the return to the student role.
4. Describe diverse learning styles.
5. Compare personal learning style with those described by theorists.
6. Develop beginning strategies for being successful in college.
7. Summarize learning resources that enhance the student's ability to be successful.
8. Discuss methods to manage time effectively.
9. Give examples of effective study skills and strategies.
10. Apply positive approaches to the educational process.

## KEY TERMS

abstract conceptualization
active experimentation
active learning
assertiveness
concrete experimentation
creative thinking
critical thinking
disintegration
diverse learning styles
diversity
educationally mobile
honeymoon

learning style
lifelong learning
mentor
re-entry process
reflective observation
reintegration
resolution
return to school syndrome (RTSS)
teaching–learning environment
time management
win/win agreement

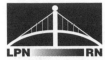

**VIGNETTE**

Sandy Martin has been an LPN for 10 years. She has always wanted to go back to school for her RN, but since her graduation from school, marriage and a full-time job at the skilled nursing facility have kept her very busy. Then she had two children, a mortgage, and all the trappings that come with life. There never seemed to be the time for herself. With her two children now in middle and high school, plus the nursing shortage at its highest in years, Sandy has decided to begin working part time and go back to school as a part-time student seeking an ADN. However, as she waits to talk to the nursing advisor about class requirements and prerequisites, Sandy is worried. Can she really meet all the obligations she currently has and go back to college part time? It is going to take her at least 3 to 5 years to finish her degree, and this is a bit discouraging. Also, will she remember enough after all these years? She remembers the struggles she had with anatomy, physiology, and pharmacology, as well as her fear of clinical rotations and assignments. Those fears will be revisited again. She also fears she will not "fit in" with students who may be much younger. She hopes the nursing advisor will be able to help her with all this.

Remember when you first made the decision to be a nurse? For many people, that desire to be a nurse revolved around wanting to help people who could not help themselves and putting caring into action. However, with your experience in the world of nursing as a licensed practical/vocational nurse (LPN/LVN), your vision and opinions of nursing may have changed somewhat. Perhaps your view of nursing differs from the views of other nurses. Your reasons for returning to school reflect changes in your life. Your reasons may include the desire to have more job opportunities, increase your job satisfaction, or expand the scope of your responsibilities, or you may be seeking self-improvement.

The fact that you are returning to school reflects the positive impact of the many changes that have occurred in your life and in society. At one time, a diploma from a school of practical/vocational nursing was seen as a terminal process; the LPN/LVN would not seek higher education. If an LPN/LVN wanted to continue her or his nursing education, it often meant starting over. Changes in the educational system have enhanced your ability to further your education and to pursue an associate or baccalaureate degree in nursing.

## Lifelong Learning in Nursing

In 1998, the National League for Nursing (NLN) convened a task force to examine competencies needed by ADN graduates. The task force identified 51 assumptions about the practice of the associate degree nurse of the future. Participation in lifelong learning was among these assumptions (NLN, 2000).

Not only advances in the healthcare industry, but also technological advances and societal trends require nurses to be continually updating their knowledge and practices. In establishing the *Scope and Standards of Practice for Nursing Professional Development*, the American Nurses Association (ANA, 2000) states the belief, "Lifelong learning is the responsibility of the nurse and is essential to maintain and increase competence in nursing practice" (p.1). Katz (1999) notes that "nursing is a career for those who want to be lifelong learners" (p. 77).

# The Re-entry Process: Overcoming Barriers and Fears

Your return to school is important, although you may be as hesitant about the prospect as was Sandy Martin. It also is a challenge and an adventure. You may have fears, whether you have been out of school for only a brief time or for many years. These fears should diminish after a few months. Returning to academic life is not easy. The thought of new risks or the return to old roles may be frightening. Other factors may relate to your desire to be highly successful in the educational process, while also wanting to be successful as an employee, a parent, a spouse, or in other roles. Although you have individual issues as you return to school, you will find you have some elements in common with others. It is time to examine what it means to return to school and to determine what strategies will best help you cope, succeed, and achieve satisfaction in the process.

Returning to the role of the student nurse involves more than taking a deep breath and mustering the courage to face what is familiar and yet completely unknown. There may be barriers and fears to overcome to make the move back to academic life. For some returning students, this section will not apply. You may not have experienced any apprehension about the re-entry process and feel well prepared to accept the challenges that lie ahead. However, for most students, some or all of this will be familiar. For this reason, common barriers and fears that are seen with the re-entry process are presented. The Thinking Critically activity in this section provides you with the opportunity to examine your own issues.

## Age

One of your perceived barriers in returning to school may be your age. You may feel that it has been too many years since you were in school. You also may fear that the other students will be much younger and you might have little in common; you will find that this is probably not the case. Related to this may be the thought that your academic ability is less than what is needed and that you haven't had to study intensively for a long time. Attaining a college degree may seem like an out-of-reach dream. The mystique that surrounds college course work can be intimidating. As an older student, you may fear that you do not have the intellectual skills to succeed or that younger students will think you are inferior.

## Ethnicity and Gender

Another barrier may be related to ethnic or gender issues. You will be joining an academic community that may differ from your LPN/LVN program. It can be emotionally difficult to look different or be different from other students, particularly in a setting in which you may already feel discomfort. Again, there may be the fear that you will not have anything in common with your classmates. However, nursing in general has become much more diverse. Ethnic and cultural diversity and the addition of greater numbers of men have made the profession of nursing more real and worldly. Academic settings also have benefited from diversity because students have more opportunities to learn from each other's experiences and world views and to relate to a more diverse client population.

The percentage of nurses who are men has increased from less than 1% in 1966 to 5% in 1996, with 12% to 13% of nursing students in 1996 being male (Katz, Carter, Bishop, & Kravits, 2000. Likewise, today's college classroom has a wider diversity of students than ever before. Crews, North, and Thompson (2001) state, "In its broadest sense, diversity includes the following: ethnicity, racial background, economic status, physical and mental ability, and the aspects of culture that include nuances of language, heritage, personal behavior, and self-identification" (p. 97). Within this diverse environment, you will find other students with whom you will have cultural values and interests in common.

## Fear of Nursing Faculty and Today's Classroom

A common fear of returning students is a dread of the nursing faculty. This may be related to previous experiences with nursing instructors or to stories you may have heard from other students. However, nursing faculties are also increasingly diverse. As with other professionals, each instructor has various strengths and weaknesses. Some may intimidate you or expect you to know more than you do. Some may treat you as a novice, whereas others will treat you as the adult learner that you are. You will undoubtedly find that you relate well with some of the faculty and have difficulty relating to others. Nursing faculty members are similar to you: unique and imperfect but dedicated to their profession.

You may also be intimidated by today's classroom environment. Perhaps your LPN/LVN program theory content was delivered in an all-lecture format. Today's ADN students are active participants in a teaching–learning environment that uses collaborative work groups, case studies, learning contracts, role playing, debates, and other interactive processes to foster critical and creative thinking.

The teacher's role is to facilitate learning, ensure relevance and inclusiveness of the diversity of learners, and assist students with attitudes and techniques to strengthen their motivation to learn (Eisen & Tisdell, 2000; Lowenstein & Bradshaw, 2000; Musinski, 1999; Ruggiero, 1998; Schoolcraft & Novotny, 2000; Ulrich & Glendon, 1999; Wlodkowski, 1999). Cerbin (2000) notes,

> I am suggesting that what is important is not just what students know, but how they think with what they know. A teacher who is attuned to students' thinking will make different decisions about what to tell students and how to support the development of their understanding, than a teacher who simply lectures according to pre-planned and inalterable syllabus. (p. 17)

As a returning student, this "new" classroom environment may make you uneasy, and it could take you several months to become comfortable in this more active student role.

# Financial and Family Constraints

Another barrier in your return to school may be financial or family constraints. The student role may require financial sacrifices. Tuition, books, and commuting costs are big burdens. The necessity to remain employed and/or find and finance child care may add to these pressures. Often children or other family members also need your time and support. Although they may support your desire to return to school, they may also want life to remain unchanged. Another related factor is that life does not stop while you are in school. Illnesses and crises may occur. Although you have planned for many things, the unexpected and unplanned may occur.

# Fear of Failure

A last barrier to returning to school is fear of failure. You have invested a lot of time and effort to be where you are today. Taking exams and being observed in the clinical area can be frightening. The fear of not being successful as a student nurse can be overwhelming. Some of this may stem from previous school experiences or from lack of self-confidence. Adult learners typically are hard on themselves because they not only want to be successful, they also want to be perfect. It often takes frequent reminders that the learning process and the transition process need not be perfect, only positive. In addition, many factors are involved as a student progresses through a nursing program, not the least of which are the multiple responsibilities.

Later in this chapter, some strategies for dealing with your fears are presented. All of these barriers and fears are real and are shared by others returning to school. For instance, as you get to know your classmates, you will find that your age, experience, and unique qualities are valuable to other class members. It may be advantageous to have had the experience of raising a family or to be of a particular culture. Your concerns about studying may be the same as a fellow student; you may find that you will be able to assist each other. You also may find that your studying skills did not disappear and that you are more organized and able to be more effective in completing the assigned work. Other students may provide insight into particular courses or instructors. Financial concerns are experienced by many, and you may find that you can share commuting costs, child care, or other resources. It is beneficial to identify your fears and concerns as you return to school. You may find they

## ▶ Thinking Critically

After reading the previous section, you may have found yourself nodding your head in recognition or wondering why your fears and concerns were not voiced. At this point, identify the barriers and fears that you face as you return to school. Include all of them, whether or not they have been mentioned. If you have determined some solutions, include those as well. As a next step, talk with a fellow student or another nurse at work who returned to school to determine if you share common concerns. You also may find it useful, as did the student in the opening vignette, to share these concerns with your nursing advisor. This is a beginning step in preparing for success upon returning to school.

are common to other students as well, and together you can find answers and solutions. It also may be reassuring to know that you are not alone.

## Returning to the Student Role: ▬▬▬▬
## "Returning to School Syndrome"

Donea Shane (1983) has identified the process of re-entry as the returning to school syndrome (RTSS). She studied educationally mobile nursing students as they returned to school and was able to identify stages that comprise an entire syndrome. Educationally mobile nurses are those who are returning to school or at least contemplating such a return. Shane's work was derived from the stories and data collected during a period of 6 years from those studying to become registered nurses (RNs). Those students were able to "share their insecurities, sorrows, failures, and anxieties as well as their triumphs, humor, and joy" (Shane, 1983, p. vii). The results of her work remain valuable today.

Shane defines RTSS as up and down emotional swings that are experienced in some way by nursing students who are returning to school. These experiences occur because returning students are familiar with their nursing roles within the work setting yet are taking on a different role by becoming nursing students again. The RTSS model depicts a series of sequential stages. "However, an individual nurse may not proceed through these phases in a linear fashion. The usual progression is an irregular one, with relapses, detours, and expressways through certain stages" (Shane, 1983, p. 73). Shane identifies three major stages within the RTSS syndrome. **Table 1-1** provides a summary of RTSS.

**TABLE 1-1**
RETURNING TO SCHOOL SYNDROME

| Stage | Description |
|---|---|
| Honeymoon | Individual is happy and delighted about being back in school; does not see any problems with the process. |
| Conflict | Characterized by high anxiety; individual feels conflict about educational process, and role changes. |
| a. Disintegration | a. Individual represses feelings of anger and hostility; may become depressed and sullen. |
| b. Reintegration | b. Person becomes outwardly hostile and angry, particularly with nursing faculty; individual is frustrated with the educational program. |
| Resolution | There are a variety of forms in the process of resolving conflicts. |
| a. Chronic conflict | a. The student nurse maintains angry feelings and fails to see anything worthwhile or valuable in the educational process. |
| b. False acceptance | b. Individual pretends to accept the changes in role but actually, does not understand or see any difference. |
| c. Oscillation | c. The educationally mobile nurse vacillates between stages; generally involves regression if a stressful event occurs; once the stressor is resolved, the person moves to a more positive resolution. |
| d. Biculturalism | d. A positive resolution in which the individual accepts the differences and role values and is challenged to grow within the professional role. |

## Stage 1: Honeymoon

Typically, the shortest and most benign stage is called the honeymoon stage. It is a somewhat blissful time, in which the reality of a situation has not quite sunk in. Individuals are generally happy about being in school and see the school experience as congenial. The end of the honeymoon usually occurs when the educationally mobile nurse is enrolled in the first clinical nursing course. At this point, the student can feel intimidated and may fear that experience is no longer of value. In particular, the dreaded clinical evaluation looms ahead and causes the individual greatly increased anxiety.

## Stage 2: Conflict

Shane suggests that the longest and most intense phase is conflict. It is a difficult time and can be emotionally exhausting and overwhelming. In general, the educationally mobile nurse experiences conflicts with beliefs, family roles, work roles, prior knowledge versus new knowledge, and nursing faculty. Such nurses may believe that there is no difference in the educational programs, that they already know what they need to know to be RNs, or that they are already better than the graduates of this program. Thus, nothing will change by continuing the educational process. Work role conflicts arise from realism versus idealism. Working nurses know and understand the real work world and dispute the idealistic presentations, or they feel guilty because they cannot practice as the ideal would have it. Other conflicts also arise, such as stressful relationships with clinical faculty or dealing with various teaching styles.

The conflict stage is subdivided into two parts: disintegration and reintegration. Disintegration is characterized by a state of anxiety in which the individual turns anxious feelings inward. This can result in several negative feelings that are potentially harmful: depression; sadness; withdrawal from friends, family, and others; and attitudes of obstinacy and gloom. It is remarkable that significant people who have contact with this person are able to overlook these behaviors or do not notice them.

Reintegration is marked by outwardly intense feelings of frustration and hostility that are directed toward those around the individual, especially the faculty. This anger is the result of the individual's frustrations with the nursing program or with the whole educational process. Although these outbursts are difficult to deal with, Shane considers them healthier than the repression of feelings that is seen in disintegration.

## Stage 3: Resolution

The third and final stage, resolution, is a variable phase because each individual has different lengths of time and outcomes. Shane (1983) presents a few of the forms that resolution can take.

1. **Chronic conflict.** This resolution is the least effective because these nurses become stuck in a quagmire of anger. They may continue with their nursing education, but they fail to recognize the value of their education or the inherent worth of the role change. They spend valuable energy and time being angry and belligerent and have little energy to put into creating a positive outcome.

2. **False acceptance**. This resolution also is not considered particularly positive. Educationally mobile nurses play games of deceit and pretense. They may claim to accept the differences in the former work role and the present educational role, and the value of the new role, but do not actually recognize any difference. They also cannot perceive the positive aspects of the education and the transition. In some regards, they become their own victims by not realizing any difference or usefulness in the process.

3. **Oscillation**. Individuals who fall into this category vacillate between the various resolutions. To some degree, their oscillation occurs because they have experienced each resolution in various forms. Fortunately, oscillation is reversible. An oscillation (most frequently a regression to a more negative state) usually occurs because of some unusual stressor, such as failure on an exam, an illness at home, or an unfortunate interchange with a faculty member.

4. **Biculturalism**. This resolution is the most positive. These educationally mobile nurses have positive feelings about their previous educational experiences. They also value their current education and their growth within the nursing profession. It is important to them to be challenged and to develop their professional roles.

The RTSS presents an interesting way to view the re-entry process. You may recognize the various emotional states. However, Shane also finds that a few educationally mobile nurses deny that any of the RTSS concepts apply to them. These nurses resent being analyzed and categorized. Behavior and role changes are not uniformly valued in the educational process. It is even more difficult to identify your own emotions and feelings. The value of understanding this syndrome is that it provides you with some insights into the conflicts and concerns that can arise when you are dealing with role change and changes in your own beliefs, and can affirm that these are normal responses.

## Diverse Learning Styles

The process of learning often seems to be formidable, particularly if the learner has not been engaged in formal learning activities for several years or if previous experiences were not especially positive. Adults have long been occupied with the tasks of return-

---

### NCLEX–RN Might Ask 1-1

The student nurse is studying about theories of adjustment to nursing school. The stage of Shane's theory that describes developing family conflicts, conflicts between the real and ideal nursing world, and feelings of being exhausted and overwhelmed is the _____ stage of the returning to school syndrome.

    A. Honeymoon
    B. Disintegration
    C. Reintegration
    D. Resolution

• *See Appendix A for correct answer and rationale.*

> ## ▶ Thinking Critically

After reading about the RTSS, consider how these phases apply to you in your own LPN/LVN to RN role transition. For example, recall your practical/vocational nursing education experience. Was it positive or negative? In thinking about the role change from LPN/LVN to RN, what do you value about this process? Have you experienced any of the emotions described in the explanation of RTSS? As you consider these questions, write down what you are experiencing and why. You may find it helpful to keep a journal as you progress through this role transition, or make a note on your calendar to review this material again after taking your first clinical course.

ing to educational settings in which they can pursue educational activities. Many adults fear that they will not be capable of learning new information or that they will not be able to focus because their other life involvements and interests will interfere too much. However, for most adults, it is a pleasant surprise when they are able to acknowledge that not only are they still able to learn, but that they also are more focused and dedicated than in previous educational endeavors.

## Adult Learning Styles

Learning styles of adults differ from those of children. Adults have a different and clearer sense of themselves, what their purpose is in a particular educational endeavor, what is worthwhile, and what is not. Adults are able to draw on their experiences to gain deeper and more meaningful understanding. There also is a greater capacity to apply theoretical concepts to practical situations. This section focuses exclusively on adult learners, with an emphasis on the value of adult experiences.

Kolb (1984) has defined learning as a process of experiential transformation. Another author develops this further by stating that learning from experience changes what we do and how we see things (Cell, 1984). From a more formal perspective, learning is an active process in which the participant engages in activities that provide knowledge, practice, and abstract skills. Styles of learning are the methods that the learner prefers to use for perceiving and processing new information (Ellis, 1994).

## Perceiving and Processing Tasks

It is advantageous to be aware of diverse learning styles to recognize that there are differences, to use strengths, and to adapt when the learning styles of others are predominant. Ellis (1994) identifies styles of learning as involving two tasks: perceiving and processing. He summarizes two methods of perceiving.

*Some people perceive by:*
    Using concrete experimentation;
    Dealing with situations with an intuitive ability to problem solve;
    Sensing and feeling; and
    Taking the initiative in unstructured settings.

*Other people perceive by:*

> Using abstract conceptualization;
> Thinking about things completely and analytically;
> Using a scientific approach to problem solving; and
> Functioning well within structured settings.
> Along with styles of perception, Ellis (1994) also has delineated two styles of processing.

*Some people process new information by:*

> Active experimentation;
> Applying new information in practical situations; and
> Seeing results despite potential risks/

*Others process by:*

> Reflective observation;
> Consideration of various points of view; and
> Presenting different ideas about a specific situation.

As Ellis (1994) emphasizes, these categories are not absolute, but they indicate extremes connected by "continuous lines between abstract and concrete, between reflecting and experimenting. In their learning styles, people can fall onto any point along those lines" (p. 53). Refer to **Display 1-1** for a review of terms used in this section.

## Four Styles of Learning

When considering the different styles of perceiving and processing, four distinct styles of learning emerge (Ellis, 1994). The following material has been adapted from Ellis' book *Becoming a Master Student*. Each learning style presented is intended as a guide for you to begin thinking about your own learning preferences.

---

**Display 1-1** **Review of Terminology**

**Abstract conceptualization:** a mode of perceiving new knowledge that entails an ability to analyze, think through, and organize theoretical material in a logical way

**Active experimentation:** a method to process information that involves a hands-on approach to be able to apply new information; implies that an individual wants to work with an idea or concept to determine if it makes sense

**Concrete experimentation:** a means to perceive new information in a more passive way; involves approaching situations in a more observational manner, preferring to look at a situation from several viewpoints and ponder various ideas

**Experiential learning:** a process of learning that evolves and is evolving as an individual matures and has a wider range of experiences; involves adaptation and growth, and increased self-awareness

**Learning style:** preferred methods to perceive and process new information

**Reflective observation:** a method of processing information that involves careful observation and a pondering about those observations; judgments occur after the individual has contemplated several alternatives

There is no hierarchal design in the four learning styles; each has validity and usefulness. It is helpful to review each style and identify the characteristics that best describe your own learning preferences. This is intended to assist you in increasing your self-awareness. You will discover that you probably draw from all four categories and that it often depends on the particular situation, the context, or your experiences.

## STYLE 1 LEARNERS

Perception of new information is best accomplished with concrete experiences. These learners prefer to find examples of how particular information applies to their world. They use reflective observation to process new learning. Characteristics may include:

- Viewing concrete situations from different points of view;
- Approaching events as observers;
- Reflecting on situations rather than taking action;
- Enjoying experiences that necessitate creation of ideas;
- Using imagination;
- Working for harmony and developing support; and
- Placing importance on concerns, caring, and trust in others.

**Goals:** being involved in important issues, bringing harmony
**Favorite questions:** Why? Why do I need to know this? Why should I attend this class? How do these concepts relate to my life?
**Skills:** valuing—brainstorming, listening, speaking, interacting, feeling, data gathering, imaging
**Preferred skill:** problem identification

## STYLE 2 LEARNERS

These learners perceive best through abstract conceptualization. Explanations through lecture style are favored, particularly if a theoretical base is included. They process new information generally by reflective observation. Characteristics may include:

- Understanding a broad range of information;
- Compiling information in a concise and logical form;
- Being interested more in abstract ideas and less in people;
- Favoring theory that is logical as opposed to practical;
- Preferring traditional learning settings that include lectures and reading assignments and do not include open-ended tasks; and
- Being industrious and goal-oriented with attention to detail.

**Goal:** understanding things on an intellectual level
**Favorite questions:** What? What is important to learn from this particular class?
**Skills:** thinking—observing, and analyzing; classifying, theorizing, organizing, conceptualizing, and testing theories
**Preferred skill:** solution identification

## STYLE 3 LEARNERS

Perceiving knowledge is best done through abstract conceptualization. Traditional modes of lecture and listening to theory are most preferred. New learning is best processed through active experimentation. Characteristics may include:

- Being skilled at applying ideas and theories for practical use;
- Answering questions and demonstrating problem-solving and decision-making skills;
- Enjoying technical tasks, as opposed to contemplating social issues;
- Discovering how things work, including experimentation and tinkering; and
- Preferring plans and schedules.

**Goal:** putting new information into use in their work and daily living tasks
**Favorite questions:** How does this thing operate? How can I use this information to make a positive difference in my life?
**Skills:** deciding—manipulating, tinkering, improving, applying, experimenting, goal setting
**Preferred skill:** selecting a workable solution from all possibilities

## STYLE 4 LEARNERS

These learners perceive information by using concrete experience. They also use active experimentation to process new information. They prefer to explore ideas to determine if they can make sense of them or apply them in a practical way. Characteristics may include:

- Learning best from hands-on methods;
- Carrying out plans;
- Being involved in new and different experiences;
- Depending on gut feelings, as opposed to logical analysis;
- Taking risks;
- Feeling comfortable in new situations;
- Encouraging others to be independent thinkers; and
- Drawing conclusions without necessarily having logical reasons.

**Goals:** bringing action to ideas; encouraging creativity
**Favorite questions:** What if? If I am learning important and accurate information, how does it apply to my own life? What else does it mean?
**Skills:** activity—modifying, adapting, risking, collaborating, committing, influencing, leading
**Preferred skill:** implementing a selected solution

Being aware of your learning preferences will assist you to have a greater understanding of your learning needs and strengths. You should not seek only situations that are conducive to your style of learning or to avoid those that are not. Instead, you should appreciate your own individuality and recognize that there are many learning styles. You will be exposed to many different modes of education and instruction. You also will care for a range of clients who will have educational needs and whose

> ### Thinking Critically
>
> After reading the preceding material and determining which characteristics apply to you, list your preferred learning styles. Identify which of the four styles is the most predominant for you. Give several examples of why that style is the most preferred. You may use examples that demonstrate when you have enjoyed or deplored a particular learning situation. Share this information with a partner, and discuss with each other observations about yourself and each other that back your selection of a learning style. It also may be helpful for you to share this with your faculty advisor.

styles of learning may be different from yours. Having the knowledge that there are various learning styles provides you not only with flexibility, but also with an ability to meet your own needs and the needs of others. The following example illustrates this truth.

## E X A M P L E

■ A student nurse is assigned to care for a client who has recently been given a diagnosis of hypertension. The client has begun a regimen of antihypertensives and a low-sodium diet. The student observes the dietitian reviewing diet pamphlets and a list of low-sodium foods with the client. She instructs the client to read the materials and to jot down any questions that he may have. After the dietitian leaves, the client tells the student that he is totally confused: None of this makes sense. Although the student feels that the instructional methods were appropriate, he asks the client what would help him to learn the information. The client tells him that it would be much easier to see the information instead of having to read about it: "I don't learn well when I just have to read about it." The student recognizes that a more visual method of instruction might be more beneficial to this client and arranges for him to view a video and to learn how to recognize low-sodium foods by reading food labels. ■

## Student Role: Strategies for Success ▬▬▬

The key to being a successful student rests with you. Methods and techniques to assist you in your endeavors are available, but only you can make them work. This will require that you assume responsibility for your academic efforts and use assertive behavior to meet your goals. Assertiveness is a positive skill because it provides you with the courage and stamina to meet your needs. Assertiveness does not mean confrontation or aggression; rather, it implies that you are able to communicate in a positive and constructive manner. Assertive behavior assists you to explore possibilities, ask for more information and clarification, consider various viewpoints, and make informed decisions.

# College Success Courses

Colleges today provide you with many opportunities to sharpen your academic skills. For instance, you may find it helpful to take courses that provide you with study skills, test-taking skills, or an improved ability to write term papers. If you have been away from an academic setting for a while or felt overwhelmed in previous academic experiences, it may be extremely beneficial to enroll in a course designed for college success. Many colleges require or strongly suggest that you take these courses. Again, you may be pleasantly surprised that some of the obstacles that you thought prevented you from being successful were not as much of a problem as you anticipated, given the right tools and college orientation. You also may discover that the relearning of various academic skills was not especially difficult and more rewarding than it was in prior experiences. In your return to school, you should take advantage of any courses that are available to assist you to be more successful in your nursing program.

# Working With a Faculty Advisor

When you are enrolled in a program of nursing, you will be assigned to a faculty advisor, most likely a member of the nursing faculty. You should introduce yourself to your advisor as early as possible so that both of you are aware of each other. Exchanging telephone numbers and e-mail addresses will help you keep in closer contact and can be invaluable in case of illness or a personal emergency. Your faculty advisor is available to you throughout the length of the program. Many students have their primary contact with their advisor when it is time to register for the next term's classes. This contact may consist of getting a signature on the registration or add-drop form. However, there are many other reasons to have contact with a faculty advisor.

Students may seek the advice of an advisor when they are experiencing academic difficulties. Faculty advisors are knowledgeable about finding appropriate resources for students to improve their academic performance. For example, if a student finds that she or he is having trouble taking multiple choice exams, the advisor may refer the student to campus resources that can teach the student ways to be successful with that type of exam or to someone who can review past exams with the student and develop methods for taking future exams. Some faculty advisors are skilled in these methods and assist the student directly.

Some students also seek assistance from faculty advisors if they feel they are not skilled at taking notes in class or that their attention to reading textbooks is not reasonable. Again, discussing these issues with an advisor may help the student focus on topics that are outlined in the study guides or that are main themes in a textbook. The advisor may refer the student to a resource for improving study and note-taking skills.

Other reasons students go to see advisors are related to personal problems at home or school. Advisors are generally skilled at listening to problems, although usually they are not trained counselors. Again, depending on the nature of the problem, the advisor may refer the student to a counselor, self-help group, or other resource. If the problem involves another faculty member, the advisor may choose not to hear that issue completely but may suggest that the student speak directly with the faculty person and then with the program administrator.

An advisor can be most helpful to you if you meet him or her as soon as possible, instead of when you have an insurmountable or overwhelming situation. Advisors can be many things, but they are not mind readers, miracle workers, or saviors. If you begin to experience academic problems, you are expected to seek help early in the process so that the difficulty can be remedied before failure. If a personal issue is interfering with your ability to be successful in the program, seek assistance before it is too difficult or overwhelming.

Advisors can help only as much as you are willing to seek help. Advisors are not always immediately available because of other academic commitments. In most instances, you will have to make an appointment to meet with your advisor. Having the assigned advisor/teacher's telephone number and e-mail address can help increase your visibility and access to this invaluable resource. If you have an urgent issue, other faculty members may need to be involved if the advisor is not available. If you find that you have difficulty relating to your advisor, you may be able to change advisors by speaking with the program administrator.

## Resource Materials

As you begin your nursing program, many different resources are available to you that will enhance your ability to be successful. The following is a brief summary of some resources usually available.

### STUDENT HANDBOOK

Usually a student handbook or pamphlet is available; these resources are designed for students at a college or university or for those in a particular program. Within these booklets is information about student policies, grading procedures, resources available on campus, and other pertinent information. It is important that you receive a copy of the handbook and familiarize yourself with its contents so that you will know how to obtain pertinent information and use campus resources.

### PROGRAM PHILOSOPHY

Faculties for each nursing program have developed a program philosophy that presents the principles, themes, and trends that drive the curriculum for the nursing program. Generally, nursing education philosophies are composed of beliefs about nursing, the education of nurses, and the various recognized levels of nursing education. They may include thoughts about the education of adults and the responsibilities of students. In many instances, the program philosophy carries out the principles stated in the college or university philosophy. You should become acquainted with your particular program philosophy to be knowledgeable about what the faculties believe about nursing and nursing education. It also is helpful to explore this in terms of your own evolving philosophy about nursing.

## COURSE SYLLABUS

A syllabus is an outline and summary of material that will be covered in a particular course. Students find this extremely useful because a brief description of the course is provided, along with expected outcomes, course objectives, teaching methods, learning activities, required texts, and course requirements, such as tests, papers, projects, reading assignments, and other assigned tasks. The syllabus becomes a study guide by defining the focus and direction of the course. You must become well acquainted with the syllabus to understand the course requirements and expected outcomes, to assist you to concentrate on the most important aspects of the course, and to be aware of how your progress and performance in the course will be assessed.

## PERSONAL PROFESSIONAL LIBRARY

Collecting nursing texts and resources often is confusing, overwhelming, and expensive. Students returning to school often are tempted to purchase all the books they can, with the hope that each book might be helpful. There are many excellent resource books, but you do not need all of them. The course syllabus generally lists required and recommended texts. Faculty selects the recommended texts because they think these are additional resources that will assist you to acquire more knowledge about a particular topic. In general, students usually should acquire a comprehensive medical dictionary, a drug resource manual, a laboratory manual, and possibly a text that assists with the nursing process and the development of care plans. Other books that students may want to purchase are those about a particular subject in which they have a strong interest. The nursing textbooks you are required to have will be valuable even after completing a course when you prepare for the National Council Licensure Examination for Registered Nurses (NCLEX-RN). Although they eventually become outdated, the information has merit for a long time. Other resources that may be helpful are pharmacology and nutrition texts, state board reviewed books, tapes, videos, and computerized programs. Before purchasing anything, you may find it helpful to discuss your choices with faculty and recent graduates of nursing programs. Your college's library will have additional resources, and many more are available via interlibrary loan, the worldwide web, and online.

## PERIODICAL SUBSCRIPTIONS AND WEB RESOURCES

Many nursing journals are available both by subscription and online. It is often difficult to choose which journals are appropriate for you. Again, talking with faculty and other students may assist you. Many nursing journals are available on campus, in hospital libraries, and online, which is a cheaper and easier way to become familiar with nursing journals as resources of information. As a student nurse, you will have many opportunities to read journal articles as part of course requirements. This will assist you to decide if you want to have a particular journal subscription. If you use an online resource, make sure it is a reputable one. Not all information on the Web is accurate. Consult your instructor or the learning resource center on campus if you are unsure of the accuracy of the website.

## UPDATING YOUR RESEARCH SKILLS

If you have not been in an academic setting for a while, you will realize that doing research has become a more technical process because most libraries now have computerized records. There also are several sources from which to obtain particular articles, journals, and books, depending on what you are researching. You must become familiar with using the library and its computer system to research a topic properly. As part of your initial orientation to academic life, make sure that a library orientation is provided. Once you begin to use the library, do not be afraid to ask the librarians for assistance. You will soon be able to access many resources, which will enable you to research a topic thoroughly. These skills will continue to be helpful if you plan to continue your education.

## Valuing Prior Learning

As stated previously, adults often return to school with the fear that they will not do well, will appear foolish, or the rest of the students will be more advanced. For LPN/LVNs, it also is difficult to be removed from an environment that values clinical skills to an environment that values different skills necessary for academic success. However, the value of your experiences as an LPN/LVN and your life experiences in general is immeasurable. You will probably find that your view of the world and of nursing has been greatly influenced by your many experiences.

Educators of adults have long recognized the value of prior learning. Malcolm Knowles (1980), who is viewed as an expert in adult learning theory, has written that adults have a wealth of experience that becomes a valuable resource for further learning. You will find that your experiences enable you to perceive course work in a different way and to place a higher value on your efforts. Ellis (1994) states:

> Being an older student puts you on strong footing. With a rich store of life experience, you've got a sound basis for choosing your educational goals. Based on that experience, you can ask questions and make connections between course work and daily life. (p. 46)

In summary, you need to value who you are. Your life, work, and education experiences provide you with a foundation for continued growth and development in your career as a nurse and as a person. You remain capable of acquiring new knowledge and of adapting to the educational process. Everything that you have learned before returning to school will serve you well. Instead of despairing about what you may not know or understand, rejoice in the knowledge that you can achieve your goals with hard work and a reliance on the skills and knowledge that put you where you are today.

## Time Management

### BALANCING PERSONAL, CAREER, AND STUDENT ROLES

One of the biggest obstacles that returning students face is a lack of time to do all roles adequately. There never seems to be enough time to manage everything and to do it well, but developing a plan will assist you to manage your time more effectively.

It is particularly helpful to plan a weekly schedule to see the entire picture. Some blocks of time are inflexible, such as work and class schedules. You also must remember to make time for other activities, such as sleeping, eating, exercising, family time, and studying. Once you have the weekly plan in place, it is helpful to formulate a daily to-do list to keep yourself organized and to be realistic about your time commitments.

It is not necessary that you do everything as you did before you started school. Involve your significant others in your scheduling plan. Try to delegate some tasks, or hire others to help. Give up some tasks until there is time to do them, and learn to be flexible so that you can take care of unexpected things. Let your family and friends know your schedule so that they have a better understanding of your needs.

Do not give up your exercise and recreation activities; you may need to modify what you do or when you do it, but continue to find time for yourself. Exercise is not only healthy, but it also reduces your stress level. Some students find it helpful to walk or jog between classes or to plan a physical activity with a friend. You also will find it beneficial to designate some periods of quiet time or down time. Students often feel guilty about taking time out, but it actually can rejuvenate you. Reading for pleasure, watching television, meditating, or going for a walk may help you to regroup and get recharged.

Returning students need to be prepared to spend 2 to 3 hours of studying for every hour spent in class. If you are carrying a full-time student load, you should spend 20 to 30 hours of study time per week. This does not need to be done in huge blocks of time and for most people is generally done best in shorter periods of time. The benefits will be realized at exam time or when a project is due because you will not have to have marathon study times to prepare or complete the work. For some students, carrying a full academic load is not feasible, and they choose to attend school on a part-time basis. This can help to alleviate the stress of multiple role responsibilities.

It also will be helpful to you to keep your employer informed of your needs and potential scheduling difficulties. Although most employers will support your decision to return to school, they also have to manage an entire staff, work schedules, and other details. It should be beneficial to both of you to maintain an open line of communication. Most students find that it is advantageous to reduce the number of work hours to the least number that is absolutely necessary to maintain financial commitments. It also may be helpful to explore various work schedules to accommodate the increased class and study time.

## REASSESSING COMMITMENTS

When you are rationing your time, consider also creating a "not-to-do" list. This list should include tasks that are not a priority and those that can be done by others while

### ▶ Thinking Critically

Track your time commitments for 1 week. Think in terms of 15-minute blocks of time so that you can account for short activities. Try to include everything, which means that you account for all 24 hours of a day. It also means that you have the plan with you all the time. At the end of the week, examine what you did, and modify your plan for the following week so that you are organizing and using your time more efficiently.

you are in school. For instance, if you serve on a committee at your child's school, consider resigning and letting someone else have the opportunity to serve. If you volunteer for a local nursing home, you may decide to take a leave of absence. When you finish school, there will always be opportunities to be a member of a board or committee or a chance to do volunteer work. One student who returned to school referred to his time in school as "the years to say 'no.'"

## USE OF THE WIN/WIN AGREEMENT

Stephen Covey (1989) has formulated a method to reach agreements in which there is mutual benefit or satisfaction from the agreement. Win/win agreements create an environment in which each party thinks in terms of cooperation, as opposed to competition. Win/win is conceived on the idea that "there is plenty for everybody, that one person's success is not achieved at the expense or exclusion of the success of others" (p. 207). Such agreements are useful in working out arrangements with significant others while you are in nursing school.

Covey has identified five dimensions that are interdependent and relational:

1. Character: This is the foundation of win/win and consists of three traits:
   a. Integrity: the value you place on yourself; a commitment to yourself and others
   b. Maturity: the maintenance between the ability to express your opinions and attitudes and the respect for the opinions and attitudes of others
   c. Abundance mentality: the notion that there is enough or plenty for everyone; requires that the individual have strong integrity and maturity
2. Relationships: Win/win involves a level of trust in the process and in the person(s) that are involved with the formulation of an agreement. It also involves an ability to listen and to communicate with respect for the person(s) and the various points of view.
3. Agreements: Win/win requires that each party have a clear understanding of the limits and scope of the process. The agreements include an understanding of the desired results, any guidelines that are needed, an awareness of all available resources, accountability by all those involved in the agreement, and an evaluation of the process with possible consequences.
4. Systems: For win/win agreements to work there must be support for the process. Each individual involved must feel equal responsibility for achieving goals and results and therefore solutions.
5. Processes: Covey suggests that win/win solutions are best achieved if each person looks at the problem from the other's perspective; this gives the other person a chance to be heard. It is then essential to name the concerns and issues that are involved. Each person next presents possible results that would be acceptable solutions to the problem. As a last step, various options could be determined for achieving the specific results.

Win/win agreements do not need to be elaborate or lengthy. The process can actually be simple, particularly if each person is committed to the process. An example of a win/win agreement within a family is illustrated in the following:

# EXAMPLE

■ When Sandy, an LPN, returned to school, she recognized that her time would be more restricted because she would be in classes 6 hours a week and clinical practice for 15 hours per week. Her study and preparation time would require 20 to 30 hours a week. She also needed to work two 8-hour shifts per week to pay certain bills and maintain benefits and seniority. Her husband works full time (9 AM to 5 PM Monday through Friday). Their son and daughter are 10 and 16 years old, respectively. Historically, Sandy has taken care of many of the household chores, particularly housecleaning, preparing meals, and the majority of errands. The other family members helped but not on a regular basis and often only with much persuasion. With classes and studying, Sandy realized that she could no longer be responsible for all of these tasks. Sandy's family developed the following win/win agreement:

Sandy will do the housecleaning in the main part of the house. The son and daughter will be responsible for the bedrooms, and the husband will be responsible for the bathrooms. They agree that these jobs will be done without reminders and in a timely way. The daughter will have Sandy's car 2 days a week, and for that privilege, will be responsible for doing most of the weekly errands and transporting her mother to and from school. The son and husband will do the weekly grocery shopping. Everyone will share in meal preparation and cleanup, with assigned days for those tasks. The children will receive compensation for their work, and the parents will put aside an equal amount so that occasionally they can have an evening out. On Sunday evenings, they will have a brief family meeting to plan for the coming week and evaluate how things are going based on the agreement. ■

The wins for Sandy are more time to devote to classes and studying and fewer responsibilities at home. The wins for the family members are that Sandy will have some time to spend with them, and everyone benefits from sharing responsibilities without having to be reminded or badgered. There also is financial and social benefit for all. The consequences also are made clear: If a person does not uphold his or her responsibilities, he or she will not receive the agreed-upon compensation. They have built in some flexibility by planning ahead each week to account for special activities and needs.

At the end of this chapter, you have an opportunity to develop a hypothetical win/win agreement to assist you to develop methods to manage your time more effectively.

## Developing Study Skills

Forming study habits and developing good study skills can be big challenges for returning students. The difficulty is often related to previous experiences in which adequate study skills were not formed or because there are many other distractions for adult learners. Another difficulty may be that past study skills involved rote memory, whereas you now will be asked to analyze, synthesize, and think critically about the material presented.

## TIME AND PLACE FOR STUDY

A first step in developing good study habits is to create study time. The specific time will depend on your other demands, but it will be most helpful if you can select a time of day in which you learn best or when you can be assured of minimal or no interruptions. Plan to study in short blocks of time (1 hour) with 5- to 10-minute breaks. Many students also plan study time between classes or between other activities.

A place to study also is essential. Generally, trying to do assigned readings while reclining on the sofa is not a good idea. Try to use a quiet area in your home or go to the library. Your family and friends need to be aware that your study time and place are off-limits so that you can study without interruption. Also, try not to be tempted by the telephone; unplug it or get an answering machine so that you can answer the calls later.

Another useful study skill is to plan your time so that you know what you want to accomplish each day. Short-term goals often are less intimidating than long-term goals. One student planned a daily task sheet for a long-term project so that he did not have to do the entire assignment during the last couple of weeks of the semester.

## READING AND NOTE-TAKING SKILLS

Other study habits are related to those that assist you to improve or strengthen your abilities. For example, in reading textbooks there are a few methods that will help to make your reading time more productive. Many educators recommend that you take a few minutes to scan a reading assignment before reading it. This enables you to get a feel for the subject and to identify the main themes of the material. You also can decide how much time is needed to complete the assignment. Some material requires in-depth concentration, whereas other texts can be skimmed. In addition, focus on reading with the course objectives in mind. The objectives are a valuable tool to help pinpoint information mastery.

Other strategies involve taking notes while you read. This can be in the form of an outline, or it can be more elaborate if the material is complex. Some students find it helpful to highlight or underline so that when they review the material, they can focus on these sections. It also may be useful to make notes in the margins or to write questions. Instructors usually start their lectures by asking for student questions; this would be a perfect time to ask for clarification of your reading materials. Make use of the chapter objectives, terminology list, summaries, and review questions. These help to clarify and reiterate certain concepts. Some students find it helpful to read aloud to maintain their focus. Finally, review your readings frequently so that the material will not look new just before an exam.

Note taking in class is another necessary skill to master. One of the most useful note-taking skills is to complete the reading assignments before attending class. In this way, the material will not sound foreign, and it may help you to reduce or simplify the notes you take. It also helps you to focus on the class content and ask questions, rather than worrying that you are missing something. Another important aspect of note taking is to sit where you will not be distracted and can focus on what you need to do. Maintaining your concentration also is related to having the proper supplies with you so that you are not worrying about paper or running out of ink. If an instructor is agreeable, taping classes can be an adjunct to note taking; you can use the tapcs to clarify certain points or as a way to review if you have a long commute. If you have solid keyboarding skills, a laptop may speed up your note-taking ability.

Other tips for note-taking are related to format and responding to clues. Note taking can be done in many forms; you probably have seen a variety of methods. Generally, whether you outline or write in narrative form, it is best to be as brief as possible. It does not matter if you use complete sentences or words as long as you write in a way that you can decipher later. Be consistent with the abbreviations that you use. Underline or star important points; instructors often emphasize or state what is particularly important and may repeat a key issue. It is useful to copy information from overheads, slides, computer presentations, or the white board, although the information does not need to be verbatim.

A final help in note taking is to review your notes within one day. Some students find it helpful to recopy or type their notes, whereas others may highlight the most important points. Get in the habit of reviewing your notes frequently so that the information remains familiar. This is especially helpful when it is time for an exam.

## PREPARATION FOR TESTS

Developing study skills also includes preparing for tests and exams. This can be stressful for many students, so it is beneficial to use methods that will help the process. Reading assignments and notes should be reviewed on a regular basis to keep familiar with the course content. This does not substitute for the big review before a test, but it enhances the process. You also may find it helpful to make study cards or something similar that helps you to focus on key points. It can help to review previous exams that you have taken for a class to learn from your mistakes and to get a feel for how the instructor asks questions.

Developing study skills is an important component of student success. Again, the process depends on you. Being a proactive student means that you accept responsibility for achieving your goals. If you are having difficulty studying or taking exams, you must seek help from appropriate sources. Asking for help is not a weakness; it is a strength.

# Cultivating Study Groups and Mentors

Forming a study group can be very rewarding. The group needs to have a spirit of cooperation, as opposed to competition, to be beneficial. The group's meeting cannot be a social gathering because the purpose must be to study. It is best to join a group with students who have goals and study habits similar to yours and who seem to have the same focus in classes as you. If the group is larger than five or six people, it probably will be too unwieldy.

The format of study group meetings should include reviewing material, comparing class notes, testing each other with review questions, or asking questions based on the readings or notes. A study group can be used for developing projects or reviewing members' written work. Nursing students find it useful to assist each other with the development of care plans to help each other understand the process.

A mentor is generally defined as a wise and trusted counselor. It is a person for whom you have respect and admiration. As you begin a nursing program, you may find that someone on the faculty, a nurse where you work, or even a fellow student is someone with whom you are able to consult or use as a role model. This relationship may provide you with the courage to explore other options or discuss new ideas. More information on developing mentors is presented in Chapter 6. At some point, you may become a mentor to someone else. This is not only flattering, but also indicates that you have achieved skills and expertise to be a role model for someone else. It also enables you to broaden your horizons.

Whatever strategies you select to enhance or improve your abilities as a student, remember that you are in college now because you met the qualifications. It is now up to you to make the most of this opportunity. Additional resources on study skills and success strategies are included in Suggested Reading at the end of this chapter.

# Conclusion

Returning to school as an adult is not easy. For as many reasons as there are for returning, there are undoubtedly many reasons to postpone or eliminate the experience. However, the strategies presented in this chapter provide you with a means to facilitate the educational process and to make the journey more successful and enjoyable; they also put you in the driver's seat.

At this point, you should not be intimidated by the process. Your prior learning and work experiences have provided you with a wonderful foundation. As an adult learner and a returning student, you have a wealth of knowledge and experience that will support your efforts. At this point, you must continue to maximize your skills and abilities. Remember Sandy Martin? She involved her job and family to meet her needs. She met with her nursing advisor and took a proactive approach to her learning experience. Together, they have built a strong foundation for her to become successful.

## Student Exercise

Consider a relationship that you have in which you feel the need to develop a win/win agreement. If possible, relate it to a time management issue.

1. Determine who is part of this relationship and who needs to be involved with determining the win/win agreement.
2. What perspectives would you anticipate that each individual has of the solution?
3. What possible solutions are there from your perspective?
4. What guidelines or resources might be necessary to carry out the agreement?
5. What are the wins for each individual?
6. What are the consequences if the agreement is not followed?

## References

American Nurses Association (ANA). (2000). *Scope and standards of practice for nursing professional development.* Washington, DC: Author

Cell, E. (1984). *Learning to learn from experience.* Albany, NY: State University of New York Press.

Cerbin, W. (2000). Investigating student learning in a problem-based psychology course. In P. Hutchings (Ed.), *Opening lines: Approaches to the scholarship of teaching and learning.* Menlo Park, CA: Carnegie Foundation for the Advancement of Teaching.

Crews, T. B., North, A. B., & Thompson, S. L. (2001). Diversity today: Challenges and strategies. In B.J. Brown (Ed.), *Management of the business classroom: NBEA yearbook, No. 39.* Reston, VA: National Business Education Association.

Eisen, M., & Tisdell, E. J. (2000). Team teaching and learning in adult education. (No. 87, Fall 2000). In *New Directions For Adult and Continuing Education 87.*

Ellis, D. (1994). *Becoming a master student* (7th ed.). Rapid City, SD: Houghton Mifflin.

Katz, J. R. (1999). *Majoring in nursing: From prerequisites to postgraduate study and beyond.* New York: Farrar, Straus, and Giroux.

Katz, J. R., Carter, C., Bishop, J., & Kravits, S. L. (2000). *Keys to nursing success.* Upper Saddle River, NJ: Prentice Hall.

Knowles, M. S. (1980). *The modern practice of adult education: From pedagogy to andragogy.* Chicago: Follett.

Kolb, D. K. (1984). *Experiential learning: Experience as the source of learning and development.* Englewood Cliffs, NJ: Prentice-Hall.

Lowenstein, A. J., & Bradshaw, M. J. (2001). *Fuszard's innovative teaching strategies in nursing* (3rd ed.). Gaithersburg, MD: Aspen

Musinski, B. (1999, January–March). The educator as facilitator: New kind of leadership. *Nursing Forum, 34*(1), 23–29.

National League for Nursing (NLN). (2000). *Educational competencies for graduates of associate degree nursing programs.* Sudbury, MA: Jones and Bartlett Publishers.

Ruggiero, V. R. (1998). *Changing attitude: A strategy for motivating students to learn.* Boston: Allyn & Bacon.

Schoolcraft, V., & Novotny, J. (2000). *A nuts-and-bolts approach to teaching nursing* (2nd ed.). New York: Springer Publishing.

Shane, D. L. (1983). *Returning to school: A guide for nurses.* Englewood Cliffs, NJ: Prentice-Hall.

Ulrich, D. L., & Glendon, K. J. (1999). *Interactive group learning: Strategies for nurse educators.* New York: Springer Publishing.

Wlodkowski, R. J. (1999). *Enhancing adult motivation to learn.* San Francisco: Jossey-Bass.

## Suggested Reading

Carter, C., Bishop, J., & Kravits, S. L. (2001). *Keys to success: How to achieve your goals* (2nd ed.). Upper Saddle River, NJ: Prentice Hall

Covey, S. (1989). *The seven habits of highly effective people.* New York: Simon & Schuster.

Dembo, M. H. (2000). *Motivation and learning strategies for college success: A self-management approach.* Mahwah, NJ: Lawrence Erlbaum Associates.

Dunham, K. (2001). *How to survive and maybe even love nursing school: A guide for students by students.* Philadelphia: F.A. Davis.

Ferguson, V. D. (Ed.). (1997). *Educating the 21st century nurse: Challenges and opportunities.* New York: NLN Press.

Gardner, J. N., & Jewler, A. J. (2000). *Your college experience: Strategies for success.* Belmont, CA: Wadsworth Publishing.

Griggs, S., & Dunn, R. (Eds.). (1999). *Learning styles and the nursing profession.* Boston: Jones and Bartlett Publishers.

Sims, R., & Sims, S. (1995). *The importance of learning styles.* Westport, CT: Greenwood Press.

Thibeault, S. (2001). *Stressed out about nursing school: An insider's guide to success.* Orlando, FL: Bandido Books.

Thorkildsen, T. A. (2002). *Motivation and the struggle to learn: Responding to fractured experience.* Boston: Allyn & Bacon.

VanBlerkom, D. L. (2002). *Orientation to college learning* (3rd ed.). Belmont, CA: Wadsworth Group.

## On the Web

**www.msubillings.edu/support101/Faculty/AdultEd.htm**: This Montana State University website has many good resources on adult learning.

**www.chaminade.org/inspire/learnstl.html**: This website includes a chart that helps you determine your learning style.

**www.arc.sbc.edu/timeschedule.html**: Sweet Briar College's website has good information on time management and includes a free downloadable calendar.

**www.lsc.cc.mn.us/programs/read/1010/internet.htm**: This Lake Superior College website has nice links to help regarding time management/reading and note taking.

# CHAPTER 2

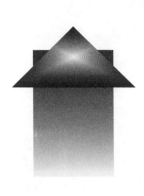

# Role Development and Transition

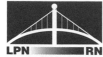

**VIGNETTE**

Ed George, LVN, is a 23-year-old bachelor who works in an outpatient clinic for the Veteran's Administration. Although he has been practicing for only 2 years, Ed has had time to become very comfortable with his role, but it doesn't offer him the challenge it used to when he first started. Part of his discontent is that Ed can help with basic assessment of the client and implementing care, but he really wants to develop his assessment and management skills. Disturbed that he isn't developing as fast as he would like, Ed is enrolled in college for his ADN. He is about halfway through his studies and will graduate next year. He finds his studies fulfilling, and he is once again excited about his new role as an RN. He is enjoying being a student, learning, and applying new theories to client care.

The notion of role development and transition is typically not a part of the decision-making process of returning to school. These terms imply a very formal mode of thinking, when actually the reasons for returning to school may be more pragmatic. However, in making the decision to pursue a degree in nursing, you already realize that a major life change is going to take place. This is the reality of role development and role transition.

# Definitions

**Role** ▼ Role is often defined as a person's particular function as it relates to others' functions. Certain behaviors must be learned so that roles and functions become a part of a whole. For example, one of your roles may be that of the oldest sibling. This role is defined by the fact that there are younger siblings. Behaviors for this role are learned: There are expectations of helping with the care of the younger children or having more responsibilities because you are the oldest. When a person is placed into a new situation, it often feels awkward and unfamiliar because of the uncertainty regarding the role and its obligate behaviors. You may recall how you felt as a newly licensed practical or vocational nurse (LPN/LVN) in your first job or how you are now feeling on your return to school. For each role, expected behaviors are learned for survival and/or success.

**Role Development** ▼ Development in a role refers to the growth that occurs as a person learns the functions, expectations, and behaviors for a particular role. In your practical/vocational nursing education, you were taught specific tasks and behaviors to function within that role. You developed the skills that were necessary to perform a specific job, and as a result, you grew and expanded your knowledge and abilities. Once employed as an LPN/LVN, you continued to expand your knowledge and skills, adding experiential knowledge.

Each person develops roles that relate to the roles of others. Shane (1983) refers to these as *role clusters*. For example, as a student nurse, you will develop in that role in relation to nursing instructors, staff nurses, and other student nurses.

You may also be a parent, a spouse, a daughter or a son, a sibling, and an employee. There are role expectations for each of these roles. These behaviors are learned as part of the role development process. In your return to school, you will learn the role expectations and behaviors needed to be a registered nurse (RN). This process will be influenced by your other roles and experiences.

Role development is not always a voluntary process. Later in this chapter, the concepts related to role development are discussed in more detail.

**Role Change** ▼ Throughout a person's life there are many role changes. Role change consists of adding a new role, dropping an old role, or modifying the behaviors associated with a role (Shane, 1983). Experiences, expected behaviors, and personal values influence development in each new change.

**Role Transition** ▼ Transition refers to a passage or shift from one place to another or from one role to another. Role transition indicates a period of change, often major change. It may involve letting go of some functions while adding others. You may have experienced the necessity of being a caregiver for a parent or grandparent. In this transition, you recognize that you have lost some of the functions of being a child and added the functions of parenting. In essence, you made the shift to your parents' shoes. The LPN/LVN role has involved certain role expectations and behaviors. In the process of acquiring the skills and knowledge needed to be an RN, you will experience changes in the way you think, act, and are. The process of role transition is individual and will not only affect you, but also may have a profound effect on others. In the transition process, it is common for a person to experience role strain or stress. These concepts are examined later in this chapter.

Refer to **Display 2-1** for definitions of role terms.

## ▶ Thinking Critically

Consider your current role change to that of student nurse. Analyze the behavior changes and expectations that you anticipate for this role. What is similar to your previous student experiences? What is different?

## ▶ *Display 2-1*   Definitions of Role Terms

**Role:** a particular function that is defined by its relationship with other functions; expected behaviors for a role are learned

**Role development:** growth within a particular role as a person learns the functions, expectations, and behaviors for that role

**Role change:** addition or subtraction of a role or the modification of behaviors associated with a particular role

**Transition:** passage or shift from one role to another; involves changing the way one thinks and acts

# Types of Roles

## Ascribed Roles

Adults are given or acquire many roles. Ascribed roles are roles that are not chosen.

### GENETIC ROLES

Many ascribed roles are genetic, such as those related to gender, age, and skin color. Previously in this chapter, the example of being the oldest sibling was used to demonstrate the necessity to learn behaviors for each role. It also is an example of an ascribed role.

### SOCIAL MILIEU

Ascribed roles also can relate to the social milieu. This includes ethnic, religious, or familial roles, which have certain functions and expectations. For example, if you are born into a family with a particular religious affiliation, you are expected to learn the particular aspects of the religion, which may include the way you dress or eat, where you go to school, or who you marry. The ascribed roles related to social milieu carry with them expectations of certain behaviors and values. Acquired and ascribed roles are differentiated in **Display 2-2**.

## Acquired Roles

Acquired roles are roles a person receives or takes on during a lifetime. These range from roles of choice, such as being a parent, to those over which there is little control, such as being an invalid. In your work as an LPN/LVN, you may have cared for clients who must adjust to a new role of being ill or disabled. It is not a role of choice, but it

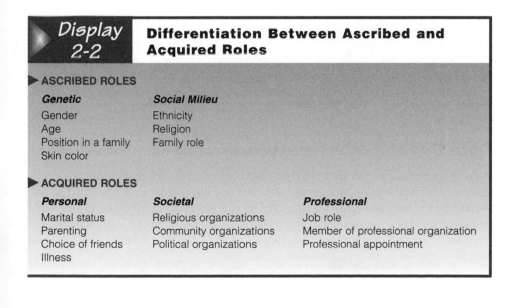

| Display 2-2 | Differentiation Between Ascribed and Acquired Roles | |
|---|---|---|

▶ **ASCRIBED ROLES**

| *Genetic* | *Social Milieu* | |
|---|---|---|
| Gender | Ethnicity | |
| Age | Religion | |
| Position in a family | Family role | |
| Skin color | | |

▶ **ACQUIRED ROLES**

| *Personal* | *Societal* | *Professional* |
|---|---|---|
| Marital status | Religious organizations | Job role |
| Parenting | Community organizations | Member of professional organization |
| Choice of friends | Political organizations | Professional appointment |
| Illness | | |

is an acquired role that involves similar issues of learning behaviors, expectations, and functions. Acquired roles can be personal, societal, or professional.

## PERSONAL ROLES

Personal roles are those you assume as an individual. They can include marital status, parenting, or choice of friends. There are learned behaviors and expectations for each of these roles. The manner in which we behave depends on the relationship. Your role functions and expectations vary on any day from being a parent to a spouse to a close friend.

## SOCIETAL ROLES

Societal roles are those you assume as a member of a group. These may involve affiliations with religious, community, or political organizations. For example, you may have certain positions within a social organization: secretary of a church committee, school board member, or a member of a political candidate's campaign organization. You are obligated to learn the expectations for each of these roles.

## PROFESSIONAL ROLES

Professional roles are those you assume related to your career or vocation. They may include job role, membership in a professional organization, or possibly a professional appointment to a committee or board. One of your reasons for returning to school is to acquire new knowledge and skills that will enhance your ability to take on new job roles and to join other professional organizations and boards. All of these roles require that certain expectations defined by a group and accepted by an individual are met.

### Thinking Critically

Consider the many roles in your life. Differentiate between your ascribed and acquired roles. In what ways do the ascribed roles influence the acquired roles? Determine if any of your acquired roles will be changed or modified as you return to school.

# Role Development

Role development is discussed briefly in the beginning of this chapter in the Definitions section. At this point, it is essential to examine this process more closely. The following text reviews concepts of role choice and personal, family, and professional development. These concepts will assist you in understanding your own role development and transition as you move from the role of an LPN/LVN to that of a professional nurse.

# Role Choice

Your decision to become an RN was not one that you made on a whim. It has been a careful process of weighing the advantages and disadvantages and determining the priorities in your life. You may have had some help with this decision, but for some, it is a lonely and agonizing time. You may have had to overcome some personal issues related to finances or child care, or perhaps your family did not support your decision to return to school. The educational road for some will be more difficult than for others. Your colleagues have different experiences and expectations. You may have noticed that strangers, some who are very different from you, who have more or less LPN/LVN experience, or who seem more or less knowledgeable, surround you. These factors may influence you in some way, but it is hoped they will not deter you.

## Thinking Critically

Review your list of ascribed roles. Consider what these roles mean to you. For example, is your age at this time beneficial? Examine the benefits or difficulties with all of your ascribed roles. How do these influence your return to school?

Acquired roles may involve choices. Your decision to continue your education has involved an active process on your part. Generally, you have not been able to sit back and let someone else make the choice for you. It is impossible to predict all the implications that returning to school can mean. You have undoubtedly experienced a variety of emotional states in your decision-making process. Now that you are actually beginning your education, it is necessary for you to contemplate two words: commitment and balance.

## COMMITMENT

Commitment is the process of pledging to assume a role, perform a job, or accomplish a goal. Your acceptance to school initiated this process. However, you also have other commitments that demand your attention. You have often heard that one must be able to set priorities. This is the establishment of balance or the maintenance of equilibrium.

## BALANCE

To be successful in a nursing program, a balance will have to be achieved. You may be compelled to let some things go or to let someone else assume some of the tasks that you normally do. Many students find that household chores must be done by a significant other, by children, or simply ignored. It may be more important that you add a physical activity, such as daily walks or swims, to relax or relieve tension and to keep your body in balance. These are the decisions that you will have to make to be successful in your nursing program.

> ### ► Thinking Critically
>
> You have already made some changes when you decided to return to school. What are those changes? How will these changes affect your life's balance? Do you anticipate other changes?

## BARRIERS

You may experience some barriers in your educational journey. Some of these barriers are internal. The following are examples of internal barriers for role development:

Fear of failure
Lack of confidence
Confusion regarding new expectations
Feelings of being overwhelmed

Palmer (1998) describes fears common to college students, including fear of failing, not understanding, being drawn into issues they would rather avoid, having their ignorance exposed or their prejudices challenged, or looking foolish in front of peers. Such fears may serve as internal barriers to your being an active participant in class discussions, seeking clinical experience, and experiencing success in the ADN program.

Other barriers to role development are external. They may include issues surrounding family needs, child care, financial concerns, job demands, and personal needs. All of these barriers have a tremendous impact on your ability to succeed. Subsequent chapters provide you with some strategies to assist in overcoming barriers.

> ### ► Thinking Critically
>
> Identify barriers to your return to school. Differentiate internal and external barriers. Design a plan of action to deal with these barriers.

## Personal and Adult Development

This section is an overview of adult developmental theory. Researchers such as Erikson, Piaget, and others have proposed theories that provide an explanation for adult development. You may recall these theorists from your LPN/LVN education. A review of these theories will assist you to examine more objectively your own development and personal journey. It will also provide you with a perspective to evaluate the development of your clients and to recognize the effects of illness on their development.

## NCLEX–RN Might Ask 2-1

The student nurse is monitoring the progress of a client with juvenile diabetes in a community clinic setting. The client is a 15-year-old girl who is having problems with her diet that stem mainly from having to eat in the high school cafeteria with others of her age. According to Erikson, this child's stage of development is

- A. trust vs. mistrust.
- B. industry vs. inferiority.
- C. identity vs. role confusion.
- D. intimacy vs. isolation.

• *See Appendix A for correct answer and rationale.*

## ERIKSON

Erik Erikson is one of the earliest theorists to delineate development in terms of phases or stages. He views these stages in terms of psychosocial development throughout the life span. Personal development occurs with passage through each of the stages. Erikson theorizes that a person develops by proceeding through developmental tasks or crises at each stage. Success or failure in resolving a crisis will influence a person's ability to deal with the next stage and may affect how he or she is as an adult.

Table 2-1 outlines Erikson's eight stages, the time in a person's life when each stage occurs, the developmental task or crisis for each stage, and the possible consequences for success or failure in resolving each task or crisis.

## PIAGET

Jean Piaget is another early theorist you may remember who examined cognitive development, the process of understanding and knowing. He identifies four stages related to intellectual development: sensorimotor (manipulation), preoperational (egocentric thought), concrete operations, and formal operations (abstract thought). Table 2-2 summarizes these four stages of cognitive development, the approximate age that each stage takes place, and what cognitive process is involved. Piaget theorizes that cognitive development occurs in a continuum from infancy on; it is an additive process in which new experiences are understood as a result of previous knowledge.

Piaget considers formal operational thought to be the highest level. To achieve this level, one must progress through the stages of manipulation and concrete thinking to consider all variables and solve problems. In his theory, this happens in adolescence. Other theorists do not agree and think that abstract thinking or formal operations develops later in life with the appropriate experiences (Stevens-Long, 1988). These concepts are important for you for two reasons. First, your thought processes are more concrete, as a result of your previous educational experiences. Shane (1983) attributes this to the rigid style used in nursing schools; formal operations may not be encouraged. These concepts also are important when considering the learning needs of your clients. Your

**TABLE 2-1**
STAGES OF PSYCHOSOCIAL DEVELOPMENT—ERIKSON

| Stage | Approximate Age | Developmental Task or Crisis | Consequences of Success or Failure |
|-------|-----------------|------------------------------|-----------------------------------|
| Trust versus mistrust | Birth–18 mo | Learn to trust others and self | Success: sense of predictability and certainty<br>Failure: sense of abandonment and distrust |
| Autonomy versus shame and doubt | 18 mo–3 y | Learn to develop sense of choice and self-restraint | Success: sense of self-control without loss of self-esteem<br>Failure: defiance, willfulness, sense of loss of control with shame and doubt |
| Initiative versus guilt | 3–5 y | Learn to have goals, develop judgment, and perceive self-behavior | Success: sense of responsibility and cooperation; ability to use positive judgment<br>Failure: lack of self-confidence; fear of doing the wrong thing |
| Industry versus inferiority | 6–12 y | Develop skills and knowledge to complete tasks; use motor and cognitive skills | Success: sense of success and competence<br>Failure: sense of inadequacy and hopelessness |
| Identity versus role confusion | 12–20 y | Develop a sense of self and abilities and an inner sense of commitment, morality, and ethics | Success: a positive sense of self and a knowledge that one has abilities and values<br>Failure: doubts about sexual and vocational identity; confusion about individual identity; can lead to identification with heroes and cliques |
| Intimacy versus isolation—early adulthood | 20–40 y | Develop intimate relationships and make commitments to work and to others | Success: intimate relationship and positive commitments to work and to others<br>Failure: avoidance of intimacy; problems with commitment |
| Generativity versus stagnation—middle adulthood | 41–60 y | Establish family and assist in the guidance of the next generation; be creative and productive | Success: feeling needed by family and helping the future generation; feeling productive and valuable<br>Failure: concerned more with self; feeling useless and without value; stagnated |
| Integrity versus despair—late adulthood | 61 y–death | Resolve that life has meaning and worth | Success: accept one's life as meaningful and fulfilling; that something has been left for the next generation<br>Failure: fear death; cannot see that life has had meaning. |

approach for teaching a specific procedure will differ depending on the age of the client and the ability of that individual to use formal or concrete operations. You also may find that some of your clients will revert to previous modes of thinking when they are faced with stress. This theory provides you with a framework to assess the learning needs of your clients and to then devise a realistic plan for teaching new information.

**TABLE 2-2**
STAGES OF COGNITIVE DEVELOPMENT—PIAGET

| Stage | Age | Cognitive Process |
|---|---|---|
| Sensorimotor | Birth–2 y | Senses and motor activity give information about the world and its objects; infant relies on totally direct experience; at the end of this stage, language skills increase, and the sense of object permanence is recognized apart from self. |
| Preoperational | 2–7 y | Time of exploration and curiosity: child is very interested in the world; explains the world so that it makes sense to self; increased language skills and imagination help child to use mental images and symbolic play. |
| Concrete operations | 7–12 y | Child uses systematic thought and is able to apply universal rules: reversibility of thought (add and subtract); classification of objects by size or mass; and consistency of quantities when physical appearance changes (i.e., pour liquid from narrow to wide container—amount remains the same). Child is able to learn in a procedural or sequential method. |
| Formal operations | 12 y–adulthood | Child is now able to think in abstract terms and to use reasoning and scientific processes; also can conceptualize the future. |

## KOHLBERG

The development of moral reasoning was researched extensively by Lawrence Kohlberg. He determined that an integral part of socialization of a child from any culture is to teach the child the difference between right and wrong. This, in essence, gives the child a sense of values. Kohlberg's concept of moral development is similar to the concepts of Erikson and Piaget. As a child identifies with parents or other caregivers, she or he is either positively or negatively reinforced for particular behaviors. If the reinforcement is consistent, a child's personal sense of values will be greatly influenced by the value system of the caregivers.

Kohlberg's stages of moral development are presented in **Table 2-3**. The first stage of preconventional moral thought signifies the beginning of value development in early childhood. The child is dependent on adults for survival and learns to view moral behavior as the avoidance of disapproval or punishment from adults. Conventional moral thought develops in the preteen years. At this time, the child is able to define the rules and expectations of society and better understands the consequences if the rules are broken. The last stage is called postconventional or principled moral thought. As the teenager moves into adulthood, she or he develops an abstract moral sense that enables her or him to determine what is just or unjust.

Nurses develop a professional value system in much the same way (Taylor, Lillis, and LeMone, 2001). Depending on your own stage of personal development and experiences, you may have some difficulty assimilating all of these factors. You also are faced with teachers, clients, and colleagues whose value systems may differ from

**TABLE 2-3**
STAGES OF MORAL DEVELOPMENT—KOHLBERG

| Stage | Definition | Characteristics |
|-------|------------|-----------------|
| Preconventional moral thought— early childhood | Obedience and punishment Action for personal satisfaction Interpersonal agreement | Believes action is right if not punished; wrong if punished Responds to bribery; will comply for personal gain Acts to please others and maintain relationships |
| Conventional moral thought—preteen | Law and order Personal values/standards | Understands and responds to authority; maintains social order Has sense of morality; protects rights of all |
| Principled moral thought—teenager to adult | Universal ethical standards | Has a conscience; respects other human beings and believes in mutual trust |

yours. As you grow and develop in your professional role, you will be more sensitive to various beliefs. Later in this text, ethical decision making is addressed. It will be helpful to apply Kohlberg's theory of moral development as you study ethical decision making.

## GILLIGAN

Carol Gilligan (1982) developed a theory of moral development from a woman's perspective. As a student of Kohlberg's and later as a colleague, she objected to the generalization of his theory to women because his theory was based on work done with males and then applied to females. The similarities in their theories are that they both identify three stages of moral development. However, Kohlberg's theory is based more on rules and justice and the development of abstract thinking, whereas Gilligan asserts that women's development is seen more in terms of relationships, caring, and connectivity. In Kohlberg's research with girls and women, he determined that women were not able to reach the higher level of moral development, concluding that women were in some way deficient. Gilligan based her research on the stories or "voices" of girls and women, finding that their sense of moral reasoning is based on relationships, responsibility, and caring.

Gilligan's three stages of moral development are as follows:

1. **Orientation to individual survival:** The individual views the moral decision as one that is necessary for her own survival in terms of herself only. There is a sense of obligation to one's own needs.
2. **Goodness as self-sacrifice:** The individual makes a moral decision based on meeting the needs and expectations of others and not hurting others. The obligation is to others and not self in this process.
3. **Morality of nonviolence:** The individual determines that the moral choice must be responsible to self and others and must involve caring and not hurting. The individual remains obligated to nonviolence.

**TABLE 2-4**
COMPARISON OF STAGES OF MORAL DEVELOPMENT—KOHLBERG AND GILLIGAN

| Stage | Kohlberg | Gilligan |
|-------|----------|----------|
| First | *Preconventional moral thought:* Child connects wrong acts with punishments; obedience through avoidance of punishment. | *Orientation to individual survival:* Child's moral decisions are based on survival of self, self-protection. |
| Second | *Conventional moral thought:* Child responds to authority to maintain law and order. | *Goodness as self-sacrifice:* Child bases moral decisions on meeting the needs of others and not causing hurt to anyone. |
| Third | *Principled moral thought:* Individual develops standards and values that determine his or her sense of morality and ethics. | *Morality of nonviolence:* The individual determines that moral choices involve responsibility to self and others and involve an ethic of caring and nonviolence. |

As the individual progresses through these stages, there is an emphasis on the relationships within a particular situation and the importance of caring, attachments, and connectedness. **Table 2-4** provides a brief comparison of the theories of Kohlberg and Gilligan.

## LEVINSON

Another theorist who advocates a stage theory approach is Daniel Levinson. He has identified various stages and phases through which a person proceeds in the developmental process. Within each phase are periods of stability and transition and certain tasks that have to be completed. **Table 2-5** shows the five stages that have been identified for adulthood, with the approximate ages involved and the tasks to be completed.

**TABLE 2-5**
STAGES OF ADULT DEVELOPMENT—LEVINSON

| Stage | Age | Task |
|-------|-----|------|
| Early adult transition | 18–20 y | The young adult begins the process of entering the adult world and leaving the security of childhood; independence is strongly desired. |
| Entrance into the adult world | 21–27 y | The young adult begins adult career paths and adapts to an adult lifestyle that involves a variety of choices. |
| Transition | 28–32 y | At this stage, the adult may choose to maintain the chosen path or to modify current life structures. |
| Settling down | 33–39 y | The adult settles in at this stage and experiences stability within work, family, and social structures; views self as an expert in many ways. |
| The payoff years | 45–65 y | Within this stage, the individual is self-directed and is able to use influence with others and assess what life has been and needs to be. |

Levinson describes three phases within each of the five stages. The first phase is referred to as the novice phase, during which the individual begins to focus on new tasks that soon become the most significant. The second phase is called the culminating phase. This is a period of stability wherein tasks are achieved and maintained. The last phase is the transition phase, in which the present tasks lose their importance and other tasks begin to take precedence. The greatest turmoil, according to Levinson, occurs in the transitional phase. He theorizes that each phase can be as long as 5 to 7 years and may involve another 5 years of modification. As a result, adults spend many years in uncertainty.

Levinson's theory again poses interesting ways to examine your personal development. Consider the tasks with which you are absorbed as you return to school. It is a time of change and transition, so it can be expected that it will be a time of turmoil, according to Levinson. You also can apply these concepts to your adult clients and determine what effect changes in health, pregnancy, or illness might have on a person's development. Does this alter or prolong the transition phase, or deter a person from completing essential tasks? Levinson's theory provides another framework to assess a client's developmental progress.

## SHEEHY

Thus far, most of the theorists presented have based their work on research studies of males, with the exception of Carol Gilligan. Other theorists view personal and adult development differently for females and males. A prominent person in this area is Gail Sheehy. In closely examining the work of stage theorists, she has noted that the developmental stages for men and women are different, and that there is more development in the adult stages than some theorists have presented. Women traditionally have been faced with more restrictions in the first half of their life cycle than have men. They have been the primary caregivers of children and aged parents and the chief keepers of the home, as well as caring for almost anything else that needs care. Although women increasingly work outside of the home, the caregiving tasks continue to be their responsibility, and frequently women choose work that compliments the caregiver responsibilities. During the second half of their life cycle, women begin to look at self-development and at this time may choose to return to school and begin or change careers. Men have typically been more active in their careers and education during the first half of their life cycle and in the older adult years are more ready to think about leisure activities and retirement.

Traditional female and male roles are becoming more similar in the 21st century. Work and leisure roles that used to distinguish men and women are no longer as clearly defined. Gender stereotypes may not be as different as they once were, but life experiences do affect individual development, and any of the theories presented are limited to the population that has been studied.

Sheehy has identified stages or predictable crises of adulthood. Based on research of both men and women, she indicates the ages when one would generally go through each stage and points out gender differences if they are very obvious. She is not so concerned with ages as she is with the sequence of the stages. **Table 2-6** outlines the stages, or crises, identified by Sheehy and their particular defining characteristics.

**TABLE 2-6**
STAGES OF ADULT DEVELOPMENT—SHEEHY

| Stage | Approximate Ages | Defining Characteristics |
|---|---|---|
| Pulling up roots | 18–20 y | The young adult experiences the need to have autonomy and also to be taken care of. At this time, the struggle is to establish an adult identity separate from parents. "The tasks of this passage are to locate ourselves in a peer group role, a sex role, an anticipated occupation, an ideology or world view. As a result, we gather the impetus to leave home physically and the identity to begin leaving home emotionally" (Sheehy, 1976, p. 27). |
| The trying 20s | The 20s | Within this stage, the adult begins to settle into life work and to attempt intimacy while continuing the process of self-identity. Sheehy refers to the establishment of life patterns in this stage, such as *locked-in, wunderkind,* or *caregiver.* |
| Catch-30 | Late 20s–early 30s | During this stage, adults question the wisdom of the choices made in their 20s. They may feel the need to change jobs or careers or to settle into marriage and start a family. On the other side, they may commit to extending their lives in the same direction they took in their 20s. |
| Rooting and extending | Early 30s | Settling in truly begins in this stage. The focus usually is on putting down roots and raising young children. |
| The deadline decade | Middle 30s–middle 40s | This stage marks a turning point in which adults recognize that they are halfway through the cycle of life. It is a time to re-evaluate where one is, what one is doing, and what one should be doing. Many adults return to school or change careers at this stage. |
| Renewal or resignation | Mid-40s on | Adults accept their lives as they are and accept that no one will ever fully understand oneself and that blame cannot be placed on one's parents. Friends are important, but this adult also values privacy. |

Sheehy believes adult development needs to be better described in terms of men's and women's experiences. She also recognized that adulthood does not represent easy work. Instead, it can be difficult and at times painful. Sheehy (1976, p. 21) states the following:

> The work of adult life is not easy. As in childhood, each step presents not only new tasks of development but requires letting go of the techniques that worked before. With each passage some magic must be given up, some cherished illusion of safety and comfortably familiar sense of self must be cast off, to allow for greater expansion of our own distinctiveness.

Sheehy's work provides a means to continue to examine your own development. Each of us progresses or develops at our own pace. Sheehy notes that the tasks for each stage are never completely done or eliminated, but we move on to the next step out of necessity or because other issues take precedence. Consider these aspects as you review the information in Table 2-6. It also is a means to assess your clients and better understand the needs of each.

## STEVENSON

Joanne Sabol Stevenson is another author who has studied adult development, particularly the middle years of the life cycle. She refers to this as *middlescence*. "'Middlescence' is a term that originated in a facetious comment about the age group in the middle. Someone considered adolescence on the one side and senescence on the other and quipped that middlescence is in the center" (Stevenson, 1977, p. 1). She delineates four stages of adult development.

**Youth or young adulthood:** 18 to 30 years
**Middlescence I (the core):** 30 to 50 years
**Middlescence II (the new middle years):** 50 to 70 years
**Late adult years:** 70 years to death

Within each of these stages are tasks that have to be accomplished. She recognizes that some tasks are in process and may overlap into a subsequent stage, secondary to individual experiences and idiosyncrasies. Stevenson uses the suffix "ing" to denote that the tasks are in operation but not necessarily complete, representing a dynamic process of development. **Table 2-7** presents each of Stevenson's stages and the tasks for each stage. Again, review the material with your own development in mind, but also consider the impact that changes in health, pregnancy, or illness might have as you think about your clients.

Stevenson is a nurse and has presented some implications in this process. She differentiates maturational crises from situational crises. Maturational crises are the turmoils or stresses that occur in developmental transitions, such as leaving home or mak-

**TABLE 2-7**
STAGES OF ADULT DEVELOPMENT—STEVENSON

| Stage | Approximate Age | Tasks |
|---|---|---|
| Youth or young adulthood | 18–30 y | Achieving relative independence from parental figures; attaining a sense of responsibility; developing roles and positions; achieving intimate relationships; beginning parenting; making personal values integral with work and social values |
| Middlescence I | 30–50 y | Assuming responsibility for self-development and for growth of associated organizations; assessing one's work roles; assisting the younger generations and older generations; involving oneself in a variety of organizations; optimizing responsibilities |
| Middlescence II | 50–70 y | Achieving ways to maintain survival; taking interest in societal changes; maintaining mutually supportive relationships with family members; enjoying increased leisure time; adapting to aging |
| Late adult years | 70 y–death | Assuming the need to share experience and wisdom; putting affairs in order; pursuing new interests; learning new skills; assessing one's life; adapting to loss of significant other |

ing the decision to have children. These crises are similar for many people. Situational crises are the remarkable events that happen only to some of us. Personal illness, a catastrophic accident, the untimely death of a parent or a spouse, or divorce are examples of situational crises. The stage at which these events occur influences a person's ability to cope. For example, an acute illness at the age of 45 years has great implications for that individual in terms of lost income, lack of support for dependent family members, and inability to meet community and work-related obligations. Continue to consider these aspects as you study this material.

## ▶ Thinking Critically

Select one of the theories outlined in the preceding material. What stage best describes your present status? Why? With what tasks are you most concerned? Do any issues remain unresolved or problematic?

# Family Development

In addition to personal development, individuals also grow and develop within the context of human relationships, which generally involve a family unit. Evelyn Duvall and Murray Bowen have studied family development.

## DUVALL

Family development is perceived by some theorists in the context of a life cycle with developmental stages and tasks similar to personal development. Duvall (1977) theorizes that if a person understands who the family members are (including age, sex, and position in the family); what the family's status is in terms of race, ethnicity, and social standing; and what stage they are in the family life cycle, much can be predicted about what is happening with the family at a particular time. Duvall describes eight stages of family development within the framework of a family life cycle (**Table 2-8**).

With each stage, she describes specific tasks that require adaptation and acquisition of new responsibilities and challenges. For example, a family with young children has the task of adapting to members of the next generation. The parents must acquire parenting skills, adapt their own relationship to make room for children, and adjust relationships with other family members, such as aunts, uncles, and grandparents.

It is obvious that not all individuals and families fit into such predictable stages. There are many variations of family units. Brief examples include:

Couples without children;
Families who have children early in a marriage and then much later;
Homosexual couples;
Children raised by grandparents or other caregivers;
Single-parent families; and
Families with a chronically ill or disabled member.

**TABLE 2-8**
STAGES OF FAMILY DEVELOPMENT—DUVALL

| Stage | Developmental Tasks |
| --- | --- |
| Marriage of young couple; no children | Growth in marital relationship; adjustment to in-laws; decision regarding having children |
| Birth of children | Growth in parenting roles; adjustment in marital relationship; resolution of conflicting roles: spouse, parent, daughter/son, sibling, employee |
| Family with preschool children | Adaptation to children who are very involved with their environment; adjustment in marital relationship; involvement of children in socialization activities, such as church and nursery school, and other activities |
| Family with school-age children | Encouragement of achievements of children in school and other activities; adjustment in marital relationship; coordination of child and adult activities |
| Family with adolescents | Promotion of teenagers' responsible independence; maintenance of communication with all family members; adjustment in marital relationship |
| Family with offspring who have left home | Adaptation to empty nest; adjustment in marital relationship; growth of relationships with married offspring and grandchildren |
| Family in early retirement | Adaptation to retirement and increased leisure activities; strengthening of marital ties; adjustment to being older |
| Family in old age | Maintenance of marital relationship; adjustment to widowhood and loss of friends; adaptation to aging |

However, Duvall's theory provides a means to begin examining family relationships and roles and the impact of individual needs on family needs. For example, if there is a sick family member during the school-age stage, it may prevent the family from participating in community and educational activities. It is not always possible to mesh individual and family needs. If a family does not quite conform to the expectations of the community, pressure may be placed on them. A young child who has the human immunodeficiency virus may be isolated, along with the family. A biracial couple may be shunned. These factors will interfere with the developmental tasks of the family. In addition, a parent or caregiver with substance abuse may place a heavy burden on other family members financially, socially, and developmentally.

## BOWEN

Murray Bowen proposes that the family is an interrelated and interdependent system that is influenced by each of its members and by external factors, such as the community, the environment, and life events. The interrelationships that exist between family members are so great that when one individual is changed, the whole family system will be affected. For instance, if a child becomes chronically ill, the parents will be focused on that child and may parent the siblings differently than they did before the child's illness. The siblings may begin to have behavior problems in school or vague physical ailments as a result of the first child's illness and the changed parenting. All of the family members are affected by the condition of one member. Bowen's approach to family therapy consists of treating the individual, not as an entity separate from the family, but rather as part of a family unit, all of whom should be involved in the counseling. In this way, family members are able to face issues and deal with them together, instead of making one member responsible.

In your work as an LPN/LVN, you have probably included family members when caring for an individual. As you move into the RN role, there will be an increased emphasis on the family unit. As healthcare delivery continues to evolve, the family plays a critical role. Not only must you assess a person, but you also must assess the family because the health status of individual members is affected by the function of the family. The family assessment will provide you with a clearer picture of the person's primary social context, family stressors, risk factors within the family, and the family's adaptation and coping mechanisms.

## ▶ Thinking Critically

Review Duvall's stages of family development. Is there a stage that describes your current status? What is the same? What is different? What impact will your return to school have on your family's development? What impact will the situations of other family members have on your development as you return to school?

# Professional Role Development

Role development is defined in the beginning of this chapter. The addition of the word *professional* requires a brief definition. To be a member of a profession, one must have special preparation and education to acquire knowledge and skills to perform a certain role. Professional role development implies acquiring the skills and knowledge that are needed to function within a particular role. Growth and development within the role are influenced by previous experiences and the expectations for that role by members of the profession and those who interface with such individuals.

## COHEN

Professional role development may also evolve in stages. Cohen (1981) has identified four stages that relate to Erikson's developmental stages (**Table 2-9**). The first stage is called *unilateral dependence*, in which a student professional begins to learn theoretical content and to practice in a limited way under the supervision of an instructor. The second stage is *negative independence*, which provides the student professional more opportunities to apply theory to practice and to internalize some of the professional role behaviors that fit with her or his own values and self-concepts. Cohen identifies the third stage as *dependence/mutuality*, in which the student professional begins to recognize role limitations to be acceptable to other professionals and to society in general. The last stage is called *interdependence*, in which the professional role seems more real. The individual is able to accept more responsibility and is able to feel that the professional role is part of her or his identity. The comfort level is much higher, and generally that person feels that the professional role is not in conflict with other roles.

| **TABLE 2-9** | | |
|---|---|---|
| **PROFESSIONAL ROLE DEVELOPMENT—COHEN** | | |
| *Stage I* | Unilateral dependence | Inexperienced student learns theoretical concepts for role development; applies theory to practice in a limited and supervised way. |
| *Stage II* | Negative independence | Student has increased opportunities to apply theory to practice and assumes more responsibility; develops confidence and takes on some of the role values; also is more willing to question traditional patterns and ways of knowing. |
| *Stage III* | Dependence/mutuality | Student is able to be more realistic about role expectations, and questions reflect a higher understanding of theoretical concepts; recognizes role limitations. |
| *Stage IV* | Interdependence | Student is able to make independent judgments and to take on the professional role; student's professional identity is more secure and not in opposition with other roles. |

Your professional role development has already begun. Your decision to become an RN initiated the process. As you progress in your academic program, you will acquire the knowledge, skills, and abilities needed to be a professional nurse.

## Thinking Critically

How has your role as an LPN/LVN affected your professional role development? Explore positive and negative effects and your present stage of professional role development. What will help or hinder you in reaching Cohen's fourth stage?

## PROFESSIONAL ROLE SOCIALIZATION

Professional role socialization is a complicated process during which an individual not only learns the necessary cognitive and motor skills for a particular role, but also gains an identity with an occupation and adopts the values and norms of that occupational group. According to Cohen (1981), four goals are associated with role socialization:

1. The student will acquire technical and theoretical skills.
2. The student will take on the values of the profession.
3. The student will modify the professional role to one that is personally and professionally acceptable.
4. The student will balance the professional role with other roles.

Several models have been developed to define the process of professional role socialization. The model developed by Hinshaw (1986) depicts three stages for socialization or resocialization for a professional role (**Table 2-10**). In the first stage, students change their concepts of role expectations from those they had anticipated to those being taught by professional role models. The second stage is a time of attachment to role models

## NCLEX–RN Might Ask 2-2

A nursing student is asked by a client what the changes to her role have been as she has gone from LPN to RN. The nurse would be *incorrect* by stating:

A. "I have acquired more advanced technical and theoretical skills."
B. "I have learned to balance my roles as wife and mother with my professional ones."
C. "I have interwoven new professional values into my existing ones."
D. "I have changed my professional roles to only what is acceptable to me personally."

• *See Appendix A for correct answer and rationale.*

within the educational and clinical settings. It also is a time when students have conflicts about incongruencies of role behaviors that were not anticipated or expected. During this time, it is essential that role models assist students to cope with these incongruencies. The last stage is the internalization of the values and standards of the new role.

In your socialization to the RN role, you will take on the values and standards for that role. As an LPN/LVN you may not recognize all the differences that exist between the two roles, except in terms of tasks. Kelman identifies three phases of value internalization:

1. **Compliance:** An individual demonstrates appropriate behaviors to receive positive feedback but has not internalized the values.
2. **Identification:** The individual is selective about the particular behaviors that are personally acceptable; this often depends on particular role models.
3. **Internalization:** The individual believes and accepts the new standards of behavior as part of her or his own value system.

**TABLE 2-10**
MODEL OF PROFESSIONAL ROLE SOCIALIZATION—HINSHAW

| | | |
|---|---|---|
| ***Stage I*** | Transition from anticipated role expectations to those that are taught | Adults who are new to a profession are committed to learning the expected role behaviors. |
| ***Stage II*** | Attachment to important role models; identification of inconsistencies | Attachments are made with significant faculty or staff members. Role models are important and essential. At this time, questions also arise regarding situations that are incongruent with those presented by role models. |
| ***Stage III*** | Internalization of role values and standards | The individual takes on the values and standards of the professional role. If the incongruencies have been significant in the second stage, the internalization of values may be affected. |

Your education to become an RN will not only provide you with new skills, but also will change the way that you think and who you are. Moving to the professional role of the RN will cause you to develop deeper analytic and critical thinking skills.

# Role Transition

Role transition means the passage or shifts from one role to another and involves changing the way one thinks and acts. William Bridges (1980; 1991; 2001) differentiates between change and transition. He defines change as a "situational shift" (getting a new boss, having a child, or returning to school). He describes transition as, "the process of letting go of the way things used to be and then taking hold of the way they subsequently become" (2001, p. 2). He notes that transition is the way we come to terms with change. Bridges further describes transition in three phases.

## Endings

The first phase of transition involves an ending. Every transition begins with an ending. We have to let go of the old thing before we can pick up the new—not just outwardly, but inwardly, where we keep our connections to the people and places that act as definitions of who we are. Bridges designates four aspects of endings.

**Disengagement:** separation from a familiar place within the social order. At various times a person voluntarily or involuntarily is disengaged from activities, relationships, places, or roles that have been important.

**Disidentification:** loss of self-definition; a process of not being quite sure of who you are. Often the old identity can interfere with transition because it is hard to let go of what you were.

**Disenchantment:** the realization that the beliefs and views in the past are no longer real. Life is a series of disenchantments in the many transitions; disenchantment may be related to the loss of a relationship or a change in career. The disenchanted person recognizes the old view as sufficient in its time but insufficient now.

**Disorientation:** the lost and confused feeling that a person experiences when in transition. There is a sense of unreality about even ordinary events; nothing feels the same.

## Neutral Zone

The second phase of role transition described by Bridges is call the neutral zone. During this phase, a person feels that she or he is "in limbo," a temporary state of emptiness or loss or an in-between state of affairs. It is a time when a person appears to be in a void but is actually contemplating important inner thoughts. The first function of this phase is one of surrender, in which a person gives in to the emptiness and does not try to escape it. A second function is one of renewal and recharging and possibly redirecting. The last function is a change in perspective about what a person has always known and how to view it differently.

## Beginnings

The last phase of transition identified by Bridges is called beginnings. There is not a clear path that can tell a person that a new beginning is at hand. Instead, there initially is just a hint that something is different. It occurs within the person, although the transition may be the result of changing jobs, changing relationships, or continuing an education. The beginning in the transition process is part of a continuum; it is a new chapter of one's life that is beginning. As the beginning becomes part of the whole, the person reintegrates the new identity with the old identity. None of us are the same as a result of a transition but are changed in many ways. Bridges' phases of transition are shown in **Display 2-3**.

### ▶ Thinking Critically

As you read through role socialization and transition, where do you see yourself? Assess the stage or phase that you are currently experiencing. What will define your new beginning?

## Role Conflict

Role conflict develops when an individual feels that she or he is faced with expectations that are incompatible with each other. Role conflict can be intrapersonal or interpersonal. Intrapersonal role conflict occurs when an individual struggles with multiple

---

### ▶ *Display 2-3* | **Bridge's Phases of Transition**

**▶ PHASE I: ENDINGS**

Four types of endings:
1. Disengagement      3. Disenchantment
2. Disidentification   4. Disorientation

**▶ PHASE II: NEUTRAL ZONE**

Three functions:
1. Surrender
2. Renewal and recharging; redirection
3. Change in perspective

**▶ PHASE III: MAKING A BEGINNING**

- A "loop in the life-journey"
- Reintegration of new identity with old identity

personal role expectations. For example, in your role as a student nurse, you may face conflict with the necessity of having to study as opposed to spending time with significant others in your life. Interpersonal role conflict occurs when different people have different expectations about the same role. An example of this type of conflict might occur in relation to others' expectations of you in your role as a nurse. You may think that your role is to spend time with a client with newly diagnosed diabetes so that you can begin teaching the process of self-care, whereas your supervisor may think that it is more important that you complete your written documentation. Role conflict is a component of role stress, in which a person realizes that role obligations are conflicting or that role demands are too difficult or impossible to fulfill. Feelings of discomfort, frustration, and anxiety can occur; this is referred to as role strain.

Several authors describe the role strain and role overload experienced particularly by women in returning to school or work while balancing this with the role of motherhood (Garey, 1999; Granrose & Kaplan, 1996; Holcomb, 1998). This phenomenon also occurs for men who are single parents or who have assumed more caregiving and parenting responsibilities in the home.

Bolton (2000) describes role overload for many women as they engage in what she calls "the third shift." In addition to dealing with concerns about work while at home, and those of home while at work, many women invest mental energy into reflecting on these two roles. They are continually assessing how well they are balancing home and work roles, which one is being compromised, and whether or not they are exercising good judgment in the choices they make each day.

Unfortunately, role conflict cannot be avoided, so it is important to develop methods to cope with conflict constructively. Five methods can be used to resolve conflict (**Display 2-4**):

1. **Avoidance:** This also is called withdrawing from or denying conflict. When this method is used, conflict is generally not resolved and may actually be perpetuated. *Example:* You checked a book out of the library and then loaned it to a fellow student. She returned it to the library late, and you were billed for the fine. You decide to pay it rather than asking the student to do so.
2. **Compromise:** This approach uses the techniques of bargaining or negotiating. There is recognition that there must be a give and take for the solution to be determined. Generally it works well, although the conflict issue may occur again. *Example:* You and your spouse arrange to accomplish household chores based on time limitations and abilities. Both of you agree that it is a good plan that will satisfy the need for a clean house and mutual responsibilities.

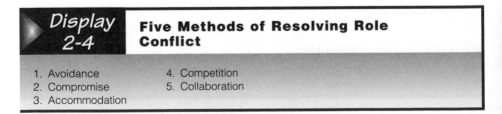

> *Display 2-4*   **Five Methods of Resolving Role Conflict**
>
> 1. Avoidance          4. Competition
> 2. Compromise         5. Collaboration
> 3. Accommodation

3. **Accommodation:** In this method, a person attempts to smooth over the conflict or to suppress the problems. Often a peaceful environment will be maintained, but one person may feel as though she or he has made a tremendous sacrifice and is inwardly angry and frustrated. *Example:* In example 2, it may be possible that one partner does not follow through on the predetermined tasks, and the other partner says that she or he understands and helps the partner to finish the undone household chores.

4. **Competition:** In this strategy, one person decides to force the issue and to put forth personal goals or desires over those of others. It sets up a conflict of power. *Example:* A group of students meet to plan for an end-of-the-year banquet and select a leader. One student spends 10 minutes describing her experience in her LPN program chairing the banquet committee, how successful the banquet was, and how grateful her classmates were for her leadership. The group agrees to let this student have primary responsibility for planning this banquet.

5. **Collaboration:** This strategy requires that all participants are willing to problem solve and to confront the issues with the intent of setting mutual goals. All participants are involved in the decision-making process. *Example:* A group of student nurses is concerned about the volume of paperwork required by clinical instructors. The instructors recognize that there is a lot of work but feel the need to validate a student's ability to be prepared for each clinical assignment. The chairperson arranges a meeting with the students and instructors to develop methods that validate student preparation without being overly burdensome.

## ▶ Thinking Critically

Consider each method of conflict resolution. Think of an example of your own for each method. Would another method have been more satisfactory?

## Conclusion

Role development and transition are complex processes that have individual and universal concepts. In this chapter, personal development is presented in relation to the work of stage theorists who perceive development in terms of stages and critical tasks that occur in a sequential pattern. Adult development is described as an ongoing and dynamic process. Family and professional role development are presented in terms of stages of development.

Concepts related to role socialization, role transition, and role conflict are presented with an emphasis on the meanings these concepts have for the LPN/LVN role transition process. Understanding the theories and concepts of role development and transition enhances a person's ability to examine her or his own experiences and assess client experiences better. The impacts of role changes and health status changes are varied and yet more predictable when all of the concepts are considered. You will find many opportunities to apply this information in your personal and work experiences, including your transition to the RN role.

## Student Exercises

1. Interview a student in your class.
2. Identify the various roles for this student.
3. Differentiate the individual's ascribed and acquired roles.
4. Select a theorist or theorists to determine the tasks with which this individual is concerned.
5. Ask the student to describe the role of her or his family and what her or his role is within that family.
6. Explore with the student what role changes are forthcoming.
7. Determine if there are role conflicts involved and what methods are used for coping.

## References

Bolton, M. E. (2000). *The third shift: Managing hard choices in our careers, homes, and lives as women.* San Francisco: Jossey-Bass.

Bridges, W. (1980). *Transitions: Making sense of life's.* Menlo Park, CA: Addison-Wesley.

Bridges, W. (1991). *Managing transitions: Making the most of change.* New York: William Bridges and Associates, Perseus Books.

Bridges, W. (2001). *The way of transitions: Embracing life's most difficult moments.* New York: William Bridges and Associates, Perseus Books.

Cohen, H. A. (1981). *The nurse's quest for a professional identity.* Menlo Park, CA: Addison-Wesley.

Duvall, E. M. (1977). *Marriage and family development* (5th ed.). Philadelphia: JB Lippincott.

Garey, A. I. (1999). *Weaving work and motherhood.* Philadelphia: Temple University Press.

Gilligan, C. (1982). *In a different voice: Psychological theory and women's development.* Cambridge, MA: Harvard University Press.

Granrose, C. S., & Kaplan, E. E. (1996). *Work-family role choices for women in their 20's and 30's: From college plans to life experiences.* Westport, CT: Praeger Publishers.

Hinshaw, A. S. (1986). Socialization and resocialization of nurses for professional nursing practice. In E. C. Hein & M. J. Nicholson (Eds.), *Contemporary leadership behavior: Selected readings* (2nd ed.). Boston: Little, Brown and Company.

Holcomb, B. (1998). *Not guilty: The good news about working mothers.* New York: Scribner, Simon, and Schuster.

Palmer, P. J. (1998). *The courage to teach: Exploring the inner landscape of a teacher's life.* San Francisco: Jossey-Bass.

Shane, D. L. (1983). *Returning to school: A guide for nurses.* Englewood Cliffs, NJ: Prentice-Hall.

Sheehy, G. (1976). *Passages: Predictable crises of adult life.* New York: Dutton and Company.

Stevens-Long, J. (1988). *Adult life* (3rd ed.). Mountain View, CA: Mayfield Publishing.

Stevenson, J. S. (1977). *Issues and crises during middlescence.* New York: Appleton-Century-Crofts.

Taylor, C., Lillis, C., and LeMone, P. (2001). *Fundamentals of nursing* (4th ed.). Philadelphia: Lippincott Williams & Wilkins.

## Suggested Reading

Clements, I. W., & Buchanan, D. M. (Eds.). (1982). *Family therapy: A nursing perspective.* New York: Wiley and Sons.

Ellis, J. R., & Hartley, C. L. (2000). *Managing and coordinating nursing care* (3rd ed.). Philadelphia: Lippincott Williams & Wilkins.

Friedman, M. M. (1986). *Family nursing: Theory and assessment* (2nd ed.). Norwalk, CT: Appleton-Century-Crofts.

Hardy, M. E., & Conway, M. E. (1988). *Role theory: Perspectives for health professionals* (2nd ed.). Norwalk, CT: Appleton & Lange.

Hill, P. M., & Humphrey, P. (Eds.). (1982). *Human growth and development throughout life: A nursing perspective*. New York: Wiley and Sons.

Leddy, S., & Pepper, J. M. (1998). *Conceptual bases of professional nursing* (4th ed.). Philadelphia: Lippincott-Raven Publishers.

Rossi, A. S. (Ed.). (1985). *Gender and the life course*. New York: Aldine Publishing.

Sheehy, G. (1981). *Pathfinders*. New York: Morrow and Company.

Valentine, P. (2001). A gender perspective on conflict management strategies of nurses. *Journal of Nursing Scholarship, 33*(1), 69–74.

Wainrib, B. R. (Ed.). (1992). *Gender issues across the life cycle*. New York: Springer Publishing.

Wrightsman, L. S. (1980). *Personality development in adulthood*. Newbury Park: Sage Publications.

*On the Web* • • • • • • • • • • • • • • • • • • • • • • • • • • • • • • •

*http://nursingworld.org.mods/mod190ceadrabs.html:* This is a CEU offering on workplace advocacy and how to handle disputes.

*www.piaget.org:* This is the website of the Jean Piaget Society.

*http://elvers.stjoe.udayton.edu/history/people/Erikson.html:* This is a Dayton University website with links to works on Erik Erikson; the site also has a picture of Mr. Erikson.

# CHAPTER 3

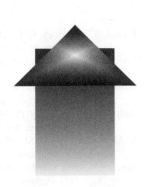

# Adapting to Change

## LEARNING OBJECTIVES

*By the end of this chapter, the student will be able to:*

1 Explore the paradoxes of change.
2 Differentiate individual and organizational change.
3 Summarize factors that motivate change.
4 Compare and contrast types of change.
5 Describe the process of planned change.
6 Outline Lewin's process of change.
7 Discuss the effects of change on individuals and systems.
8 Apply theoretical effects of change.
9 Describe methods for adjusting to change.
10 Give examples of positive outcomes of change.

## KEY TERMS

| | |
|---|---|
| adaptation | general adaptation syndrome |
| ambivalence | individual change |
| autonomy | loss |
| biotechnology | organizational change |
| change | paradox |
| change agent | resistance |
| conflict | resonance |
| crisis | restraining forces |
| distress | self-actualization |
| driving forces | stakeholders |
| eustress | transactional change |
| flexibility | transformational change |

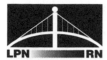

## VIGNETTE

Deborah Pogwist is a 54-year-old LPN who has worked in the mental health unit of a state hospital for the past 25 years. She is taking her first clinical nursing course for her associate degree. After having difficulty with the clinical component in a hospital setting, she is meeting with her nursing adviser, John Tercha, to discuss her problems with adjusting to change.

**Deborah:** I feel so inadequate! I remember being in the hospital setting years ago, but why do I need to go through this again when there is a job opening where I have worked for 25 years? I just feel that I'm jumping through hoops!

**Advisor:** I hear what you're saying and I understand. It is often very uncomfortable for adults to be in a new environment. It sounds as if you feel frustrated and are not sure whether the concepts you are learning are applicable to your professional work.

**Deborah:** Yes, you are right! Do I really have to do all of this?

**Advisor:** Yes, you will have to complete the clinical objectives for the courses. However, I can assure you that the newness will wear off, and even though you cannot see the relevance of what you are learning, it is part of the bigger picture. This picture includes making you become more flexible, more well rounded, more educated, and more of a critical thinker. Change is a very difficult process, but it is necessary. Let's review what specific difficulties you are having and review some change theory and how it can help you through this first clinical course transition.

## Change Defined

William Bridges (2001, p. 1), a leading author on change and transitions, identifies several change paradoxes that define its dynamic state (**Display 3-1**). A paradox is a statement that seems absurd or contradictory but is based on fact.

Change is ever present in our daily lives. With change, each person, group, or organization has the opportunity to develop, grow, and adapt. Change is inevitable and dynamic. Each of us copes with change in unique ways. Our responses to change are affected by what is occurring in our lives, what needs we have, and what our experiences have been.

---

### *Display 3-1*  The Paradoxes of Change

- To achieve continuity, we have to be willing to change.
- Change is the only way to protect whatever exists, for without continuous readjustments, the present cannot continue.
- The very things we now wish that we could hold onto and keep safe from change were themselves originally produced by changes.

# The Process of Change

Examining the process of change is particularly important for student nurses for several reasons. First, you are experiencing personal change by your return to school. Second, you will be presented with many aspects of change within the nursing curriculum. For instance, in issues related to trends in healthcare, the faculty may present you with current methods of delivering care and have you explore how the future in healthcare delivery will be affected by biotechnology or economic concerns. Third, as you prepare for your own role transition, you will learn about the new roles nurses have today and will have in the future. It is essential to understand that change is inevitable. Change occurs even when you think societal and work roles and values are stable or resistant to change.

# Individual and Organizational Change

When differentiating between individual and organizational change, remember that change always implies the alteration or modification of behaviors or functions. Within the individual, change may occur without any plan at all, or it may be the result of much planning. Later in this chapter, types of change are described. Organizational change also results in behavior or function alterations but has the potential to have a greater impact on parts of an organization and its individuals. **Display 3-2** compares individual and organizational change. Change within an organization involves modifying working practices and procedures, causing individuals to work in different ways. This can produce a great deal of fear among employees. Carter and Alfred (1999, p. 28) note that, "Change, by its very nature, represents breaking with the past. Ironically, it is most successful when the process honors and respects institutional history and tradition."

# Factors That Motivate Change

Many factors motivate change. If you were to examine your reasons for desiring a change from your role as a licensed practical/vocational nurse (LPN/LVN) to that of a registered nurse (RN), you may identify some aspects that are described in the following text. You also may recognize some factors that have played a part in other life changes.

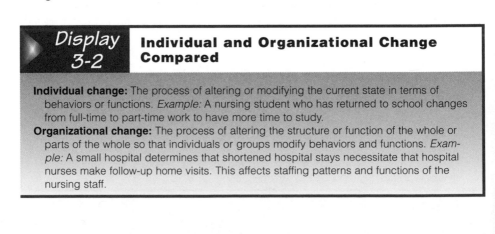

**Display 3-2** | **Individual and Organizational Change Compared**

**Individual change:** The process of altering or modifying the current state in terms of behaviors or functions. *Example:* A nursing student who has returned to school changes from full-time to part-time work to have more time to study.

**Organizational change:** The process of altering the structure or function of the whole or parts of the whole so that individuals or groups modify behaviors and functions. *Example:* A small hospital determines that shortened hospital stays necessitate that hospital nurses make follow-up home visits. This affects staffing patterns and functions of the nursing staff.

# Crisis

One factor that can precipitate change is a crisis—a turning point or a critical time in the course of an event. As discussed in Chapter 2, a situational crisis involves an unexpected event, such as a natural disaster, loss of a loved one, illness, or divorce. This type of crisis can motivate an individual to make other changes. For example, a 40-year-old nurse who had recently been through a divorce recognized a need to further her education and develop a career. This may not have happened if she had remained in the marriage.

# Conflict

Another factor that can influence the process of change is conflict. There is always a sense of battle or opposition when the term *conflict* is used. In relation to change, it also denotes a struggle or variance with a particular situation or person. Conflict may result in change because an individual feels frustrated with the current circumstances. An example is that of a man who has not been happy in his position as a nurse in a local hospital. He wants to practice nursing in a more holistic way and feels that the fragmented care system is not adequate. Although he has spoken to his boss many times, he has been unable to make any changes in the care delivery system. Finally, he decides that he cannot deal with the conflict within himself and his job, so he resigns. He subsequently is hired by a community health agency that practices a more holistic approach. Conflict motivated him to make a change.

# Disappointment

Disappointment can be another motivator for change. Everyone has experienced disappointment at some point. Disappointment is related to a sense of failure for not meeting expectations or fulfilling certain plans. A nursing student who has done poorly in math has avoided working on math problems. After failing her first quiz, she meets with her advisor, spends time with the class tutor, and purchases a step-by-step nursing math review text. This student nurse has vowed to change her practice habits so that she will pass the next quiz and her clinical performance will be accurate and more satisfying.

# Lack of Rewards

Another stimulus for change is lack of reward in the current circumstances. An individual may be in a position that affords little recognition or reward. This situation can motivate the person to take courses or advanced training or to change jobs to gain more rewards and prestige.

# Desire for Autonomy and Self-improvement

The last factor that can activate change is the desire for autonomy and self-improvement. A person may feel stagnated and powerless in a particular position and thus may take appropriate steps to change the situation. For instance, a certified nursing assistant may enjoy the work but not feel able to influence policy or procedures. She or he also may desire to learn more and take on more responsibility. This sense of powerlessness and need for self-improvement is a potent factor for making a change.

### Thinking Critically

Identify factors that have caused you to make a change in your life. Give examples of changes that you have made. Analyze the results of these changes and how certain behaviors or functions were affected.

## Types of Change

There are various types of change with which an individual or organization can be faced. From your own experiences, you probably can delineate some of these. The following text defines some of the types of change that are generally encountered.

### Forced Change

Forced change is a type of change that is imposed on an individual or organization that requires action, often of an immediate or emergent nature. An example would be a fire in a person's home, in which the entire home and its contents are lost. Family members are forced to consider rebuilding the home, replacing lost items, and realizing that everything is forever different.

### Spontaneous Change

Spontaneous change refers to change that is impulsive or effortless and often is random or unpredictable. For example, when a person begins a new job, she or he may take on the characteristics of other co-workers. This may involve buying the same types of clothes or becoming interested in similar activities. In retrospect, it may seem like a planned response, but in reality it occurred spontaneously and without forethought.

### Developmental Change

Developmental change is change in which a person proceeds through stages in a fairly predictable order. Tasks are identified for each stage that must be accomplished to complete a stage. Examples of this type of change are described in Chapter 2.

### Unplanned Change

Unplanned change can refer to positive or negative, desired or undesired change that was not planned. The three types of changes described in the preceding material are types of unplanned change. An example of positive unplanned change would be an unexpected promotion within an organization. A negative unplanned stage might be unannounced layoffs at a place of employment.

# Planned Change

Planned change involves advanced strategy by a change agent. Ellis and Hartley (2000) describe a change agent as a champion who is responsible for leading the group to change. Members who are affected by the change are referred to as stakeholders. In an organization, anyone can become the change agent and present ideas to the stakeholders. For example, a planned change is your return to school; you probably made careful plans to achieve your goals. These plans may have included child care or other personal issues, revision of work schedules, or a change in daily activities. Other planned changes may have occurred in your workplace. Schedule changes are an example. Some healthcare settings have opted to have their employees work 12-hour shifts. To establish that schedule, an implementation plan is developed so that the transition to the new schedule is as smooth as possible. This is the process of planned change. There are several types of planned change.

## INCREMENTAL CHANGE
Planned change develops incrementally, in steps or stages. This type of planning is often applied to long-term projects, such as hospital mergers or curriculum changes. Some of you may have planned your return to school in increments. You may have taken all of your general education courses first as the initial stage of your education. The second part of the process involves completing the nursing courses. In this way, you are able to continue working or have greater ability to care for a family.

## RAPID CHANGE
Change that is planned quickly may or may not be successful. For instance, rapid plans may need to be developed in rescue situations to assist people quickly and to change a precarious situation. Rapid change also can mean the implementation of an organizational plan without considering all of the ramifications. As an example, a nursing organization recognizes that staff positions need to be eliminated fairly quickly because of reduced census or revenue shortfalls. The plans are made to eliminate positions based on seniority, without considering what units have the highest staffing needs and how staff might need to be transferred and oriented. The plan is implemented quickly but without considering all of the ramifications.

## TRANSACTIONAL CHANGE
Transactional change occurs for mutual benefit. For example, nursing faculty and students determine that a change is needed in clinical experiences so that all seniors have an opportunity for a leadership experience. Representatives of both groups meet to plan the best method to accomplish this goal. The plan is formed so that all parties are able to transact an appropriate and mutually agreeable plan.

## TRANSFORMATIONAL CHANGE
Transformational change occurs within the process of planned change. In your return to school, a change will occur as you progress through ADN course work. With this process of change will come not only new knowledge and skills, but also a new way of thinking and being. Transformation implies that there is a radical difference in an individual or a group as a result of change.

## NCLEX–RN Might Ask 3-1

The nurse is taking care of a large group of clients in a community care setting. Because of the high influx of new clients, the nurse manager independently decides to make a radical change in the way clients are assessed and processed. This type of radical change would be most consistent with

    A.  transactional change.
    B.  transformational change.
    C.  unplanned change.
    D.  spontaneous change.

• *See Appendix A for correct answer and rationale.*

### ▶ Thinking Critically

Review the types of change that have been described. Think of experiences that have involved change in your life. Categorize these changes according to the previous descriptions. Consider these changes in terms of individual, group, and organizational changes. Are any of them transformational in nature? Why?

## The Stages of Planned Change ▬▬▬▬▬▬

The process of change is complex because it involves the modification of behaviors. Unplanned change is, obviously, less structured and more haphazard than planned change. When change is planned, there will be a more systematic approach that entails problem solving, decision making, and deliberate steps. Kurt Lewin is a social scientist credited with doing the first work in change theory. The following text outlines his theory of planned change. **Display 3-3** summarizes Lewin's three stages of planned change (1951).

### Unfreezing

The first stage Lewin (1951) identified is referred to as the *unfreezing* stage, in which a person, group, or organization is motivated to bring about a change. There is a need

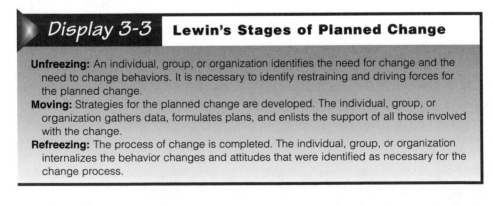

| *Display 3-3* | **Lewin's Stages of Planned Change** |
|---|---|

**Unfreezing:** An individual, group, or organization identifies the need for change and the need to change behaviors. It is necessary to identify restraining and driving forces for the planned change.
**Moving:** Strategies for the planned change are developed. The individual, group, or organization gathers data, formulates plans, and enlists the support of all those involved with the change.
**Refreezing:** The process of change is completed. The individual, group, or organization internalizes the behavior changes and attitudes that were identified as necessary for the change process.

to learn new behaviors. This stage is one of imbalance and disequilibrium and is very unsettling. During this stage, two types of forces are present: one against and one in support of change.

## RESTRAINING FORCES

Restraining forces are those that inhibit change. For example, as you have become motivated to return to school, you undoubtedly have encountered some restraining forces. For example, some of the restraining forces may have been related to family concerns, loss of income while in school, or lack of confidence in your ability to succeed.

## DRIVING FORCES

Opposing such restraining forces are driving forces. These are the forces that encourage and sustain change. For example, your motivation to return to school may have been supported by such forces as your desire for more decision making, increased clinical skills, more recognition, or the encouragement and support of a family member, mentor, or friend.

# Moving

The second stage is called moving. During this stage, plans are detailed and initiated. It is important to collect data and supplemental information from as many sources as possible. In addition, it is helpful if all people involved are in agreement that change is desirable. For example, you entered the moving stage after you began making plans to return to school. At this time, you formulated plans for child care or alternative work schedules. You also may have obtained information about financial aid and scholarships. You gathered as much information as possible to assist you in your plans. You may have enlisted the advice of a colleague who had been through this process. It may have been necessary for you to persuade those around you that this was an important move for you to make and that you needed their support and understanding.

It is during this second stage of change that transitions occur, as described in Chapter 2. Letting go of the past (i.e., accomplishing endings) becomes essential to make room for new beginnings. Role conflict may increase as both you and others around you work to put old roles behind you to prepare for new ones.

# Refreezing

The last is called *refreezing*. The change has occurred and is an integral part of the individual, group, or organization. Refreezing implies that there is commitment to the change and that the restraining and driving forces have stabilized. There is a change of behaviors and attitudes within the change process. In continuing with the same example, as you re-enter school, one change has already occurred: You are a student nurse again. You have internalized the value of continuing your education and have made the commitment to become an RN. This change is part of who you are.

> ## Thinking Critically
>
> Recall a planned change with which you were recently involved. Critique your change as viewed through the three stages of planned change described by Lewin. What steps were taken to initiate the change? What were the restraining and driving forces? What was your role in the planned change? What role conflict did you experience? When were you aware that you had made a transition and were prepared for the refreezing stage?

# The Effects of Change

Change can have many effects. Some are expected and some are not. As previously stated, individuals cope with and adapt to change in unique ways.

## Stress, Distress, and Eustress

Stress, distress, and eustress are terms defined by Hans Selye (1976) to describe various conditions that humans experience. Stress is a universal response to any situation or factor that disturbs a person's equilibrium. It has become a familiar term to all of us and may be a term that you will use frequently while in nursing school. Selye calls the side effects of stress *distress* and *eustress*. Distress is the negative or maladaptive effects of change or stress, and eustress represents the more beneficial effects.

With any stress or change, nonspecific bodily changes occur. If a person is able to cope effectively with change, the side effects will be kept to a minimum, but poor adaptation to stress or change results in damaging side effects, or distress. Physical signs of distress can include prolonged elevated blood pressure, increased gastric acid secretions, and decreased urine output. Emotional signs may include insomnia and hyperexcitability. There also may be behavioral changes, such as depression or anger. Selye (1976) believed that some conditions (e.g., hypertension, ulcers, and some emotional disturbances) represent diseases of adaptation. Although many researchers and physicians argue differently, the concepts of distress and eustress are interesting and provide a means for you to evaluate the typical coping patterns of your clients.

## General Adaptation Syndrome

As the preceding paragraphs indicate, a common effect of any change, planned or unplanned, is stress, which disturbs an individual's equilibrium. Selye (1976) was the first person to describe a nonspecific general response to stress, which he called *general adaptation syndrome*. He differentiated stress as a condition of the body that is characterized by the changes that occur within the body. A stressor is defined as any factor that upsets the equilibrium and results in stress. For example, a student may experience nausea before making a class presentation. The stressor is the presentation; the stress is the condition of nausea.

Selye (1976) delineates three stages that occur in the general adaptation syndrome: alarm reaction, resistance, and recovery or exhaustion. **Table 3-1** shows these stages.

## ALARM REACTION

The first stage of the general adaptation syndrome is the alarm reaction. The body responds to a particular stressor, such as an extreme in temperature, infection, verbal abuse, or other conscious and unconscious factors. With this process, the defense mechanisms of the mind and body are activated. The autonomic nervous system releases large amounts of hormones into the body. Blood volume is increased, and blood glucose levels rise to meet energy needs. Increased epinephrine results in a higher heart rate, more blood flow to muscles, better oxygen intake, and greater mental alertness. Norepinephrine is released in greater quantities to decrease blood flow to the kidneys. Increased rennin secretion will result in more angiotensin production, thus elevating blood pressure. This process initiates the fight or flight response and may last for a short period to many hours. A person is ready for action during this phase.

## RESISTANCE

The second stage is called the *resistance* stage. During this stage, the alarm reactions stabilize. The hormone levels and cardiac functions return to previous levels. The person attempts to adapt to the stressor or to cope more effectively with its effects. For example, if a person has sustained a fracture, the body responds by beginning the process of healing at the site of the fracture. This would be considered recovery. If the stressor is more difficult, such as hemorrhage, adaptation may be impossible, and the outcome is exhaustion. In both cases, the individuals enter the next stage.

**T A B L E   3 - 1**
**STAGES OF THE GENERAL ADAPTATION SYNDROME**

| Stage | Body Responses |
|---|---|
| Alarm reaction (fight or flight) | Increased release of hormones by the autonomic nervous system:<br>• Increased heart rate<br>• Increased oxygen intake<br>• Increased blood sugar<br>• Increased mental acuity<br>• Increased blood flow to muscles<br>• Increased blood pressure<br>• Decreased flow to the kidneys<br>• Decreased urine output |
| Resistance | Stabilization:<br>• Hormone levels return to normal<br>• Cardiac functions return to previous levels<br>• Adaptation to stressor(s) |
| Recovery or exhaustion | Defense mechanisms described in alarm reaction stage are exhausted<br>Decreased energy levels<br>Fatigue<br>Decreased ability for adaptation<br>Death |

## RECOVERY OR EXHAUSTION

The third stage is referred to as the stage of *recovery* or *exhaustion*. The body will either recover or find it can no longer cope with the stressor, having exhausted its ability to defend itself. The effects of stress may involve the entire body. A person who experiences psychological trauma will enter a state of exhaustion and demonstrate physical and emotional symptoms, such as abdominal pain, insomnia, or depression. If the state of exhaustion is severe, such as the state that follows unchecked hemorrhage, death may occur.

The concepts of stress and adaptation may be familiar to you from your LPN/LVN program. One's ability to adapt to stress also describes the ability to adapt to change. Adaptation involves a person's capacity for change as she or he is faced with new experiences. Understanding how you adapt to change can assist you with some of the stress you may encounter as you return to the student role.

### ▶ Thinking Critically

Recall a situation that has created stress for you. Review the stages of the general adaptation syndrome. Determine what physical, emotional, or behavioral changes occurred. What was the outcome of the change that took place? What is your general response to stressful situations? How do you adapt?

## Ambivalence

Another effect of change is ambivalence. This term pertains to opposing views an individual may have for a particular situation, person, or other factor. For instance, some claim to have experienced a love–hate relationship with a particular person. This means that within one's self are conflicting emotions of love and hate.

Feelings of ambivalence can occur when a person is experiencing change. During the change process, a person may have mixed feelings about what the change will

### NCLEX–RN Might Ask 3-2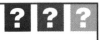

The nurse is caring for a client in the emergency room after an automobile accident. Although there are no visible signs of injury, the client's heart rate, blood pressure, and respirations are elevated. The client's peripheral oxygenation level is 100%, the blood glucose level is slightly elevated, and the client is answering questions appropriately. The nurse knows that this stage of the general adaptation syndrome is

   A. normal.
   B. alarm reaction.
   C. resistance.
   D. exhaustion.

• *See Appendix A for correct answer and rationale.*

involve. At some point, you may have decided to change your hair style or facial hair. Halfway into the change, you may have been tentatively pleased, yet also appalled about this new look. This is ambivalence.

### Thinking Critically

Consider changes that you have experienced, for example, a marriage, divorce, or change in living arrangements. Analyze ambivalent feelings you had about these changes.

## Resistance

Resistance has been defined as conduct that tries to preserve the status quo. "People prefer things with which they are familiar and have a natural tendency to resist change, especially if it requires a change in values or beliefs or if it will require something extra" (Ellis & Hartley, 2000, p. 277). This effect of change is common throughout a change process. There always is comfort in the way things are. Fear of the unknown or a lack of self-confidence can hinder a person's ability to welcome change. Other factors that may be involved include the following:

- Experiences with change have not been positive. *Example:* An employee who resists change states that previous job changes always meant loss of job or pay.
- Resistance to change is higher if an individual or group has not participated in the decision to make the change. *Example:* The head nurse in an intensive care unit decides to implement the use of computerized standard care plans. The equipment that is purchased is very labor-intensive to learn and not nurse-friendly. Many of the staff nurses are irate and refuse to comply with the change.
- Lack of communication throughout the change process increases resistance. *Example:* Employees of a medical clinic are informed that there will be a change in the management structure to make the organization more efficient and less costly. They are told that more information will be coming soon. After several weeks of hearing nothing, some of the employees are disgruntled. Rumors are rampant, and many of the employees are now vehemently opposed to any change that may occur, although initially they recognized a need.
- Passive resistance may occur, and may be manifested as inefficiency, lethargy, failure to complete tasks, increased errors in job performance, or poor attitudes. *Example:* A nurse at a small hospital is unhappy about being floated to a similar medical-surgical unit. Although she goes to the assigned unit, she barely speaks to the other staff nurses and displays a sullen attitude when she sees the supervisor.

Resistance to change is not only important to consider from a personal or organizational point of view, but also from the perspective of clients. Many of your clients will experience change, much of which may be undesirable and unwanted. These clients may resist the efforts of the healthcare system to accomplish the needed changes.

## CULTURAL RESISTANCE FACTORS

Predictability and linearity of change is basically a Western phenomenon. Looking at change from the Eastern perspective can help us learn much. Taoist and Confucian philosophies view change as cyclic and ongoing, rather than as having an endpoint. Life is a quest for balance and harmony within an ever-changing environment. Resistance may occur when needed changes are incompatible with cultural beliefs. For example, some people of Hispanic background believe that illness is caused by diet imbalance and that certain foods in combination restore balance, even though some foods may be contraindicated in some conditions.

## SOCIAL RESISTANCE FACTORS

Resistance also may occur when needed changes are not seen as normal within a social group. For example, a woman with chronic bronchitis does not change from her weekly social routine of playing bingo, even though the game is played in a smoke-filled room, which aggravates her bronchitis.

## PSYCHOLOGICAL RESISTANCE FACTORS

Finally, resistance to change may occur when needed changes produce anxiety secondary to fear of the unknown, lack of confidence, loss of control, and fear of being a burden. For example, a client with newly diagnosed diabetes is afraid to give himself injections because he is afraid that poor technique will make the disease worse.

### ▶ Thinking Critically

Consider a change that has occurred in your workplace or within another organization. Review the factors that increase resistance to change. What methods of resistance did you observe? What methods were used to overcome the resistance? Was the change a success or a failure? Why?

You must assess your clients' feelings and attitudes about a particular change. You also must not impose change without regard to a person's cultural, social, and psychological beliefs. According to Creasia and Parker (2001), change is better perceived if a client/stakeholder is actively involved in the change process (**Display 3-4**).

### ▶ Display 3-4 | Improving Reception to Change

Change will be better received if a person perceives a need for change, is open to change, has the ability to have choices regarding the change, and commits to the change process.

# Loss

Change frequently involves some type of loss. The death of a spouse is an obvious example of loss. However, other changes can induce a sense of loss. Many recent graduates report a sadness or grief when they complete a program of study. This is often related to leaving school, leaving friends, and beginning something new and unknown.

## INDIVIDUAL LOSS AND CHANGE

Elisabeth Kubler-Ross (1969) developed a model of death and dying that describes stages when dealing with loss and change. The first stage is denial, in which an individual refuses to believe that anything has happened or is different. Others may believe that everything is under control. In the second stage, the person experiences anger and is mad at everyone and everything. The third stage is the bargaining stage, in which a person attempts to barter or deal to make things better or to delay reality. Depression is the fourth stage; the person fully recognizes the impact of the loss and frequently withdraws and is mournful and lonely. The last stage is acceptance, in which the individual is more at peace with the loss and has come to terms with the situation.

## ORGANIZATIONAL LOSS AND CHANGE

Perlman and Takacs (1990) have developed a model based on Kubler-Ross' model to describe the phases that are seen within an organization that is involved with change. These phases can be used to depict the emotions that one may experience with any change. The following is a brief description of each stage:

**Phase 1: Equilibrium**—A person is happy with current conditions, feels that everything is in balance, and experiences anxiety if the status quo is threatened.

**Phase 2: Denial**—When change becomes apparent, the person attempts to act as if nothing has changed or will change; the person may choose to ignore what is happening or not participate in activities that help prepare for change.

**Phase 3: Anger**—Within this stage, the individual actively resists change by being visibly angry, disgruntled, and uncooperative. The person typically blames others and wants everything fixed.

**Phase 4: Bargaining**—A person tries to negotiate to keep things from changing. The person is willing to make some concessions in an attempt to maintain as much of the status quo as possible.

**Phase 5: Chaos**—The person feels powerless to stop the change or to make it better. She or he feels insecure and disoriented because the change does not make sense.

**Phase 6: Depression**—The individual grieves and feels tremendous sorrow for the loss or change. She or he also experiences self-pity and emptiness.

**Phase 7: Resignation**—The individual is lethargic and mechanical; the change is passively accepted.

**Phase 8: Openness**—Within this stage the individual becomes more engaged with the change and is more willing to be involved in the activities needed to complete the change.

**Phase 9: Readiness**—The individual continues to be more engaged and enthusiastic about the change; she or he is more willing to participate in necessary activities.

**Phase 10: Re-emergence**—The person now values the change and is willing to make a personal investment in the change process.

## NCLEX– RN Might Ask 3-3

The nurse is caring for a client who has had a radical mastectomy. The client refuses to look at her operative site and be involved in dressing changes. This client's behavior best describes which stage of grieving?

    A. Depression
    B. Denial
    C. Bargaining
    D. Acceptance

• *See Appendix A for correct answer and rationale.*

The models by Kubler-Ross and Perlman and Takacs are compared in **Table 3-2**. These models will assist you to contemplate what change can mean for an individual or a group. It is helpful to consider these aspects when you are experiencing personal changes or when your clients are forced to adapt to a new situation. As with any stage theory, the phases may not be as clear or sequential, but the emotions that can accompany any change will be similar. The following critical thinking activity requires that you role play the part of a client and imagine the stages of changing that this client will experience.

### ▶ Thinking Critically

Mr. Fleming is 40 years old. He is a lawyer in a prominent law firm. He is married and has two young sons. Last weekend he was on a long bicycle ride and was hit by a truck. His injuries included a severe traumatic injury to his left foot, resulting in a below-the-knee amputation. His other injuries were not as severe. Consider the stages or phases of change shown in Table 3-2 and explain in each stage or phase what you might observe in terms of his behavior and emotions.

**T A B L E   3 - 2**
A COMPARISON OF MODELS OF STAGES OF INDIVIDUAL LOSS AND CHANGE (KUBLER-ROSS) AND PHASES OF ORGANIZATIONAL CHANGE (PERLMAN AND TAKACS)

| Stages of Individual Loss and Change (Kubler-Ross) | Phases of Organizational Change (Perlman and Takacs) |
| --- | --- |
| | Phase 1: Equilibrium |
| Stage 1: Denial | Phase 2: Denial |
| Stage 2: Anger | Phase 3: Anger |
| Stage 3: Bargaining | Phase 4: Bargaining |
| | Phase 5: Chaos |
| Stage 4: Depression | Phase 6: Depression |
| | Phase 7: Resignation |
| Stage 5: Acceptance | Phase 8: Openness |
| | Phase 9: Readiness |
| | Phase 10: Re-emergence |

# Resonance

The term *resonance* is generally used to define the reflection of sound or the reverberation of sound. However, it also describes the response of a system to changes from within and without the system. For example, if an individual has a cold, not only are the nasal passages affected, but also malaise, fever, and general discomfort occur. Likewise, the individual who is depressed also will be fatigued and disengaged from day-to-day activities. An entire system is affected by what is happening to a part or parts.

General systems theory is often used to explain the interrelatedness of parts of a system and the resonance response. When one part of a system experiences change, the whole system responds. The system can be a human, a family, an organization, or a community. Although the parts may be defined as separate, each part has a function that contributes to the total function of the system. A change in one part resonates throughout the system.

The nursing profession has always held a holistic view of wellness and illness. Within this holistic view, change within one part affects the entire system. The whole is considered greater and different than its parts. In using the holistic perspective, a person constantly experiences change internally and externally. These changes resonate within the entire system. An open system must be maintained for the exchange of energy, information, and matter to occur.

Following are examples of changes that occur to a part in which the entire system responds.

### EXAMPLE 1

■ Alice dives into a cold pool. She experiences a sense of shock as she hits the cold water. She also feels other sensations related to internal changes, such as blood vessel constriction, an inability to focus on anything except the immediate sensations, and a feeling of discomfort. Alice experiences other changes depending on how long she remains in the pool. Her internal environment responds to the changing external environment. ■

### EXAMPLE 2

■ There are four members of the Allen family. The parents both work outside of the home. Two teenage daughters go to the local high school. The father has not been home from work on time for many weeks. When he arrives home, it is obvious that he has been drinking. The parents frequently fight about this situation. The oldest daughter is frequently having headaches and stomach aches. Her grades at school have dropped. Her teachers are concerned about the change in her demeanor—she is withdrawn, quiet, and inattentive. ■

### EXAMPLE 3

■ A respected resident of a small town dies suddenly as the result of a heart attack. Members of the community experience shock, dismay, and grief after this event. ■

In all of these examples, a part of the system is affected by a change in the internal or external environment; the change resonates within the system, and the entire system responds in some way to the change that has occurred. The concepts related to general systems theory present a holistic approach to the effects of change. Nurses are able to intervene more effectively and holistically if they recognize how change in one part affects change of the whole.

> ### Thinking Critically
>
> Develop your own examples of resonance that have happened to you, within your family, work setting, or community. Consider how change to one part affected the whole. Determine how a holistic approach is helpful in examining the effects of change.

## Adjusting to Change

In the process of adjusting to change, turmoil exists. Adjusting to change is not always an easy task. Emotions vary widely, from despair to joy, with much tension and doubt in between. You probably have learned through experience how to adjust more readily to change.

### Attitude

The primary method for adjusting to change is often related to the attitude one has about the change. The manner in which one approaches change can have a major effect on the ability to adapt. For instance, an employer informs a nurse who has been employed full time by a community health agency for 7 years that only full-time nurses will be taking emergency calls in the future. The nurse can approach this change in several ways. The first is to endorse the change as positive for continuity of care for the clients who are seen by the agency. The second approach would be to lament to the employer that this is not a fair system and that everyone should have to take calls. This nurse has some control over her adjustment to change, depending on which attitude she adopts.

In other changes that are more sudden or in which an individual has less control, it may be more difficult to have the appropriate attitude. If a loved one dies suddenly, a positive attitude will assist a person to adjust, but other strategies are generally used. For instance, one person may solicit the support of other family members and friends. Others may benefit from joining a support group consisting of people who are experiencing a similar situation. Some people plunge into work or other activities so that they can get on with the business of living and avoid dwelling on the loss.

### Flexibility

Maintaining an approach that incorporates flexibility also assists with successful adaptation to change. Katz and associates (2001) note that especially during rapid change or unplanned change, flexibility can help you shift priorities quickly to minimize negative results and move ahead. Flexibility allows you to discover unforeseen opportunities and to grow.

## Coping Strategies

Coping strategies vary and often depend on the circumstances and previous coping methods used. When faced with change, one person may try to avoid it, whereas another faces it directly. A third person may try to enlist the support of others or gather more information to deal with the change more effectively. All of these methods may be effective in the adjustment to change.

In your return to school, you must identify what strategies will assist you in being successful. Obviously, a positive attitude is extremely beneficial, not only for yourself, but also for your student colleagues. It often is useful to develop a support system within the student nurse group. A small group of colleagues will provide support and guidance for many issues that you encounter while in school. Some find that it helps to study together or to socialize away from school to adjust more effectively to the changes caused by returning to school.

### ▶ Thinking Critically

In your return to school, consider the strategies that are useful for you as you adjust to the changes that school necessitates. Summarize methods that help you cope with change. Compare these methods with those of another nursing student and assess alternative methods you each could use.

McKenry and Price (1994) emphasize that successful coping depends on both our perception of change (i.e., how we approach it will determine the amount of stress it poses) and our ability to adapt to change. They note that families under stress rely on both internal family system resources and external community resources.

## Positive Outcomes of Change

Change has the possibility of many outcomes. Within any change process, the positive aspects of the change should be visualized. In examining positive outcomes of change, the following relates to your process of returning to school and the changes that will occur.

The possible positive outcomes that will occur are as follows:

1. You will acquire more education and knowledge. Although the educational process at times can be overwhelming or frustrating, the benefit will be an increased ability to integrate theory with practice and to be more informed regarding client care and healthcare issues.

2. One of the reasons that you returned to school may have been related to a desire to increase responsibilities and a greater scope of practice. The RN role will provide more opportunities for career mobility and flexibility and more ability to develop within the professional nurse role.

3. Another positive outcome of change will be monetary rewards. Salaries for RNs have improved in the last decade. The potential for financial growth continues to be greater within the professional roles, even with the uncertainty of future healthcare reform.

4. With any additional education, there is a greater potential for increased prestige. Although such recognition may not seem important or may seem to have elitist overtones, being recognized for increased knowledge and abilities and associated achievements reaps the reward of educational changes. The associate degree in nursing and the title of RN bestow a distinct and honorable recognition and provide opportunities for increased decision making.

5. Along with increased prestige comes increased self-confidence and self-esteem. Maslow identified a hierarchy of basic needs. According to his theory, after physiologic, safety and security, and love and belonging needs are met, an individual has needs of esteem and self-esteem. Esteem needs include respect from others, recognition, prestige, and importance. Self-esteem needs encompass those related to achievement, competence and independence, and self-worth. Advanced education provides a greater means to achieve a belief in your own abilities and thus to have self-confidence and self-esteem.

6. A final positive outcome of change is self-actualization. Maslow theorized that the highest level of needs occurs when the other basic needs have been met. Self-actualization is the need to be all that you can be through self-fulfillment and reaching your potential. In your return to school, you are fulfilling a dream or a goal. You also are increasing your ability to solve problems, broadening your means to deal with various situations, and developing greater power to cope with stress. The positive outcomes of change are varied. Each change with which you are faced provides the opportunity for positive outcomes. In the following critical thinking activity, you are asked to consider some positive outcomes of change.

## Thinking Critically

Critique an organizational change that has occurred in your workplace or within a community organization with which you are involved. Compare the positive outcomes experienced with that change, both for the organization and for yourself. Examine similarities and differences.

## Conclusion

Change is a dynamic and ongoing process. Many of the changes that we face are not of our choosing. However, we also have the ability to affect our own change and to plan for and deal with the results. Nurses must understand the dynamics of the change process. Not only do nurses face the challenges of personal changes, but they also encounter the changes that face their clients. The processes of stress and adaptation are key to understanding the coping strategies that individuals may use. Nurses also are involved with organizational changes, which can involve complex processes personally and collectively. The effects of change are varied and often depend on individual and group coping mechanisms.

Nursing and healthcare in general is ever changing. Although it is impossible to predict what changes will occur in the future, it is certain that change will be continuous. You must recognize these dynamics and determine how your experience will assist you to adapt and be part of the change process.

## Student Exercises

Recruit another student, peer, or friend to assist you with the following exercises.

1. Create a change situation that involves role playing a client who is faced with a new diagnosis of heart disease.

2. Determine what factors may motivate this client to change her or his lifestyle.

3. Develop a plan that will assist the client to make changes.

4. Discuss the possible effects of change related to the impact of the diagnosis and the need for a change in lifestyle.

5. What are the possible negative and positive effects?

6. While role playing, follow Perlman and Takacs' phases of change.

## References

Bridges, W. (2001). *The way of transition: Embracing life's most difficult moments*. Cambridge, MA: Perseus Publishing.

Carter, P., & Alfred, R. (1999). *Making change happen*. Ann Arbor, MI: Consortium for Community College Development, University of Michigan.

Creasia, J., & Parker, B. (2001). *Conceptual foundations: The bridge to professional nursing practice* (3rd ed.). St. Louis: Mosby.

Ellis, J., & Hartley, C. (2000). *Managing and coordinating nursing care* (3rd ed.). Philadelphia: Lippincott Williams & Wilkins.

Katz, J., et al (2001). *Keys to nursing success*. Upper Saddle River, NJ: Prentice Hall.

Kubler-Ross, E. (1969). *On death and dying*. New York: Macmillan.

Lewin, K. (1951). *Field theory in social science*. New York: Harper and Row.

McKenry, P. C., & Price, S. J. (1994). *Families and change: Coping with stressful events*. Thousand Oaks, CA: Sage Publications.

Perlman, D., & Takacs, G. (1990). The ten stages of change. *Nursing Management, 21*(4), 33–38.

Selye, H. (1976). *The stress of life* (Rev. ed.). New York: McGraw-Hill.

## Suggested Reading

Johnson, S. (1998). *Who moved my cheese?* New York: G.P. Putnam's Sons.

Lancaster, K. (1999). *Nursing issues in leading and managing change*. St. Louis: Mosby.

Mauksch, J. G., & Miller, M. H. (1981). *Implementing change in nursing*. St. Louis: C.V. Mosby.

Morrison, M. (1993). *Professional skills for leadership: Foundations of a successful career*. St. Louis: C.V. Mosby.

Peters, T. (1998). *Thriving on chaos*. New York: Alfred Knopf.

Redman, G., Riggleman, J., Sorrel, J., & Zervil, L. (1999). Creative winds of change: Nursing collaborating for quality outcomes. *Nursing Administrative Quarterly, 23*(2), 55–64.

Salmond, S. (1998). Managing the human side of change. *Orthopaedic Nursing, 17*(5), 38–51.

## On the Web

*www.unl.edu/stress/mgmt/concept.html*: An excellent outline on stress.

*www.unl.edu/stress/255N*: Good resource for physiologic stress.

*www.top-education.com/Management/ChangeManagement.asp*: Excellent source on change theory.

*www.muskingum.edu/~psychology/psycweb/history/lewin.htm:* More for those interested in Lewin's change theory.

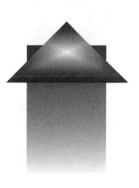

# Transitions Throughout Nursing's History

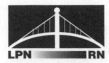

**VIGNETTE**

Joan Chin and Lucy Braveheart are two students who have formed a study group and are meeting over coffee in the student center to discuss the upcoming lecture.

**Joan:** Today we are supposed to discuss the history of nursing. History is something I've never been really good at. I think it's because I find it boring.

**Lucy:** I think it all depends on how it is presented. Rumor has it the professor has a unique way of presenting this topic. The fourth semester students say that she dresses up like Florence Nightingale and helps students learn her thinking through a monologue. Some say you can imagine what it was like back then.

**Joan:** I guess I remember those history lessons in school where we were lectured to about historical battles and such.

**Lucy:** Being a Native American, I have always been interested in history. My people say: 'You can never tell what it was like until you walk in someone's moccasins.' I guess we'll be walking in Florence's today.

**Joan:** Yes, my folks are third generation Chinese. They value what the elders say. I guess it's so we won't repeat the same mistakes.

The history of nursing is rich and tumultuous. In many respects, the history of nursing is a reflection of society in general and of women in particular. Although it may not seem important to know and appreciate nursing history, it is crucial to understanding and appreciating the world of nursing today. Depending on your perspective, nurses have existed in some form since there have been people on this earth. However, nursing as it is known today is a relatively young profession.

The workplace for nurses has changed radically in the last 2 decades, and significant changes continue. There is no doubt that nurses will always be challenged by changes in society, technology, and the healthcare industry. There should continue to be greater opportunities and rewards in nursing. The issues that confront nurses today will continue to be the foundation for the profession and practice of nursing tomorrow, just as those that came before us brought us to where we are today.

# Development of Nursing

The history and origins of nursing are rich and multifaceted. The evolution of nursing from ancient times through the ages was particularly influenced by Christianity. The Nightingale reform had a significant impact on the development of nursing in the United States, as did the evolution of nursing as a profession, the formation of professional nursing organizations, and the women's movement.

## Ancient Origins

There have always been humans who have required care when they were sick, injured, with child, elderly, or dying. Women, as demonstrated by cave drawings of women caring for sick children or preparing a brew of herbs and bark to aid an ill person, have generally done this work. However, little is known about nursing as a specific entity in ancient times.

In ancient Egypt, there were identified physicians or healers. Usually they were priests who were responsible for healing diseases. The priests acted as the link between humans and the gods. It was believed that people had to keep the gods happy to have good health and peace of mind. The priests or physicians did not interfere with the process of childbirth and infant care and left that work to midwives and wet nurses. These women probably had developed special skills and abilities to assist friends and neighbors.

The ancient Israelites were important in the development of modern medicine in that they formulated strict codes for personal hygiene and cleanliness. They instituted careful handwashing techniques, boiling of water, meat inspection, and other sanitation measures. Some of their practices are still followed by Orthodox Jews today.

Hindu Indians had a team concept approach to the care of the sick. The team consisted of a patient, a healer (physician), and a nurse, who was male. Each person had identified duties and functions. It is still probable that within the home, women cared for the young, sick, and elderly. The Hindus described the use of various instruments and surgical techniques that were used during ancient times. Many of the treatments that used herbs, plants, or animal parts were discovered by accident or trial and error.

Ancient China is known for the use of acupuncture, drug therapy, massage, hydrotherapy, and exercise to treat and prevent illness. Many of these same procedures and techniques are used today. The Chinese believed that a balance between Yang (the male elements of light, life, and optimism) and Yin (the female elements of dark, lifelessness, and cold) kept the body in harmony and health. In other ancient cultures, such as those in South America, there is evidence that hygiene, diet, and herbal medicine practices were important. Not much is known about nursing care specifically, although it appears that women were esteemed for their knowledge of medicines. As with other ancient cultures, the emphasis usually was on the balance between good and evil spirits and the appeasement of the gods.

## Christian Origins

With the advent of Christianity came a renewed focus on the value and dignity of human life. Bishops of the church were charged with caring for those in need, but the services were actually rendered by deacons and deaconesses. Men and women committed themselves to the care of the poor and sick. Women, and in particular, deaconesses, matrons, widows, and virgins, especially took care of the sick in their homes. Phoebe, the first deaconess, is cited by Paul in the New Testament as providing nursing care. She also is called the first visiting nurse (Ellis & Hartley, 2001).

The deaconesses of the early Christian church were required to be unmarried or widowed only once to serve in that capacity. These were often wealthy women of culture and education who were from fine homes and backgrounds. "These dedicated young women practiced 'works of mercy' that included feeding the hungry, clothing the naked, visiting the imprisoned, sheltering the homeless, and burying the dead. The deaconesses were the early counterparts to the community health nurses of today" (Ellis & Hartley, 2001). They carried medicine and food in baskets to people's homes. **Display 4-1** highlights several women credited for their contributions to nursing in the early years of Christianity.

As Christian churches were established, orders were formed that provided care for the sick, injured, poor, orphaned, widowed, and elderly. In early Christian times, men and women were considered equal, and there were more opportunities for single women to serve within these orders than had ever been available before. Within the religious orders, there was an established hierarchy of rank. This hierarchy demanded that there be absolute discipline and adherence to maintaining the rank and order. Some of the doctrines of faith, charity, servitude, and discipline of the early religious orders have continued to be a part of modern nursing influencing today's healthcare arena.

During the rise of Christianity, there was tremendous turmoil and chaos as battles and wars raged. Many men were killed, leaving many widows. Survival of widows during these troubled times was not a priority of society in general. For this reason, many of these women became interested in the various religious orders as a means of survival. Eventually, the Order of the Widows was formed. These women no longer had home responsibilities and were able to devote themselves to the care of the poor. As the church placed more value on purity of the body, the Order of the Virgins evolved. They later were called *nuns non-nuptaeor*, meaning "not married" (Zerwekh & Claborn, 1997). Convents were built to provide safe shelter for these women. However, they continued to care for the poor and the sick within these shelters.

The Middle Ages (approximately 500–1500) occurred after the fall of the Roman Empire. The development of medical science and nursing care halted as the Christian church advocated little concern for its growth and instead focused on preparing for the afterlife. Europe was divided into many kingdoms, which were continually at war with each other; poverty, illness, and starvation were widespread. Religious orders grew even stronger, particularly as deaconesses lost favor and decreased in great numbers. Monks and nuns of various religious orders assumed control of hospitals. However, they were more concerned with spiritual, rather than physical, care of the ill.

---

> ## Display 4-1   Early Nursing Leaders

**Phoebe:** First deaconess; carried letters for Paul; credited with being the first visiting nurse

**St. Marcella:** Established the first convent for women in her own palatial home; interested in the care of the sick; known as "mother of nuns"

**Fabiola:** After converting to Christianity, she established the first public hospital in Rome and devoted herself to the care of the sick and poor; she personally nursed many of them and was revered in Rome

**St. Paula:** A student of Marcella's; traveled to Jerusalem and used her money to found hospitals and inns for pilgrims traveling to the Holy Land; in Bethlehem she also established a convent and built hospitals for the sick and hospices for the pilgrims; the first to teach nursing as an art

# Military Origins

In the latter part of the Middle Ages, the Crusades occurred, lasting for about 200 years (approximately 1090–1290). The Crusaders were generally men of religious and military orders: priests, brothers, and knights. Their mission was to reclaim the Holy Land for the Christian faithful. As they traveled throughout Europe and the Near East, they gathered new information, learned new ways of doing things, and obtained different products and goods. The Crusaders were interested in the organized facilities for the sick that the Moslems used. As a result, similar hospitals were built near battlefields, and the men were sometimes assigned to fighting and sometimes assigned to caring for the sick and injured. Eventually, military nursing orders evolved.

An example of a military nursing order was the Knights Hospitalers of St. John, located outside Jerusalem. These men staffed two hospitals and in addition to caring for patients, frequently had to defend the hospital and the patients. They wore habits with a suit of armor underneath and the Maltese cross on top. Many nurses today wear pins that designate the school from which they graduated. One of the symbols used by some schools is the Maltese cross or another form of a cross. The Nightingale School designed a badge that used the Maltese cross. Other symbols also are used, and many represent the military origins of earlier centuries. In addition, military nursing orders advocated strict discipline and hierarchical lines of authority that emphasized devotion and obedience. These characteristics have extended to modern nursing, and in some settings can be problematic.

As the Crusaders returned to their homes, they brought with them a vision of improvement. Religious and secular groups organized hospitals and clinics that were better able to meet the needs of the sick and injured. The organizations became structured and ordered. The caregivers, or nurses, wore white robes and were given a hood on completion of a novitiate period. They remained responsible to a director or *maitresse*. During this time, nursing care was valued, although advances in medical science were not. Nursing care generally involved providing comfort measures and hygiene. There was no scientific basis for the nursing care. Toward the end of the Middle Ages, many countries were faced with rampant diseases and plague. The need for advancements in medicine was acute.

# Protestant Reformation

Various Protestant churches were created as church leaders took issue with the Roman Catholic Church. In countries where the reformation was widespread, the care of the sick suffered because there were not enough nuns to provide that care. Deaconesses were urged to take on this work. However, the standards that had marked military and nursing orders were not maintained; thus, the quality of care greatly diminished. In addition, Protestant women had religious freedom, but they did not have other freedoms, such as being able to work outside of the home. Society expected them to remain at home to provide care for children and the elderly and assume other domestic responsibilities. As a result, the caliber of nurses was diminished. In countries such as England, nurses in the 1800s were generally considered to be drunkards or thieves; women

## NCLEX–RN Might Ask 4-1

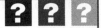

A nurse is explaining the relevance of various changes in the history of nursing. The nurse is aware that symbols, organization, strict discipline, and hierarchical lines of authority have

   A. ancient origins.
   B. Christian origins.
   C. military origins.
   D. Protestant origins.

• *See Appendix A for correct answer and rationale.*

chose to do their jail time serving within a hospital setting. Conditions in hospitals were deplorable, and the mortality rates greatly escalated.

In the 15th to 19th centuries, medical progress was more profound. Many advances were made in the knowledge of anatomy and physiology, the use of pharmaceutical agents, and surgical techniques. For example, the vaccination for smallpox was developed, the microscope was invented, and pasteurization was developed. However, the practice of nursing did not advance until after the mid-1800s.

## The Nightingale Reform

In 1836 in Kaiserwerth, Germany, a young Protestant minister named Theodore Fliedner strove to revitalize the deaconess movement by starting a training institute for deaconesses. As part of this institute, he and his wife started a nursing course that included hands-on training and some lectures by physicians. Fliedner's work and the formation of other secular and religious groups once again laid the foundation for the growth of nursing.

Florence Nightingale was born in 1820 to a family of wealth and social standing. With her culture and education, she was expected to marry and continue the traditions of English society women. However, she had a strong desire to be a nurse. Her family considered this ambition absurd, but she nonetheless managed to learn about hospital reforms and public health issues and became an expert in these areas. In her travels and through information from friends, she learned about the institute at Kaiserwerth. Because this was a church-sponsored institution, she was allowed to attend the nursing program. She spent 3 months there learning as much as she could about nursing.

After she returned to England, she continued her own studies and served on a committee that oversaw the Establishment for Gentlewomen During Illness. Although her family was not happy about her continued interest in nursing and in hospitals, she was later appointed superintendent of this organization. Her work in that capacity resulted in general acknowledgment of her expertise about hospitals and the need for educated nurses. She was asked to take a group of nurses to the Crimean War battlefields to improve the conditions there. Thirty-eight nurses who met Nightingale's standards accompanied her to Scutari. The work that was accomplished there was nothing short of miraculous. When they arrived, the conditions were filthy and unsafe. Through Nightingale's extraordinary efforts and with the assistance of powerful English friends, the situation improved dramatically. Sanitary and hygienic measures were instituted and maintained, nutritious food was provided, and conditions radically improved. She was especially concerned about the welfare of the soldiers and was able to obtain sick pay benefits for them, along with other benefits that improved their health and well-being. The mortality rate was reduced from 50% or 60% to approximately 1% or 2%. Nightingale became known as the lady with the lamp and the ministering angel because of her late night rounds to ensure that all was well.

Improving conditions at the battlefields was not without its own conflicts. The physicians and military officers resented Nightingale's intrusion, and some of the nurses who were involved argued with each other and disagreed with Nightingale. She tended to be controlling to accomplish her mission and was known to be stubborn, obstinate, and strong-willed (Barritt, 1973). During her service in the Crimean War, she became ill with what was called the Crimean fever and came close to death. However, she recovered and remained in service until the end of the war.

When Nightingale returned to England, she essentially became a recluse, secondary to health problems. However, she still was able to exert a powerful influence on the development of nursing because of the widespread fame that she attained as a result of her accomplishments in the Crimean War. She wrote many books and reports that demonstrated her ability to use research and statistics. Many refer to her as the first nurse researcher. Nightingale also continued to work on the development of nursing education and on improvement in the conditions for soldiers, particularly those in foreign lands. She established the Nightingale Fund, which was later used to establish a training school for nurses, and was awarded the Cross of St. George by Queen Victoria.

## Nightingale System of Education

Nightingale established a training school for nurses in 1860. It was founded in St. Thomas' Hospital as a 1-year program. Women between the ages of 25 and 35 years were selected based on qualifications relating to their character, conduct, and desire to be a nurse. The nursing program was highly structured and rigorous. See **Display 4-2** for Nightingale's ideas on the education of nurses.

The Nightingale system of education is considered to be the beginning of modern nursing education and the start of professional nursing. Nightingale's insistence on discipline and high moral character had a profound effect on the growth of modern nursing and the education of nurses, effects that continue to influence nursing education today. Within the first two decades after the Nightingale Training School opened, there were graduates that became superintendents in hospitals throughout Europe, Asia, and the United States. A whole new system of professional nursing was introduced throughout the world.

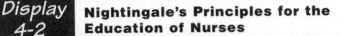

> **Display 4-2**   **Nightingale's Principles for the Education of Nurses**
>
> 1. Nursing is an art and a science.
> 2. The student must be taught to treat the patient as a total human being, not a disease, and there must be compassion and empathy for each individual.
> 3. The emphasis must be on education, not service. For this reason, a school of nursing should be independent from the hospital.
> 4. Graduate nurses should always continue their education.
> 5. Nurses must be taught to take care of the sick and must not do the laundry, clean, run errands, and other such chores that take them away from their nursing responsibilities.
> 6. Education for nurses should be a combination of theory and practice.

### ▶ Thinking Critically

Consider the following statement from Nightingale's (1992) *Notes on Nursing: What It Is and What It Is Not*:

"I use the word nursing for want of a better. It has been limited to signify little more than the administration of medicines and the application of poultices. It ought to signify the proper use of fresh air, light, warmth, cleanliness, quiet, and the proper selection and administration of diet— all at the least expense of vital power to the patient." (p. 6)

What is the relevance of this statement to nursing, as you know it today?

## Nursing in the United States

The growth of nursing in the United States was stimulated in particular by the Civil War. Before this war, there was no organized method for caring for the sick, especially during times of war. Women were the primary caregivers in the home or in the homes of neighbors. There were few formal educational programs available, except those that were within Catholic sisterhoods.

The Civil War began in 1861. The obvious need for nurses prompted many women to volunteer to care for the wounded soldiers. Although they were not trained as nurses, they demonstrated great compassion and concern. The Union Army appointed Dorothea Dix, a woman who had championed causes for the mentally ill, to be the superintendent for these nurses and to provide some training for them. Women from religious orders also volunteered in the North and the South, and other women assisted but never were trained nurses. In the South, fewer women volunteered because it was not socially acceptable. Many hospitals were built during the Civil War to house the large numbers of wounded soldiers. The nurses of this time experienced multiple difficulties: The working conditions were poor, the Army medical staff did not always think highly of them, and they were generally poorly treated. However, they persevered, and in some areas their work was well received and respected.

After the Civil War, there was a recognized need for educated nurses. The popularity of Florence Nightingale in England and the proliferation of educated Nightingale nurses also helped to promote the growth of nursing in the United States. In 1869, the American Medical Society proposed that the issue of trained nurses should be investigated. As a result of that study, three schools for the training of nurses opened in 1873: the Bellevue Training School in New York City, the Connecticut Training School, and the Boston Training School. Although these training programs were theoretically modeled after the Nightingale system, the major thrust was service, as opposed to education. Eventually, many schools of nursing opened. Hospitals realized that there was economic value in having student nurses deliver the bulk of patient care and other tasks. Essentially, the student nurses provided a free labor force for the hospitals. Despite the hardships, these programs were popular because they provided young women with the eventual means to earn a living. The choices for young women during these times were limited. Nursing was considered an acceptable alternative to traditional female roles and provided a slightly higher income than any other occupation available to women.

Uniforms and caps were not originally a traditional characteristic of training schools. In 1875, the first cap was used to cover long hair and particularly long and dirty hair. Its function was practical, not decorative. Later, a student at Bellevue Training School designed a student uniform. Eventually, caps, uniforms, and school pins came to signify a particular school or particular accomplishments within the school and have continued to be a part of nursing heritage.

In the early 1900s, nurses were expected to be submissive within a hospital organization and to the dominance of physicians. As reported by Zerwekh and Claborn (1997), there was a similar expectation for women in the male-dominated society. The woman was esteemed by her husband and had limited power within the confines of the home and society. She was expected to be hard working and able to maintain harmony, while at the same time be submissive to the demands of her husband. However, some women of this time worked hard for reform and laid the foundation for societal changes for women in general and nurses in particular. These issues are examined later in this chapter.

The first licensure laws for nursing did not exist until 1903, and even with the first law's passage, licensure was not mandatory or enforced. Hospitals continued to promote their own needs and not those of nurses or students. A few nursing programs moved to an educational setting, but the education continued to be practice driven and involved many long hours. There were many objections to nurses being overeducated and overtrained. Physicians in particular did not perceive a need for nurses to have increased education. Two important factors in the development of nursing in the United States were the upgrading of the Johns Hopkins School of Nursing in 1918 and the opening of the Yale School of Nursing in 1924. The first stressed the need for improved education of public health nurses, and the second was the first to be a separate university department with its own dean.

From the early decades of the 20th century emerged many of nursing's important leaders.

- **Linda Richards:** Called American's first trained nurse, she moved from one hospital to another to establish new training programs and to upgrade the quality of nursing services.

- **Isabelle Hampton Robb:** She graduated from Bellevue Training School after having been a teacher. She was instrumental in improving conditions for student nurses and founded the program at Johns Hopkins. When she married and resigned her position, she still maintained an active interest in nursing. She authored nursing textbooks, helped in the formation of the first nursing organization, and was one of the founders of the *American Journal of Nursing*.
- **Adelaide Nutting:** She was a graduate of the Johns Hopkins program and later a principal of that school. She obtained the funding to improve the education for public health nurses and was a strong advocate for reform in nursing education. Nutting later developed the nursing department at Teachers College, Columbia University. She was able to establish a 3-year nursing program and to reduce a student nurse's workday to 8 hours.
- **Lavinia Dock:** She was an early graduate of Bellevue Training School and later an assistant to Isabelle Hampton Robb. She was an early organizer of what is now known as The National League for Nursing (NLN). She wrote *History of Nursing*, which remains a classic on that subject.
- **Lillian Wald:** She founded the Henry Street Settlement in New York in 1893. This marked the beginning of public health nursing in the United States. She was particularly interested in the ability of nursing graduates to provide high quality care to people within their homes.

These are only a few of the women who helped to change the course of nursing. The changes that occurred in the 20th century reflect the hard work and dedication of women who were compelled to advocate reform in nursing. Although the women's movement has often ignored their work, their accomplishments did affect the changes women have experienced in general.

The presence of African Americans and men in nursing is not well documented. The first African American graduate of a training program was Mary Mahoney in 1879. She was dedicated to the promotion of excellence in the care of private duty patients and the acceptance of African Americans within the nursing profession. Although African American nurses were not accepted for military service until World War II, Adah Thomas fought for the acceptance of African American nurses in World War I and was effective in getting African American nurses to work for the American Red Cross. The prejudice against men in nursing also was high, and essentially, men were not influential in nursing until after World War II.

# Professional Nursing Organizations ▬▬

The formation of nursing organizations initiated the process of using cooperative efforts to achieve common goals and missions. Nurses found that a collective voice was much more likely to have an impact on the development of nursing.

## National League for Nursing (NLN)

The first nursing organization in the United States was established in 1893. The group initially was called the American Society of Superintendents of Training Schools for

Nurses in the United States and Canada. These nurses gathered for the purpose of improving and standardizing the education of nurses. In 1912, they changed the organization's name to the National League of Nursing Education. Membership was originally limited to nurses, but in 1943, the League decided to open membership to lay members. There continues to be two levels of membership: individual and agency. Schools of nursing and other agencies that provide nursing services are eligible for membership as agency members.

In 1952, a major reorganization took place, along with another name change. The League became the NLN and actually merged seven organizations into one. These groups were the National League of Nursing Education (1893), the National Organization for Public Health Nursing (1912), the Association of Collegiate Schools of Nursing (1933), the Joint Committee on Practical Nurses and Auxiliary Workers in Nursing Services (1945), the Joint Committee on Careers in Nursing (1948), the National Committee for the Improvement of Nursing Services (1949), and the National Nursing Accrediting Service (1949). Although in some respects, these were very diverse groups, they were able to formulate a common mission of promoting and providing for quality healthcare through effective nursing practice and education.

The National League for Nursing Accreditation Commission (NLNAC) provides accreditation processes to schools that choose to participate. Accreditation by the NLNAC is a voluntary process for schools of nursing, involving the writing of a self-study report according to established criteria. Representatives of NLNAC then visit the school to evaluate and assess the nursing program according to the established standards. These visitors make recommendations regarding accreditation of the program. Graduation from an NLN-accredited program provides for national recognition and the acceptance of credits from another NLN-accredited program if a graduate chooses to continue her or his education. Not all schools participate in the process, which is labor intensive and costly. However, all schools participate in the accreditation/approval process conducted by their State Board of Nursing. That process is mandatory in most states.

Another important contribution the NLN makes to nursing is high quality publications. The official journal of the NLN is *Nursing and Health Care Perspectives*. This journal presents many current issues related to education, practice, administration, changes in healthcare delivery, research, and other relevant topics. In addition, NLN produces many books, publications, and multimedia and maintains a website at *www.nln.org*. All of these demonstrate the League's commitment to the promotion and development of nursing.

# American Nurses Association (ANA)

The Nurses' Associated Alumnae of the United States and Canada was organized in 1896 by a group of nurses who thought group action would be more beneficial. In 1903, Canada's name had to be removed from the name of the organization to be able to incorporate, according to the laws of New York. The name of this organization was changed in 1911 to the American Nurses Association (ANA), and Canadian nurses formed their own national organization. The ANA is known as the professional organization for registered nurses (RNs) and limits its membership to RNs. There have been numerous changes throughout ANA's history, but it has always maintained a commitment to individual nurses and in turn to the public, as recipients of the work nurses do. A significant change occurred in 1982, when the ANA adopted a federation model of membership. With this model, individual members join state nurses associations (SNA) and the SNAs are members of the ANA. This was done in hopes of strengthening the state organizations and possibly increasing membership. Unfortunately, only a small percentage of employed nurses belong to their state organization. However, despite the relatively low membership, the ANA has been a powerful voice in nursing issues. The official journal of the ANA is the *American Journal of Nursing*, and the organization's website is *www.ana.org*.

The ANA comprises a number of councils that represent specialty areas. Standards of practice have been developed by each council, whose function is to be a forum for discourse related to continuing education, consultation, and other issues that pertain to that council's interests. There also are two congresses, one for nursing practice and the other for nursing economics, whose function consists of setting policies, standards, new programs, and other related responsibilities. Other activities of the ANA include:

- Advanced certification of RNs;
- Accreditation of continuing education programs;
- Participation in public policy issues;
- Development of an economic and general welfare program;
- Promotion and support of research activities; and
- Publication of journals, pamphlets, and multimedia.

Several areas of controversy have been prevalent in ANA's recent history and may account for some of the reasons that nurses choose not to belong to this organization. One issue is ANA's position on entry into practice. In 1965, an ANA position paper advocated that the entry level for professional nursing should be the baccalaureate nurse. This issue has caused and continues to cause a great deal of conflict within nursing. Another area of conflict began in 1974 with the passage of the Taft-Hartley Act. This act legislated that professional nursing organizations also could be labor unions. Nurses in management positions or nurses who disagree with professionals being represented by a bargaining unit frequently choose not to support the ANA. Other areas of conflict have related to ANA's legislative activities, in which there can never be total agreement. The ANA maintains an active involvement in national and state health policy issues.

Other organizations that are related to the ANA include:

- American Nurses Foundation: This organization is a tax-exempt and nonprofit organization that is committed to supporting research related to nursing. It provides analysis and research related to public policy, supports a group of nurse scholars who are involved with public policy and journalism endeavors, and funds research activities.
- American Academy of Nursing: The ANA established an honorary association to recognize nurses who have made a meaningful contribution to the nursing pro-

fession. Nurses so honored are called fellows and use the title Fellow of the American Academy of Nursing (FAAN).

- International Council of Nurses: This is the international organization for professional nurses. The ANA is one of the national nursing organizations with membership in the Council. There are 98 national members. The Council's headquarters are in Geneva, Switzerland.
- National Student Nurses Association (NSNA): Students in schools of nursing started this organization in 1952. Their organizational structure is similar to ANA's in that there are national, state, and local chapters. It is closely associated with ANA but is a completely separate operation. The quarterly journal *Imprint* is published by NSNA.

## Other Nursing Organizations

There are many organizations for and about nursing. Many clinical nursing specialties have their own organizations. There also are organizations for nurses that are related to educational, religious, ethnic, and other interests. All of these groups have recognized the importance and value of collective effort and action.

### ▶ Thinking Critically

Before the Civil War, women's organizations did not exist on a national level. Nurses formed the first professional organizations for and by women. What impact did this have for women in general? What impact did this have for nurses specifically? What significance does this have for you as a female or male entering registered nursing?

## The Evolution of Nursing as a Profession ■■■■

In the development of nursing as a profession and nurses as professionals, it is necessary to assure the public that the title of nurse represents a defined responsibility and obligation to professional standards and criteria.

### NCLEX–RN Might Ask 4-2    ？ ？ ？

A nursing student is discussing information on nursing organizations with her clinical preceptor. The nurse is aware that the agency that endows nursing schools with accreditation is the

    A. American Nurses Association (ANA).
    B. American Medical Association (AMA).
    C. National League for Nurses (NLN).
    D. National Student Nurses Association (NSNA).

- *See Appendix A for correct answer and rationale.*

# Qualities of a Professional

Certain qualities are considered necessary to be professional (Leddy & Pepper, 1998).

1. Intellectual characteristics: Professional practice is based on a body of knowledge gained from research and experience. The education is a combination of general and specialized courses.
2. Service to society: Professional service entails ethical commitment and legal responsibility to the public. Within this service, the public must be guaranteed the competence of professional nurses by a licensure or credentialing system. Ethical obligations are defined by a code of ethics. The ANA's (2001) *Code of Ethics for Nurses* is discussed later in this chapter.
3. Autonomy: By definition, autonomy means that the individual has self-determination over functions within the workplace. A professional must be responsible and accountable for her or his actions. Nurses have had more difficulty achieving autonomy because of the hierarchal nature of nursing organizations and the continued dependence on the medical profession.
4. Shared personal values: Many values are important to the growth and development of a professional, just as characteristics of commitment, accountability, responsibility, ethical and moral standards, and caring are important to the maturation of the profession as a whole.

The move toward mandatory licensure, the development of a social policy statement and a code for nurses, and the growth of nursing theory have promoted nursing as an independent profession. There have been major advances in the practice and profession of nursing during the past several decades.

# Licensure

In the late 1800s, there was a move in the United States to license nurses. Nursing leaders of that time believed that a mechanism should exist to assure the public that nurses were competent to practice nursing according to defined standards. Licensed nurses would be titled registered nurses. These early leaders recognized that the great variance in nursing education programs did not guarantee adherence to any standards. The organizations that preceded the NLN and the ANA supported the licensure of nurses. Although it was a difficult battle, licensure was eventually achieved. See **Display 4-3** for more information about the history of nursing licensure.

The early licensure laws granted permissive licensure, which means that the person is "permitted" to be licensed if requirements are met (Ellis & Hartley, 2001). Licensure was not required for a person to practice nursing. For that reason, employers made a distinction between registered nurses and nurses. North Carolina, New Jersey, New York, and Virginia first granted permissive licensure in 1903. Mandatory licensure later was advocated as additional insurance to the public that all nurses were registered and

## Display 4-3   The History of Nursing Licensure

1867: Dr. Henry Wentworth Acland first suggests licensure for nurses in England.

1892: American Society of Superintendents of Training Schools for Nurses organized and supported licensure in the United States.

1901: First nursing licensure in the world: New Zealand.

1903: First nursing licensure in the United States: North Carolina, New Jersey, New York, and Virginia (in that order).

1915: ANA drafted its first model nurse practice act.

1919: First nursing licensure in England.

1923: All 48 states had enacted nursing licensure laws.

1935: First mandatory licensure act in the United States: New York (effective 1947).

1946: Ten states had definitions of nursing in the licensing act.

1950: First year the same examination used in all jurisdictions of the United States and its territories: State Board Test Pool Examination.

1965: Twenty-one states had definitions of nursing in the licensing act.

1971: First state to recognize expanded practice in the nursing practice act: Idaho.

1976: First mandatory continuing education for relicensure: California.

1982: Change to nursing process format examination: National Council Licensure Examination for Registered Nurses (NCLEX-RN).

1986: First state to require a baccalaureate degree for initial registered nurse licensure and associate degree for licensed practical nurse licensure: North Dakota (effective 1987).

1994: Computer-adapted testing initiated nationwide.

1998: Mutual Recognition Nurse Licensure Compact finalized. Utah is the first state to become part of the Compact.

Reprinted with permission from Ellis, J. R., & Hartley, C. L. (2001). *Nursing in today's world: Challenges, issues, and trends* (7th ed.). Philadelphia: Lippincott Williams & Wilkins.

thus met specific criteria and standards. In 1938, the first mandatory licensure law was passed in New York.

Nurse practice acts evolved as licensure laws were enacted. The purposes of these acts are to

- define nursing;
- stipulate the qualifications to practice nursing;
- outline the methods of obtaining licensure, licensure renewal, and interstate endorsement or reciprocity;
- establish and maintain rules and regulations of nursing;
- delineate unlawful acts, misconduct, or disciplinary actions; and
- name the state agency (and its functions) that will oversee the nurse practice act (for most states this is the State Board of Nursing, made up of nurses, other professionals, and consumers).

By 1923, all states had some form of a nurse practice act. Since then, nurse practice acts have changed to reflect the changes in nursing and the advent of mandatory licensure. It is imperative that licensed nurses are familiar with the nurse practice act for the state in which they practice.

# American Nurses Association's Social Policy Statement

Defining nursing has historically been problematic for the nursing profession. There are many viewpoints related to philosophical and practice perspectives. In 1980, the ANA formulated and published *Nursing: A Social Policy Statement*. The purpose of this document was to assist nurses in conceptualizing their practice; to provide direction to educators, administrators, and researchers within nursing; and to inform other health professionals, legislators, funding bodies, and the public about nursing's contribution to healthcare (ANA, 1980).

Within this policy statement, the ANA incorporated the use of the nursing process and the diagnosis and treatment of human responses. This defined the autonomous and unique practice of nursing. The statement also stipulated that nurses are responsible and accountable to society for their actions, which may be in a variety of settings for clients of all ages. The ANA asserts that nurses must include preventive health measures in their practice. This policy also included a section about specialization in nursing practice, spearheading the move toward advanced nursing practice.

The *Statement* has been important to the development of the nursing profession in that responsibility and professional accountability are viewed as an essential element of nursing practice. Obviously, as knowledge and roles change, changes also must be made in the responsibilities. However, the accountability to the public remains unchanged; nurses accept defined responsibilities for providing care at a particular level. They are always accountable and must practice according to state rules and regulations, standards of practice, and the *Social Policy Statement*. In 1995, the *Social Policy Statement* was revisited and updated to meet contemporary practice of the profession.

# American Nurses Association's Code of Ethics for Nurses

A professional code of ethics is a guide for ethical behavior of practitioners in that professional field. A professional code does not have any legal authority, but it does advocate ethical and moral behavior for practitioners of that profession.

The American Nurses Association (ANA) developed a *Code for Nurses* in 1985. The ANA began a process to review and revise the code in 1995, culminating in the new *ANA Code of Ethics for Nurses With Interpretive Statements* in 2001. The new code had extensive review and input from practicing nurses and nursing organizations. As shown in **Display 4-4**, the ANA's 2001 *Code of Ethics for Nurses* clearly expresses nursing's own understanding of its ethical standards, commitment to society, and the ethical obligations and duties of every individual entering the profession.

# North American Nursing Diagnosis Association

Since the mid-1960s, the concepts related to the nursing process have become more common in the nursing world. In most educational and practice settings, some form of the nursing process is used. This involves assessing the client, making nursing diagnoses,

## Display 4-4   ANA Code of Ethics for Nurses

1. The nurse, in all professional relationships, practices with compassion and respect for the inherent dignity, worth and uniqueness of every individual, unrestricted by considerations of social or economic status, personal attributes, or the nature of health problems.
2. The nurse's primary commitment is to the patient, whether an individual, family, group, or community.
3. The nurse promotes, advocates for, and strives to protect the health, safety, and rights of the patient.
4. The nurse is responsible and accountable for individual nursing practice and determines the appropriate delegation of tasks consistent with the nurse's obligation to provide optimum patient care.
5. The nurse owes the same duties to self as to others, including the responsibility to preserve integrity and safety, to maintain competence, and to continue personal and professional growth.
6. The nurse participates in establishing, maintaining, and improving healthcare environments and conditions of employment conducive to the provision of quality health care and consistent with the values of the profession through individual and collective action.
7. The nurse participates in the advancement of the profession through contributions to practice, education, administration, and knowledge development.
8. The nurse collaborates with other health professionals and the public in promoting community, national, and international efforts to meet health needs.
9. The profession of nursing, as represented by associations and their members, is responsible for articulating nursing values, for maintaining the integrity of the profession and its practice, and for shaping social policy.

From American Nurses Association. (2001). *Code of Ethics for Nurses with Interpretive Statements.* Washington, D.C.: American Nurses Publishing. http://nursingworld.org/ethics/chcode.htm.

formulating and implementing plans of care, and evaluating the client to determine the effectiveness of the care plan. Later in this text, in-depth information about this process is presented. It is mentioned here because one component of the nursing profession has been the development of a separate nursing diagnostic taxonomy. This means that diagnoses are classified and ordered based on a set of principles. The North American Nursing Diagnosis Association (NANDA) has guided the development of this process.

In 1976, NANDA was formed as an organization made up of individual and group RN members. Its purpose is to provide a forum to discuss information and issues related to nursing diagnoses and to develop uniform language for nursing diagnoses. The group's website is *www.nanda.org*. Members may propose new problems or diagnoses by preparing appropriate research and documentation and submitting them to NANDA for consideration. Committees review the proposals and then present them to the membership at a national convention that is held every 2 years. The organization provides and promotes this taxonomy as a common language for nurses.

## Transitions in Nursing Education

You may be well aware that nursing education has made many transitions since the late 1800s. Again, the history of nursing can often be told in part by the educational methods that are used. Florence Nightingale believed that the education of nurses should be a separate function from the service to patients. However, in this country, hospitals and physicians found it beneficial to have nurses educated within a hospital setting to essentially provide the bulk of the labor force. It took many years and hard effort to change this mentality, and undoubtedly some people would prefer that nursing education continue to be provided in the slave labor mode.

## Educational Program Similarities

With the many educational options that are now available, nurse educators from the various programs recognize that in some regards, there are as many similarities among programs as there are differences. For example, the student bodies generally have a large variance in age. The average age often is around 30 years or more. Many students are married or have partners. Many have children, and single parents and mixed families are common. More men are entering nursing, and the profession comprises a wide array of ethnicities. Often students are entering nursing as a second or third career. For some, it is the first time in higher education, and for others, it is a return to school after having earned other degrees. Most students work at least part time to pay rising tuition costs and support themselves and their families.

To meet the needs of older students and students with family and work responsibilities, evening, weekend, part-time, and self-study programs are available. A challenge for nursing programs has been the increased cost of nursing education and the challenge to provide quality education at a greatly reduced cost in nontraditional formats. Nursing education programs are among the most costly of programs on college campuses and often struggle for adequate financing to provide high-quality, relevant, technologically advanced instruction.

Other similarities revolve around program essentials. The State Board of Nursing or other designated state agency must approve all programs. Many schools seek NLN accreditation. All programs require that the faculty have or seek graduate education. Clinical education is a common component of all nursing programs in that students receive a portion of their education in various clinical settings. The challenges to nursing students and faculty are many. There are three basic modes of entry to becoming an RN.

## Diploma Programs

The oldest form of education is the diploma program. The first programs began in 1873 and initially were similar to on-the-job training programs. Traditionally, these were strict and structured modes of instruction, practice, and conduct. Most diploma programs continue to be located in hospitals and require 3 years to complete. The program includes basic theory courses along with structured clinical experiences. Many diploma programs are now affiliated with local colleges, so students may receive college credit for general education courses. Graduates of diploma programs are prepared to function as primary caregivers in hospital and ambulatory care settings. They are not educationally prepared for administrative, school nursing, or public health positions. There has always been a fierce loyalty to diploma education, but in the last 2 decades, the number of diploma programs has declined, partly because of the increased costs for the programs and partly because of the advent of associate degree education.

## Associate Degree Nursing Programs

Associate degree nursing (ADN) programs were instituted in the 1950s as a result of Mildred Montag's published doctoral dissertation in 1952 entitled "Education for Nursing Technicians." She proposed that technical nurses could be educated in 2 years within a community or technical college and work as RNs. Although there was much opposition to this mode of education, the postwar need for nurses was an impetus for the start of these programs as an additional mode of entry to registered nursing practice. Seven programs were initially started. They were so successful that many community colleges started similar programs. ADN education was designed to have a balance between general education and nursing courses, without affiliation to a particular hospital, but rather clinical nursing experiences in one or more agencies for "hands-on" training to accompany collegiate theoretical classes. These programs are generally 2 years in length and are usually located in community and technical colleges. However, some programs are found in 4-year colleges and within hospitals. ADN graduates are prepared to be direct caregivers in hospitals, long-term care facilities, and ambulatory care settings. They are not prepared educationally for nursing administrative, school nursing, public health nursing, or nurse educator positions, although some may work in these settings as part of a "tiered, team approach" to healthcare delivery.

## Baccalaureate Degree Nursing Programs

Baccalaureate of science in nursing (BSN) programs were first established in 1909 at the University of Minnesota. They are the third mode of entry to registered nursing. Early programs were 5 years long; most programs are now 4 to 5 years. The early programs were greatly opposed by most nurses and physicians, who did not see the need for women and nurses to have higher education. BSN programs today generally begin with 2 years of liberal arts and science education. Nursing courses are concentrated in the last 2 years. Clinical education is similar to that of ADN programs but also includes the use of research in the practice setting. BSN graduates are prepared to care for clients in a variety of settings, including administrative, school, and public health settings.

## Masters Degree Programs

Another option that is available to prospective nursing students are master's degree programs that lead to an initial degree in nursing at the master's level. These programs are open to students who hold bachelor's degrees in other majors and decide to become RNs. Generally the programs last 2 to 3 years and involve a combination of undergraduate and graduate level courses. Graduates of these programs are similar to entry-level BSN graduates but have broader ability in research-related nursing activities, case management, and preparation for teaching.

# Career Mobility Options

Career ladder programs provide several opportunities for nursing education. They are sometimes called multiple entry/exit programs. For example, a person who is already a licensed practical or vocational nurse may enter the second year of an ADN program after completing prerequisite general education courses and a transition course. Alternatively, a person may enter a 2-year ADN program and exit at the end of the first year after completing a practical vocational nursing program option. These types of programs are popular because a student can better meet her or his needs in terms of education and work.

Other career mobility options are related to people who are already RNs but are seeking a higher degree. Many baccalaureate programs provide direct articulation agreements with local community colleges. Essentially, this means that all credits or most of the credits transfer directly to the 4-year program so that the student does not lose any time or credits in the move to obtain a BSN. Other BSN programs provide a challenge process so that students may take challenge examinations for credit in lieu of taking the entire course. This entails self-discipline and determination.

A final option is the availability of external degree programs, in which courses that are required for a BSN may be taken at a local community college or on a self-study basis. Often a student must have a preceptor or advisor for this process. There are benefits in that the student has more flexibility and can eliminate some of the problems related to traveling and work schedules. Drawbacks are that the student does not always have the benefit of learning from other students' experiences and must be able to succeed in an independent study model.

The initial entry to becoming an RN is important, no matter which route is taken. However, the business of nursing education is not terminated with the initial process. Nursing must always include a dedication to lifelong learning. Continuing education is now mandatory for relicensure in most states. Many programs are available to nurses through work and professional organizations. There also are options available for seeking higher degrees as a way to continue your education. Advanced practice roles require a master's degree or doctoral degree, as do many jobs in specialty areas and education. Many nurses also seek advanced certification in a specific practice area through the ANA or other professional organizations. Continuing education in nursing is absolutely essential for remaining current in nursing practice.

# Factors That Have Influenced Trends and Transitions in Nursing

Throughout history and continuing to today, influences outside the realm of nursing have had a major impact on the growth and development of nursing. Nursing does not exist in a vacuum, and as technology and communication advance, so does the influence of society on the profession and practice of nursing. In the following section, a brief examination of some of the historic and societal trends are presented.

# Impact of War

The impact of war has been mentioned several times in this chapter. In theory, nursing education was born in the United States as a result of the Civil War. When the Spanish-American War occurred in 1898, injured soldiers required the services of nurses from training schools, although the military physicians were greatly opposed. There was less opposition after the war, but it was 1901 before the Army Nurse Corps was created. The Navy Nurse Corps was founded in 1908.

World War I initiated a new dimension for military nurses; injuries caused by shrapnel and gas were now evident, and there were massive numbers of casualties. This war also created a great demand for nurses, which prompted quicker training programs to satisfy some of the demand. After this war, a nursing shortage continued, secondary to the return to longer training programs.

World War II created more demand for nurses and more need for them to be at the battlefront. Educational programs were not providing the necessary numbers, so the Cadet Nurse Corps was created, in which students received tuition and living costs in exchange for serving as a military or civilian nurse for the duration of the war. The curriculum for these programs was shortened, which prompted all nursing programs to reevaluate the length of programs. Eventually, nurses in the military achieved officer status, but it took longer for male and African American nurses to gain equal status.

The Korean War initiated the use of the mobile army surgical hospital units. Nurses were in greater demand than ever. The Vietnam War and the Persian Gulf War emphasized the great role that nurses have in wartime. However, nurses still struggle to achieve full recognition for their efforts.

# Women's Role in Society

Although nursing and the women's movement have frequently ignored one another, they are closely aligned. Nursing has been, and continues to be, a female-dominated profession. The work that women and nurses do has traditionally not been valued. The women's movement initially devalued women's work in an attempt to promote gender equality in traditional men's work. Nurses were seen as doing traditional women's work and thus were not valued. In part, this was because nurses have had difficulty defining nursing.

In the last decade, there has been more recognition from women and nurses that the work that women do is important and undervalued. This also includes the work that nurses do. Although generally nurses have not received their fair worth (as women have not), conditions have improved, and society in general is less opposed to gender equity issues.

# Societal Trends

Other societal trends have had, and continue to have, an impact on nursing. Several of these are summarized here.

## AGING POPULATION

The population is getting older; there are increasingly greater numbers of elderly people who require healthcare services. The inclusion of elder care and gerontologic concepts in nursing curricula is increasing. Emphasis is being placed on individualizing care for the old; very old; and very, very old. Emerging concepts in caring for the well, frail elderly are being included in nursing curricula. Family-centered care for four- and five-generation families is also prevalent.

## SHORTENED LENGTHS OF STAY IN HOSPITALS

Acute care settings have seen a shift to clients who are more critically ill than before but are staying in the hospital for shorter periods. Fewer hospitalized patients are ambulatory. There is also a greater need for high-technologic and highly skilled care in long-term and home care settings. Outpatient nursing services also are in greater demand. Nursing education has to continue to be creative in preparing graduates for this new environment.

## MULTICULTURALISM

Ethnic diversity has increased greatly in the United States, resulting in a growing need for caregivers who are multiculturally sensitive and who value diverse perspectives, views, and values. In some areas of this country, two of three clients are of minority populations, and in a few states the new majority is persons of color. Therefore, the need for nurses who reflect this cultural diversity to better meet client needs is acute. Educators need to prepare nurses to think and act from a multicultural perspective, and nursing school recruitment, admission, and retention practices need to address this challenge of increasing the ethnic diversity of student and graduate nurses.

## ACQUIRED IMMUNODEFICIENCY SYNDROME (AIDS)

The AIDS epidemic has greatly influenced the world of nursing. Implementation and maintenance of Standard Precautions can minimize the danger of AIDS and other blood-borne pathogens, but healthcare workers continue to have some risks. It has prompted some nurses to leave the profession and possibly has deterred others from seeking a nursing education. In other ways, the workplace has become a safer environment for healthcare workers if all precautions are practiced.

## ADVANCING TECHNOLOGY

Technologic changes and the growing trend toward specialization have changed the educational needs of nurses. In some settings, nurses are highly skilled technicians, well trained to perform necessary functions. Computer-based documentation and high-technologic caregiving equipment demand new skills from nurses. As advances continue in medical care, the need for highly specialized nurses will also continue to increase. The technology in home care and long-term care settings also has escalated. This has an obvious impact on families and healthcare providers in those settings.

## HEALTHCARE REFORM

Today's political agendas surrounding healthcare reform emphasize access, primary preventive care, cost containment, and choice in caregivers. There is also more emphasis on primary preventive care that is more community based. The primary care provider will serve as a gatekeeper in the continuum of healthcare needs. The functions of acute care centers will change; they will provide only acute, intense care. Other illness care will be provided in community-based settings. Cost-containment efforts will emphasize quality care in more reduced and efficient ways. Communities will see that services are integrated and consolidated so that costly duplication is eliminated. The work that nurses, and especially advanced practice nurses, do now is held in high esteem because of nursing's holistic and preventive tradition. The quality of care and the reduced cost of that care will be greatly influenced by the work that nurses do.

## MANAGED CARE

The expansion of healthcare systems and health maintenance organizations (HMOs) caused by mergers and cost-saving strategies is affecting nursing and how clients receive care. In addition, the use of preferred provider organizations (PPOs) and diagnostic related groups (DRGs) in an effort to contain skyrocketing inflation in healthcare costs has an impact. Use of unlicensed assistive personnel to defray costs causes nursing to be concerned with the quality of the care being given.

## QUALITY OUTCOMES

Efforts to incorporate quality assurance (QA), total quality management (TQM), and continuous quality improvement (CQI) practices are adding work to already overworked nurses. Although these initiatives are designed to ensure accountability for quality-based outcomes, the increased management of patient/client care is removing nurses from the "soft skill" side of promoting health patient education and meeting psychosocial needs.

## HEALTHCARE ADVOCACY AND SERVICE LEARNING

The need for social healthcare reform (i.e., prevention of cancer, AIDS, teenage pregnancy, etc.) poses new roles and challenges for nursing. Palmer and Savoie (2001) note the explosion of service learning curricular strands in college educational programs. Service learning experiences provide an opportunity for students to develop civic responsibility by working with individuals and agencies in the community to improve qualityof life. The "fit" of this curriculum with nursing's need for more community-based learning experiences is evident.

## HOLISTIC AND SPIRITUAL CARE

The current attention to holistic, spiritual care in nursing is noted by Wilt and Smuker (2001). The impact of providing spiritual care amidst the increasing complexity of multiethnic client populations poses new challenges for nurses.

## INFORMATICS AND NURSING ENTREPRENEURISM

Informatics and nursing entrepreneurism are two new areas of practice emerging in today's information society. Chaska (2001) notes the need for nurses to assist clients in the new knowledge-based economy, in which individuals are able to have a greater voice in the selection of healthcare providers and services.

## SOCIAL POLICY AND POLITICAL ADVOCACY

Deloughery (1998) and Catalano (2000) both cite the need for nurses to become active in the development of legislation and social policy as they encounter complex ethical dilemmas. Critical and creative thinking is needed to address such issues as biomedical technology, genetic engineering (cloning), robotics, and bioethical decision making.

### ▶ Thinking Critically

Select one of the societal trends above. How do you think it will affect your practice as a RN in the future? How will clients be affected?

The impact of societal trends on nursing cannot be underestimated. There will always be a cause-and-effect trend on nursing education and practice. The evolution of nursing is a reflection of society in general. Nurses must have an understanding of their roots and societal trends to understand the future better and prepare for tomorrow's challenges.

### Student Exercise

Choose an event in the history of nursing that interests you. Research that event more thoroughly and then consider the following points:

1. What was the general tone in society at that time?
2. What was the role of women?
3. What were the functions of nurses, even if not defined in a formal sense?
4. What drew you to this particular event?
5. What impact did this event have on the future of nursing?

## References

American Nurses Association (ANA). (1985). *A code for nurses.* Kansas City, MO: Author.

American Nurses Association (ANA). (1980). *Nursing: A social policy statement.* Kansas City, MO: Author.

American Nurses Association (ANA). (1995). *Nursing: A social policy statement.* Kansas City, MO: Author.

American Nurses Association. (2001). *Code of ethics for nurses with interpretive statements.* Washington, D. C.: American Nurses Publishing. http://nursingworld.org/ethics/chcode.htm.

Barritt, E. R. (1973). Florence Nightingale's values and modern nursing education. *Nursing Forum, 12*(1), 7–47.

Catalano, J. T. (2000). *Nursing now: Today's issues, tomorrow's trends.* Philadelphia: FA Davis.

Chaska, N. L. (2001). *The nursing profession: Tomorrow and beyond.* Thousand Oaks, CA: Sage.

Deloughery, G. (1998). *Issues and trends in nursing* (3rd ed.). St. Louis: Mosby.

Ellis, J. R., & Hartley, C. L. (2001). *Nursing in today's world: Challenges, issues, and trends* (7th ed.). Philadelphia: Lippincott Williams & Wilkins.

Leddy, S., & Pepper, J. M. (1998). *Conceptual bases of professional nursing* (4th ed.). Philadelphia: Lippincott-Raven Publishers.

Nightingale, F. (1992). *Notes on nursing: What it is and what it is not.* (A commemorative edition of the first edition published in 1859.) Philadelphia: JB Lippincott.

Palmer, C. E., & Savoie, E. J. (2001). Service learning: A conceptual overview. In G. P. Poirrier (Ed.), *Service learning: Curricular applications in nursing.* Sudbury, MA: Jones and Bartlett.

Wilt, D. L., & Smuker, C. J. (2001). *Nursing the spirit: The art and science of applying spiritual care.* Washington, DC: American Nurses Association.

Zerwekh, J., & Claborn, J. C. (1997). *Nursing today: Transition and trends* (2nd ed.). Philadelphia: WB Saunders.

## Suggested Reading

Chitty, K. (2001). *Professional nursing: Concepts and challenges* (3rd ed.). Philadelphia: WB Saunders.

Kelly, L. Y. (1992). *The nursing experience: Trends, challenges, and transitions.* New York: McGraw-Hill.

*On the Web* • • • • • • • • • • • • • • • • • • • • • • • • • • • • • • • • •

*www.aahn.org/calendar:* American Association for the History of Nursing

*www.nln.org*: National League for Nurses

*www.ana.org*: American Nurses Association

*www.florence-nightingale.co.uk*: Florence Nightingale Museum Trust

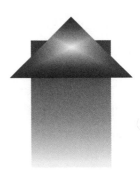

# Learning at the ADN Level

## LEARNING OBJECTIVES

*By the end of this chapter, the student will be able to:*

1  Describe learning concepts related to the adult learner.
2  Apply adult learning concepts to one's self.
3  Describe the differences between medical and nursing conceptual models.
4  Give examples of learning activities in each of three learning domains: cognitive, affective, and psychomotor.
5  Discuss the roles of licensed practical/vocational nurses (LPN/LVNs) and associate degree nurses related to nursing process and nursing diagnosis.
6  Differentiate among the six cognitive learning achievement levels: knowledge, comprehension, application, analysis, synthesis, and evaluation.
7  Differentiate between passive and active learning processes.
8  Identify learning strategies to maximize success in an associate degree nursing (ADN) program.
9  Describe the differences in transition needs of LPN/LVNs entering ADN programs as advanced placed generic, straight-through LPN to ADN students, and time-out LPN to ADN students.
10  Differentiate between ADN students and LPN/LVN practice roles.

## KEY TERMS

active learning
affective learning domain
cognitive learning domain

conceptual model
experiential knowledge
generic ADN student

learning achievement levels:
  –knowledge
  –comprehension
  –application
  –analysis
  –synthesis
  –evaluation

nursing diagnosis
nursing process
proxemics
psychomotor learning domain
self-actualization

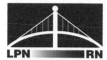

## VIGNETTE

George Dobian is fearful of his first nursing course, which he will take in the fall. He has heard from others that nursing school is very different from when he attended LVN school 10 years ago. George was never good at taking tests, and that fear has haunted him through his adult life. He is afraid of being embarrassed because his employer is paying for his education. He is wondering if he has the wrong study skills or if he has a learning disability. He has talked about his fears to his friend John Scott, a student in George's anatomy and physiology class. John has taken a "Success Strategies for the Returning Student" seminar at the community college. John speaks openly about his professor's introduction to skills in learning. George is impressed when John says his test scores and overall memory of materials improved when he began rewriting his notes, discussing course content with others, experiencing problems firsthand during clinical sessions, and participating in teaching projects. George is on his way to sign up for the summer "Success" seminar and has made an appointment to talk with a counselor about determining if he has a learning disability.

## Adult Learning Theory

Much has been written about adult learning theory. The knowledge and life experiences you bring with you to the ADN program are valuable assets as you move to the registered nurse (RN) role. Perhaps you find yourself in a situation like George's. George has a clear understanding of what his goals and motivation mechanisms are but really needs help with his transition process. As an adult learner, you need a clear understanding of your goals, learning style, motivational mechanisms, and desired societal roles to aid you in the transition process.

Adult learners draw on a wide variety of life experiences as they pursue additional education. These experiences are a resource and support adults in acquiring knowledge. Adults are generally self-motivated and self-directed and have developed a particular learning style. Unlike the child's learning environment, which is structured and directed by the teacher, the milieu for the adult learner must provide opportunities for self-established goals and learning techniques. Adults are motivated to learn when they see the meaning and relevance of learning in fulfilling societal roles or solving daily problems faced at home or on the job. The key characteristics of adult learners are provided in **Display 5-1.**

## Display 5-1 — Characteristics of Adult Learners

Adult learners:
- Draw on a variety of life experiences in the educational process.
- Are motivated to learn when they see that such learning solves problems confronting them.
- Are motivated to learn when such learning is needed to fulfill social roles.
- Are self-motivated and self-directed and seek learning to fulfill self-established goals.
- Learn best when the program of learning addresses the individual learning styles they have developed with time.

# Experiential Knowledge and the Adult Learner

As an LPN/LVN and an adult with a wide variety of life experiences, you bring to the ADN program a great deal of knowledge, including expertise in specific content areas of the curriculum. This extensive experiential knowledge enhances the educational process in several ways.

First, having both theoretical and practical knowledge, skills, and abilities provides you with the self-confidence to tackle new areas of learning and venture into new clinical experiences.

Second, your areas of expertise will be a rich resource to peers, as theirs will be to you, as you participate in learning activities and work in groups to fulfill course objectives and meet clinical competencies at the RN level.

Third, your rich experiential background provides a wealth of information for making connections between prior learning experiences and new ones, problem solving, and analyzing and synthesizing new theoretical and practical content.

# Meaning and Relevance of New Knowledge

Adult learners are motivated to learn when what they are learning is relevant and useful in their work and home lives. The LPN/LVN who returns to school to pursue an ADN often does so for monetary reasons or for increased autonomy or career mobility. However, once in the transition process, this same nurse discovers the increased ability she or he has to plan and implement individualized care to clients.

The ability to make nursing diagnoses, solve problems, and work collaboratively with physicians and other healthcare workers to provide comprehensive client care supplies additional motivation and incentive to continue pursuit of this increased scope of practice. The increased independence and ability to solve problems and accept new challenges in their everyday world creates even greater motivation for LPN/LVNs to further their learning.

## ▶ Thinking Critically

Reflect on an experience when some new knowledge had particular meaning and relevance to you in your personal or work life. How did this motivate you to learn even more?

# Personal and Professional Achievement and Self-actualization

A parallel but different motivational force in adults pursuing learning is self-fulfillment or self-actualization. To self-actualize is to realize fully one's potential (*Random House Webster's Dictionary,* 2000). Whether for personal or professional achievement, one motivation for LPN/LVNs to seek ADN education is to realize their potential as nurses, to acquire the knowledge, skills, and abilities to practice at the RN level.

> ## Thinking Critically
>
> Reflect on the factors that have motivated you to pursue an ADN. When things get tough from time to time throughout the program, how can you draw on these resources to maintain that motivation?

# Self-directed, Individualized Learning

In addition to a wealth of experiential learning, the adult learner has gained insight into the means by which she or he learns best. Individualizing your approach to new content can offer many possibilities for maximizing the learning process.

The adult learner is self-directed and seeks learning to fulfill self-established goals. The LPN/LVN who sets personal goals related to the accomplishment of competencies and objectives of the ADN program is more likely to experience success than are those who are not self-directed.

# Practical/Vocational and Associate Degree Nursing Education: A Comparison

Although the educational programs for the LPN/LVN and the ADN student may appear to be similar, close examination reveals major differences between the two.

## Philosophies and Conceptual Models

Each nursing program is built on a philosophy developed and shared by the nursing faculty. Although both levels of nursing programs set forth beliefs about the practice of nursing in their philosophy statements, the ADN program philosophy generally provides greater depth in its view of nursing, defining such central concepts as man (client or person), health, environment, nursing, caring, teaching, and learning.

The conceptual model is the template of theoretical concepts and principles that is a basis for developing the curricular content for the nursing program. The conceptual model is derived from the program's philosophy and guides the development of course objectives and competencies. Many LPN/LVN programs are built on a medical model, in which the LPN/LVN operates as a member of the nursing profession, providing care to clients with medical disorders or dysfunctions. As a directed care provider, the LPN/LVN carries out physicians' orders and contributes to the planning, implementation, and evaluation of care to clients based on nursing diagnoses. The LPN/LVN programs that use a nursing model (i.e., based on nursing theory and nursing diagnoses, rather than medical diagnoses) often choose a human needs approach because this model fits well with the directed scope of practice of the LPN/LVN. ADN programs often use an integrated nursing model for their conceptual framework, drawing on the research of nurse theorists and incorporating nursing diagnoses to guide the developing autonomous practice of the RN student. These models allow for the nurse with an associate degree to practice both independently and collaboratively with other healthcare providers, within their scope of practice.

## Curricular Frameworks

The curricular frameworks for each of these levels of nursing programs are consistent with their nurse practice acts, National Council of State Boards of Nursing Test Plans, and competencies identified by such professional organizations as the National League for Nursing. Each state's Nurse Practice Act outlines the educational preparation needed for the LPN/LVN and RN practice levels. Each nursing school's curriculum must be approved by the state board of nursing to be accredited so that program graduates will be eligible for licensure through the licensing exam after completion.

The National League for Nursing (2000) has identified eight core components of nursing practice for graduates of ADN programs. These components are essential to the work of the entry-level registered nurse and inherent in the three roles of professional nursing practice (provider of care, manager of care, and member within the discipline of nursing). The eight core components are professional behaviors, communication, assessment, clinical decision making, caring interventions, teaching and learning, collaboration, and managing care (**Display 5-2**). These core components provide the framework for organizing educational outcomes of graduates of ADN programs.

## Curricular Content and Learning Domains

In the mid-1900s, Benjamin Bloom and others (1956) identified three learning domains into which curricular content falls and from which educational objectives are written. The *cognitive* domain is the area of learning in which you acquire knowledge. The *affective* domain is the area of learning involving values and attitudes. The *psychomotor* domain is the area of learning in which you develop manipulative skills in the discipline.

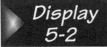

| | |
|---|---|
| *Display* 5-2 | **Core Components of Nursing Practice for Graduates of ADN Programs** |

| | |
|---|---|
| 1. Professional behaviors | 5. Caring interventions |
| 2. Communication | 6. Teaching and learning |
| 3. Assessment | 7. Collaboration |
| 4. Clinical decision making | 8. Managing care |

## NCLEX–RN Might Ask 5-1

**? ? ?**

The nursing student is teaching a client with a colostomy about irrigation of the stoma. The type of learning domain the student would use to teach the client is

    A. cognitive.
    B. psychomotor.
    C. affective.
    D. communicative.

• *See Appendix A for correct answer and rationale.*

### Thinking Critically

To gain a better understanding of the three learning domains, think about the last time you attended a nursing in-service at work. What cognitive learning took place? What words, procedures, and rules did you need to learn and apply to participate in the in-service? What affective learning took place? What attitudes did you need to change or develop? How did your beliefs or views about nursing and the type of people involved change? What psychomotor learning took place? What hands-on skills did you need to learn?

Both LPN/LVN and ADN education programs contain curricular content in all three learning domains. For example, both programs require knowledge of body structure and function (cognitive domain), an appreciation for the self-image changes confronting the aging individual (affective domain), and the ability to take accurate vital signs (psychomotor domain). However, more in-depth content in each of the three domains is included in the ADN program curriculum. A review of the curriculum content in each of the two program levels reveals that additional content or coursework is required for the ADN program in such areas as the biological and behavioral sciences; computational, communication, and language skills; advanced medical–surgical nursing; psychiatric nursing; and management skills.

## Learning Achievement Levels

Within the cognitive domain, Bloom and others (1956) identified six learning achievement levels that continue to guide curricula today and that differentiate the practice of LPN/LVNs and RNs. These six cognitive learning achievement levels, as shown in **Display 5-3**, are knowledge, comprehension, application, analysis, synthesis, and evaluation. Competencies at the LPN/LVN level include the knowledge, comprehension, and application of content within the scope of practice of the LPN/LVN. Competencies at the ADN level include all six cognitive learning achievement levels. The ability to analyze, synthesize, and evaluate data is essential to the RN in establishing nursing diagnoses, designing nursing care plans, and managing client care. Curriculum content and learning activities in the ADN program support learning achievement at these three higher levels of thinking.

> **Display 5-3**  **Cognitive Learning Achievement Levels**

1. Knowledge
2. Comprehension
3. Application

4. Analysis
5. Synthesis
6. Evaluation

## Nursing Process and Nursing Diagnosis

Taylor, Lillis, and LeMone (2001) describe the nursing process as a systematic method that helps the nurse and client develop a plan to meet the client's needs. Nursing process progresses through its scientific steps in five phases: assessment, diagnosis, planning, implementation, and evaluation. Both the LPN/LVN and the RN participate in the nursing process within their respective scopes of practice. However, the roles played by each differ. **Table 5-1** provides a comparison of the roles played by LPN/LVNs and RNs with regard to nursing process and nursing diagnosis. The LPN/LVN collects data, assists with patient assessment, contributes to the planning phase, implements basic therapeutic and preventive measures outlined in the plan, and evaluates the effectiveness of such measures. The RN collects data and performs patient assessment, analyzes and groups data, draws conclusions and uses judgment in establishing diagnoses, designs a plan of care collaborating with other healthcare providers, develops an implementation plan with short- and long-term goals, and provides outcomes of the plan, redesigning as needed.

The *Test Plan for the National Council Licensure Examination for Practical Nurses (NCLEX-PN)* (National Council of State Boards of Nursing, 1999) outlines the role of this practitioner in relation to the nursing process, stating

> The entry-level practical nurse acts in a more dependent role when participating in the planning and evaluation phases of the nursing process and acts in a more independent role when participating in the data collecting and implementing phases of the nursing process.

In contrast, the *Test Plan for the National Council Licensure Examination for Registered Nurses (NCLEX-RN)* (NCSBN, 2001) recognizes the role of the RN in all five phases of the nursing process, including the analysis (nursing diagnosis) phase. Because of the independent role played by this level of practitioner in the five phases and the importance of each phase according to the job analysis study by Hertz, Yocom, and Gawel (2000), the *Test Plan* designates an approximately equal percentage of items in each phase.

## Differences in the Learning Process

As you enter the ADN program, you may discover differences in the learning process from that encountered in the LPN/LVN program you attended. These differences may be attributed partly to the length of time between the programs, especially if it has been

TABLE 5-1

COMPARISON OF THE ROLE PLAYED BY LICENSED PRACTICAL/VOCATIONAL NURSES (LPN/LVNs) AND REGISTERED NURSES (RNS) IN NURSING PROCESS AND NURSING DIAGNOSIS

| Nursing Process Phase | Role of LPN/LVN | Role of RN Beyond LPN/LVN Scope of Practice |
|---|---|---|
| *Assessment* | Gathers data<br>Performs patient assessment<br>Identifies patient strengths | Gathers more extensive biopsychosocial data<br>Groups and analyzes data<br>Researches additional data needed<br>Identifies client resources |
| *Nursing diagnosis* | Not applicable | Draws conclusions<br>Uses judgment<br>Makes diagnoses |
| *Planning* | Contributes to development of care plans | Sets short- and long-term client goals<br>Establishes priorities<br>Collaborates and refers |
| *Implementation* | Provides basic therapeutic and preventive nursing measures<br>Provides client teaching<br>Records client information | Manages client care (performs and delegates)<br>Provides client and family teaching<br>Provides referrals<br>Records and exchanges client information with health team |
| *Evaluation* | Evaluates effects of care given | Evaluates effectiveness of overall plan; analyzes new data<br>Modifies, redesigns plan<br>Collaborates with other health team members |

many years since your participation in the LPN/LVN program. However, even if you just recently completed the LPN/LVN program, you will encounter differences attributable to the areas discussed in this chapter: program philosophies; conceptual models; curricular frameworks; curricular content within learning domains; addition of the analysis, synthesis, and evaluation learning achievement levels; and role in nursing process and nursing diagnosis.

Because the goal of the ADN program is to enable you to function in the independent and interdependent (collaborative) modes, use higher level thinking skills, and make nursing diagnoses using analysis and judgment, you will experience two key differences in the educational process: (1) an active learning process will mostly likely be the mode of operation, and (2) learning activities will include a focus on developing your ability to analyze and synthesize curricular content.

Active learning is the act or process of acquiring knowledge or skill (by being) engaged in action or activity (*Random House Webster's Dictionary*, 2000). In addition to traditional lecture, laboratory, and clinical experiences, learning activities in the ADN program include classroom exercises and out-of-class assignments that require active participation. Such exercises are designed to build self-confidence, develop communication skills, develop analytical skills, and foster critical thinking to prepare you for the autonomous professional role you will be expected to assume after graduation. No longer will the correct response be to report findings to the RN or physician. You will now need to analyze information, use judgment, establish diagnoses, confront issues, take action, manage client care, and delegate interventions while maintaining responsibility for clients under your care. The active learning process in the ADN program and learning activities that focus on developing your ability to analyze and synthesize curricular content will prepare you for these new challenges.

# Learning Strategies for Success

As an adult learner, you can adopt learning strategies that will maximize your success in the ADN program by increasing your self-awareness, establishing self-directed goals, becoming an active learner, and adopting techniques to stimulate your thinking.

## Self-awareness

### ADDRESSING YOUR LEARNING STYLE

In Chapter 1, you learned about learning styles and how individuals have different ways they best learn in an educational setting. You reflected on this material to determine your own learning style(s) or ways you learn best. Are you an auditory or a visual learner? Do you need to role play or in other ways "experience" the content you are trying to learn? Exploring new forms of study habits or redesigning group study sessions to address your learning style(s) will enhance your success. In addition, make sure your instructor knows how you learn best. Stitt-Gohdes (1999) stresses the need for teachers to be aware of learning styles so they can focus on teaching students first and subjects second.

### ACCOMMODATING FOR DISABILITIES

Many individuals with physical, mental, or learning disabilities have experienced success in pursuing a career at the ADN level. The law requires all educational institutions to provide reasonable accommodation to individuals with disabilities, but it is up to the individual to request such accommodation.

Some students may have experienced difficulty in school without knowing they had a learning problem or learning disability. Several indicators of possible learning problems or learning disabilities are shown in **Display 5-4**.

The key to success is first to identify and understand any learning problem or disability you may have; second, seek accommodation for the disability to succeed in the ADN program. Each college provides support services and referrals for students who have been identified as having a disability.

### ADDRESSING AGE, GENDER, AND CULTURAL DIFFERENCES

LPN/LVNs enrolling in ADN programs may experience barriers to achievement of course objectives and competencies because of age, gender, or cultural differences in relation to other students or social roles, as described in Chapter 1. The re-entry nurse may feel uncomfortable if classmates or peers in study or clinical groups are much

| Display 5-4 | Indicators of Possible Learning Problems or Learning Disabilities |
|---|---|

▶ **VISUAL PERCEPTUAL PROBLEMS**

- Reverses letters and order of letters
- Omits endings of words
- Cannot edit own work
- Mismarks computerized scoring sheets
- Loses place while reading (marks place with finger or piece of paper)
- Has difficulty lining up numbers correctly (uses graph paper to do math)
- Is confused by complex visual fields (when doing a work sheet, blocks out all but essential item)

▶ **AUDITORY PERCEPTUAL PROBLEMS**

- Cannot differentiate sounds (e and i, m and n)
- Has difficulty sounding out unknown words
- Is poor at spelling
- Is highly distracted by background noise
- Cannot locate stress in words or sentences

▶ **SPATIAL PERCEPTUAL PROBLEMS**

- Has trouble differentiating left from right
- Has trouble following directions (gets lost easily)
- Is slow to learn dance routines

▶ **VISUAL–MOTOR PROBLEMS**

- Miscopies information
- Has poor handwriting

▶ **INTEGRATION PROBLEMS**

- Understands concepts but forgets facts, dates, names
- Frequently has difficulty recalling commonly known words
- Is poor at spelling (cannot remember order of letters)
- Understands mathematical concepts but cannot remember the order of steps to solve math problems
- Has poor organizational skills

▶ **ATTENTION DEFICIT**

- Has trouble sitting still for an extended time
- Is highly distractible
- Is unable to concentrate for an extended time
- Jumps from task to task

younger. The male student who acquired his LPN/LVN through military service may be participating for the first time in an educational setting where peers and instructors are predominantly female. He or his peers may be uncomfortable in group learning activities, or he may be called on in the clinical area to help move patients, thus detracting from his ability to work on clinical objectives and competencies in his student role.

Cultural mores also may hamper success in the program. The dependent role of women in some cultures may prevent such female students from developing autonomy, the ability to collaborate with physicians, and management skills. Cultural views of time, acceptable verbal and nonverbal communication skills, and proxemics (comfort in special relations) may prevent the student from meeting clinical competencies involving these areas of interpersonal skills and responsibilities.

Strategies for success for students experiencing difficulties because of age, gender, or cultural differences include:

1. identifying situations that generate discomfort;
2. discussing these areas with the instructor(s);
3. sharing and confronting such issues openly in class discussions and clinical conferences; and
4. exploring successful coping and accommodation strategies that have been used by other students and nurses.

See **Display 5-5**.

## SELF-DIRECTED GOALS

A second strategy for maximizing success is to establish self-directed goals. Breaking up reading and other learning activities into smaller time blocks and scheduling time in advance for study are milestones in the goal-setting process. Doing research online or preparing questions for discussion before a study group session will enhance your learning at the session. Seeking clinical skills during each clinical session will ensure completion of clinical skill checklists by the end of the term.

# Active Learning

The ADN program will include learning activities for students to work with peers and other healthcare professionals in a variety of ways. Through this active learning process, the student will develop the ability to apply curricular content, analyze and problem solve, think critically, and perform independently in the eight core components outlined by the National League for Nursing (2000).

A variety of active learning activities may be included in the design of the ADN educational program. Commonly found are such activities as brainstorming, small group discussion, role playing, and formal debates. The student who takes a proactive

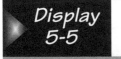

**Display 5-5**

**Strategies for Success for Students Experiencing Difficulties Because of Age, Gender, or Cultural Differences**

1. Identify situations that generate discomfort
2. Discuss these areas with the instructor
3. Share and confront such issues openly in class discussions and clinical conferences
4. Explore successful coping and accommodation strategies that have been used by other students and nurses

approach in creating her or his own active learning activities will enhance success. Forming study groups, posing problems to solve, writing study questions to exchange with peers, and designing care plans in a collaborative process are examples of ways you can strengthen the learning process for yourself and peers.

## Techniques to Stimulate Thinking

A similar learning strategy for success is to develop techniques to stimulate thinking about curricular content in each of the three learning domains. One of the best strategies for stimulating thinking is to continually ask yourself questions about the learning being acquired (the what, where, why, who, how, and what if questions). Example questions follow for each of the three learning domains.

### COGNITIVE DOMAIN

What is the meaning of this content? How does it relate to last week's learning? How does it relate to prior content or courses? How would I explain this to someone else? How would I apply this in practice? How would this apply to clients of different ages, the opposite gender, different cultures, or those who are disabled? What are opposing viewpoints to this content?

### AFFECTIVE DOMAIN

How would I feel if I were experiencing this disorder, dysfunction, or difficulty? How would I react if this were happening to someone close to me? How do I value this type of response or behavior? How might someone experience this who is of a different age, gender, or cultural background? What values or beliefs underlie this patient's or nurse's comments? What ethical dilemmas might arise in this situation, and how would I confront them?

### PSYCHOMOTOR DOMAIN

What are the principles underlying this procedure (aseptic techniques, ethical considerations, protection of privacy, body mechanics, energy conservation, resource conservation, therapeutic effect)? How else could this be performed while maintaining these principles? How would I teach this to a client? How could this be done in a home environment? What verbal and nonverbal communication is taking place? What shortcuts can I take to save time or supplies, while maintaining the principles involved?

In addition to these learning strategies for success, you will want to take into account your individual uniqueness. Chapter 6 provides you with an opportunity to draw on these strategies and others in designing your own individualized learning plan. Chapter 9 provides you with more information on critical thinking. See **Display 5-6** for information on adult learning.

## Transition Needs Unique to the LPN/LVN to ADN Student

Thus far in this chapter you have been learning about the process of transitioning from the LPN/LVN role to the ADN student role. As an LPN/LVN, you are entering the ADN program in one of three entry patterns. Transition needs of LPN/LVNs vary among the three patterns.

**Display 5-6**   **Things to Think About When Learning**

Adults remember:

10% of what we read.
20% of what we hear.
30% of what we see.
50% of what we see and hear.

60% of what we write.
70% of what we discuss.
80% of what we experience.
95% of what we teach.

From Dale, E. (1969). *The core experience.* Indianapolis: Merrill.

## LPN/LVNs Entering a Generic ADN Population

The generic ADN student starts at the beginning of the ADN program and progresses through the curriculum to completion of the program. Generic ADN students are provided with an orientation at the start of the program and learn about the history and development of ADN and registered nursing in general. An overview of the program philosophy, conceptual model, and curriculum framework is usually presented, and the student is socialized into the role and expectations of the RN scope of practice.

The LPN/LVN who enters a generic ADN class is usually advance-placed 25% to 50% of the way through the program. She or he may be a lone enrollee or may be accompanied by others advance placed at this point of entry. The orientation and socialization (transition) process varies according to nursing program policies and practices, but most programs provide only a minimal orientation/socialization process. Material and student exercises presented in this text are designed to enhance the success of students who have or who have not been provided with a formal transition course or process.

The unique needs of LPN/LVNs entering a generic ADN population center around socialization not only into the program culture, but also into the class culture. These cultures include all the unwritten and written rules and acceptable behaviors of student participants. The LPN/LVN who takes a proactive approach in seeking assistance from faculty and classmates in getting to know the ropes and trying to fit in with study groups increases her or his chance of success.

## Straight-Through LPN/LVN to ADN Students

The straight-through LPN/LVN to ADN student is one who has participated in the school's LPN/LVN program and has continued on, directly into the ADN program (usually at the second year level). When large groups of students are involved in this entry pattern or if the college offers only a career ladder (LPN/LVN to RN) program and no generic program, the transition may be smoother. The culture of the school will be familiar, including instructional support areas (e.g., library, computer lab, skills center), and the student may know faculty in the program. The ADN program generally provides a formalized orientation or transition course for these students. This text's design allows for its use in this entry pattern.

The unique needs of LPN/LVN to ADN students in this entry pattern center on the role transition required to move to the registered nursing scope of practice. The learning environment may shift from a more passive to a more active learning process. Performance that was considered acceptable and competent in the LPN/LVN program is suddenly inadequate, as faculty foster independent thinking, problem solving, and self-directed learning in these students.

## Time-out LPN/LVN to ADN Students

The time-out LPN/LVN to ADN student completes an LPN/LVN program and then works (or not) before embarking on the ADN program. The time out may be as short as 1 year or as long as a decade or more. Thus, the needs of these students are individualized according to the length of time out, whether the individual worked as an LPN/LVN and in what job role, and whether the individual is attending the same or a different school. This text is organized to enable the time-out LPN/LVN to ADN student to meet her or his individual needs.

# Differentiating ADN Student and LPN/LVN Practice Roles

A difficulty encountered by most LPN/LVNs returning to school to pursue the ADN is the role confusion that emerges in the clinical setting. Issues of liability, legal parameters, and the level of autonomy can be confusing and problematic for the ADN student who is an LPN/LVN.

## Issues of Liability

As a student in the ADN program, the LPN/LVN is bound by contract language in the agreement between the school and clinical agency, policies of the clinical agency, policies of the ADN program, and course-by-course objectives and competencies in the curriculum. For example, the LPN/LVN may work at an agency other than that of the clinical assignment as an ADN student. Differences in policies, standardized procedures, and protocol between the two agencies may cause frustration for the student, particularly if she or he is employed on alternating days with the student experience and thus is operating out of two different agencies. As a second example, procedures the LPN/LVN performs regularly in her or his licensed practice because the LPN/LVN has had additional training (e.g., intravenous therapy) may be beyond the curriculum level or contract language for the course in which she or he is enrolled in the ADN program and not allowed. Keeping in close contact with the instructor at the clinical site and verifying interventions planned is essential when dealing with liability issues and helps to minimize frustration.

## Legal Aspects

In addition to these liability issues, several legal aspects must be considered by the LPN/LVN in the ADN student role. While in the student role, the LPN/LVN is not functioning as a licensed person, but rather as a student in the ADN program. As such, she or he practices as all other program students within the legal parameters of that role. Handling controlled substances and signing for insulin, blood, and narcotics should be performed by the LPN/LVN in the student role under the same guidelines as such procedures would be performed by other ADN students.

## Autonomy and Parameters for Instructor Supervision

LPN/LVNs in the ADN student role also may experience a feeling of loss of autonomy. In particular, the time-out LPN/LVN to ADN student who has gained clinical expertise and has been given increasing responsibilities in the practice setting may experience this loss the greatest. Patient assessment and nursing interventions that the LPN/LVN has been performing independently may now have to be done under the supervision of the instructor. The LPN/LVN to ADN student must have a clear understanding of the level of independence allowed in relation to nursing care activities according to program policies and each course's clinical guidelines and must discuss areas of role conflict with the instructor.

## Conclusion

This chapter is built on information presented in Chapter 3 about ADN education programs. This chapter also examines adult learning theory and how you as an adult learner can enhance your success in the ADN program. The LPN/LVN and ADN education programs are compared in the areas of philosophies and conceptual models, curricular frameworks, curricular content and learning domains, learning achievement levels, nursing process and nursing diagnosis, and differences in the learning process.

Learning strategies for success are covered, including addressing your learning style; accommodating for disabilities; addressing age, gender, and cultural differences; establishing self-directed goals; engaging in active learning activities; and adopting techniques to stimulate thinking. Transition needs unique to a variety of LPN/LVNs pursuing ADN education also are addressed, including a discussion of the difference in the licensed versus student roles played by these LPN/LVNs entering an ADN program.

---

## NCLEX–RN Might Ask 5-2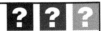

The LPN to RN student nurse is assigned to a client in an ambulatory surgical setting. The LPN in this setting is held to the legal accountability of a(n)

    A. layman.
    B. student.
    C. LPN.
    D. RN.

• *See Appendix A for correct answer and rationale.*

## Student Exercise

Obtain a school catalog with course descriptions of the curricula for the ADN program you are planning to enter (or have entered). Review nursing and non-nursing course titles, course descriptions, and breakdown of lecture and laboratory spent in each course. In the space below, write key concepts or phrases from the course descriptions that indicate learning you will gain in each of the three learning domains as you complete coursework for the program.

| Learning Domain | Course No. | Key Concepts/Phrases |
|---|---|---|
| **1.** Cognitive domain (knowledge) | | |
| **2.** Affective domain (values, attitudes) | | |
| **3.** Psychomotor domain (skills) | | |

# References

Bloom, B. S. (Ed.). (1956). *Taxonomy of educational objectives: The classification of educational goals.* New York: David McKay.

Dale, E. (1969). *The core experience.* Indianapolis: Merril.

Hertz, J., Yocom, C., & Gawel, S. (2000). *Linking the NCLEX-RN national license examination to practice: 1999 practice analysis of newly licensed registered nurses in the U.S.* Chicago: National Council of State Boards of Nursing, Inc.

National Council of State Boards of Nursing (NCSBN). (1999). *Test plan for the National Council Licensure Examination for Practical Nurses (NCLEX-PN).* Chicago: Author.

National Council of State Boards of Nursing (NCSBN). (2001). *Test plan for the National Council Licensure Examination for Registered Nurses (NCLEX-RN).* Chicago: Author.

National League for Nursing. (2000). *Educational competencies for graduates of associate degree nursing programs.* Sudbury, MA: Author, Jones and Bartlett Publishers.

*Random House Webster's dictionary.* (2000). New York: Random House.

Stitt-Gohdes, W. L. (1999). Teaching and learning styles: Implications for business teacher education. In P. G. G. Villee & M. G. Curran (Eds.), *The 21st century: Meeting the challenges to business education.* Reston, VA: National Business Education Association.

Taylor, C., Lillis, C., & LeMone, P. (2001). *Fundamentals of nursing: The art and science of nursing care* (4th ed.). Philadelphia: Lippincott Williams & Wilkins.

# Suggested Reading

Bloom, B. S. (Ed.). (1974). *The taxonomy of educational objectives: Affective and cognitive domains.* New York: David McKay.

Bonner, J. (1982). Systematic lesson design for adult learners. *Journal of Institutional Development, 6*(1), 34–42.

Browne, M. N., & Keeley, S. (2000). *Striving for excellence in college: Tips for active learning.* Upper Saddle River, NJ: Prentice Hall.

Carter, C., Bishop, J., Bixby, M., & Kravitz, S. L. (2001). *Keys to study skills: Opening doors to learning.* Upper Saddle River, NJ: Prentice Hall.

Carter, C. (2002). *Keys to college studying: Becoming a lifelong learner.* Upper Saddle River, NJ: Prentice Hall.

Daloz, L.A. (1999). *Mentor: Guiding the journey of adult learners.* San Francisco: Jossey-Bass.

DeTornyay, R., & Thompson, M. A. (1982). *Strategies for teaching nursing* (2nd ed.). New York: John Wiley and Sons.

Dunn, R.S., & Griggs, S.A. (1998). *Learning styles of the nursing profession.* New York: NLN Press.

Kelly, L. Y. (1985). *Dimensions of professional nursing* (5th ed.). New York: Macmillan.

Knowles, M. S. (1970). Gearing adult education for the seventies. *The Journal of Continuing Education in Nursing, 1*(1), 11–16.

Knowles, M. S. (1980). *The modern practice of adult education: From pedagogy to andragogy.* Chicago: Follett.

Leddy, S., & Pepper, J. M. (1998). *Conceptual bases of professional nursing* (4th ed.). Philadelphia: Lippincott-Raven Publishers.

Mast, M. E., & Van Atta, M. J. (1986). Applying adult learning principles in instructional module design. *Nurse Educator, 11*(1), 35–39.

Musinski, B. (1999). The educator as facilitator: A new kind of leadership. *Nursing Forum, 34*(1), 23–29.

National League for Nursing: Council of Associate Degree Programs. (1990). *Educational outcomes of associate degree nursing programs: Roles and competencies.* New York: Author.

National League for Nursing: Council of Practical Nursing Programs. (1999). *Entry-level competencies of graduates of educational programs in practical nursing.* New York: Author.

Nugent, P. M, & Vitale, B. A. (2000). *Test success: Test-taking techniques for beginning nursing students* (3rd ed.). Philadelphia: FA Davis.

Sides, M., & Korchek, N. (1998). *Successful test-taking: Learning strategies for nurses.* Philadelphia: Lippincott Williams & Wilkins.

Smith, C. E. (1978). Planning, implementing, and evaluating learning experiences for adults. *Nurse Educator, 3*(6), 31–36.

Tarnow, K. G. (1979). Working with adult learners. *Nurse Educator, 4*(5), 34–40.

Tileston, D. W. (2000). *10 best teaching practices: How brain research, learning styles, and standards define teaching competencies.* Thousand Oaks, CA: Corwin Press.

Wlodkowski, R. (1985). How to plan motivational strategies for adult instruction. *Performance and Instruction, 24*(9), 1–6.

*On the Web* · · · · · · · · · · · · · · · · · · · · · · · · · · · · · · · · · · · · · ·

*www.ncsbn.org*: National Council of State Boards of Nursing
*www.nlnac.org*: National League for Nursing Accreditation Commission
*www.nsna.org*: National Student Nurses Association

# Individualizing a Plan for Role Transition

## LEARNING OBJECTIVES

*By the end of this chapter, the student will be able to:*

1 Assess preparedness for the student role based on information learned in previous chapters.
2 Describe learning style(s) based on information learned in previous chapters.
3 Assess own uniqueness as an adult learner based on information learned in previous chapters.
4 Identify prior cognitive, affective, and psychomotor learning achieved through formal education and experience.
5 Design a personal educational plan to enhance success in the associate degree nursing program.
6 Apply concepts learned to establish an effective instructor–student partnership.

## KEY TERMS

experiential learning
feedback mechanism
instructor–student partnership
mentor
mutual goal setting
nonstandardized test

personal education plan (PEP)
proactive learner
standardized test
strategic learner
student success strategy
time management

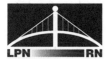

# VIGNETTE

Sherry Williams is an LPN in her first semester of ADN school and is meeting with her nursing advisor. Sherry has opted to take an advanced placement course via the Internet and isn't sure where to start with a needs assessment that has been assigned to her to perform.

**Advisor:** Hi, Sherry. Thank you for scheduling an appointment with me. I enjoy seeing my students, but sometimes they don't come in until after the first exam. How can I help you?

**Sherry:** I see you have sent me a needs assessment. I'm not sure why we are doing this, and I'm a little intimidated with how long the form is. Can you help me understand why I'm doing this and how to do it?

**Advisor:** Since you have opted to take the advanced placement course for LVNs on the web, we the faculty want to tailor your course so that it concentrates on your needs. For example, if you're a whiz at math, we want to spend less time on that and more on, say, nursing planning—especially if your exposure to that has been minimal in your current position.

**Sherry:** So this is similar to how we deal with teaching a patient with diabetes. If the client and family know about insulins and can return-demonstrate an injection, we might concentrate more on their diet, especially if blood sugars aren't under control.

**Advisor:** Exactly. We realize that our students in this course come from a wide variety of backgrounds. Some haven't been in school in years, some have been away for a few years, and some are fresh out of LPN school.

**Sherry:** I guess I didn't realize that. I guess it is sort of like a new employee working at our nursing home. Everyone comes with different experiences, and being new, you have to get adjusted. We have learned a lot from people just out of school and other workplaces.

**Advisor:** And so you will with this course. I will send everyone a list of course participant e-mail addresses so that even though you won't meet each other face to face, you can 'talk' to each other online. I hope this will help you share experiences.

**Sherry:** OK, now on to the assessment...

**Advisor:** The reason this is so in-depth is that it makes you think about what you are good at. Perhaps you are an expert at administering tube feedings or inserting urinary catheters but need more help with fluid and electrolytes or medication theory. Then we can concentrate more on these topics, and you may want to attend the sister course that meets here on campus for more hands-on work in the lab or more classroom work.

**Sherry:** I see now. It's all falling into place...I think I can take it from here.

**Advisor:** Great. Let's do the first page together. You can either finish outside my office and hand it in now, or you can mail it or e-mail it to me in a day or two.

**Sherry:** I have to pick my kids up now, so I will e-mail it to you by tomorrow. Thanks for your help.

Throughout Unit I, you have explored the concepts of transition and change. Chapter 1 discusses lifelong learning and your return to school. Chapter 2 examines role development and transition, including the phases of role transition and how they apply to you as you move from a licensed practical/vocational nursing (LPN/LVN) role to a registered nursing (RN) role. Chapter 3 discusses the process of change, the effects of change, and how to adjust to change. In applying these concepts to your LPN/LVN to RN role transition, you have looked at the positive outcomes you will experience in the change process.

Chapter 4 provides you with a historical account of the transitions that have been experienced in the discipline of nursing, including the evolution of associate degree nursing (ADN). Chapter 5 focuses on learning at the ADN level.

In Chapter 6, you are given the opportunity to apply knowledge gained from the preceding chapters to yourself, assess prior knowledge and experience, and design an educational plan specific to your individual needs. You will assess your preparedness for the student role, examine your learning style, and reflect on the unique characteristics and needs you bring to the ADN program.

Several methods for assessing your theoretical and experiential knowledge and abilities are discussed in this chapter, and you will design a personal education plan (PEP; see Display 6-1 at end of chapter) to enhance success in the ADN program and on the National Council Licensure Examination for Registered Nurses (NCLEX-RN), which you will take after you complete the ADN program.

Also presented in Chapter 6 is a discussion of the instructor–student partnership. Strategies for fostering a successful partnership are explored, as are techniques for individualizing your learning activities and strengthening your clinical practicum in the ADN program. Such concepts as mutual goal setting and feedback mechanisms are presented.

# Assessing Preparedness for the Student Role

The first step in individualizing a plan for role transition is to examine your preparedness for the student role, as discussed in Chapter 1. If you just recently completed the LPN/LVN nursing program or you have been recently completing course work and receiving academic advising in preparing for the ADN program, you may already feel comfortable with or settled into the student role. In assessing your preparedness for the student role, four areas of preparedness should be examined:

1. the re-entry process,
2. the school setting,
3. student success strategies, and
4. time management.

# Re-entry Process

For those who have been away from the educational setting for some time or acquired their LPN/LVN license in a pathway other than formal education (e.g., military or other service experience), moving into the student role may feel awkward and uncomfortable. It is important to find out the demographics of the ADN program you plan to enter to know how your characteristics and biases will fit with the class you will enter. What have the age, gender, and cultural distributions of classes been during the last few years at this nursing school? How many other LPN/LVNs will be entering this class, and what percentage of the class as a whole will be represented by the LPN/LVN constituency? Are the LPN/LVNs in this group advance placed, straight-through, or time-out students (as described in Chapter 5)?

## ▶ Thinking Critically

On a sheet of paper, write how you are similar to and how you are different from the typical student in the ADN program you will enter. Consider age, gender, ethnicity, and nursing experience. In areas in which you are different, cite strengths you will bring to the class to enhance others' learning and identify actions you can take to develop comfort with the re-entry process. (Save this information for use in designing your PEP.)

# The School Setting

Feeling prepared to enter (or re-enter) the school setting develops self-confidence and comfort in the student role. Knowing the ropes or knowing where to find things on campus and how to function within the processes and systems of the school, can assist you in this process. Chapter 1 describes strategies for success in the student role. Ask yourself these questions: Do you have a campus map? Do you know the location of such areas as counseling, registration, student services, the health center, child care services (if needed), nursing office, library, and bookstore? Do you know how to register for classes, apply for financial aid or scholarships, and seek assistance for disabilities? Do you know how to use the library, research a topic, use online systems and the *Cumulative Index for Nursing and Allied Health Literature* (CINAHL) to locate periodical (journal) articles? If you do not have a computer, do you know where on campus you can access one to complete an assignment? Do you know where and how to access copying services? Are there any orientation sessions, printed materials, or student success courses you can take to prepare yourself better for the school setting?

## ▶ Thinking Critically

Take a moment to reflect on the previous questions. On a piece of paper, write several actions you can take to prepare yourself better for the student setting. (Save this information for use in designing your PEP.)

# Student Success Strategies

As described in Chapter 1, many strategies can be used to support your success in the ADN program. Preparing for the student role involves identifying student success strategies that meet your individual needs and with which you feel comfortable.

## LEARNING TECHNIQUES

Have you developed effective learning techniques and study skills to be successful in this more complex ADN course work? Meeting objectives and achieving competencies identified for this program will necessitate that you not only gain knowledge, comprehension, and the ability to apply content learned, but that you also analyze data, draw conclusions, use judgment, synthesize information, and make decisions by thinking critically about course content during learning activities. Critical thinking and clinical decision making are discussed later in this text. What learning techniques do you possess and what resources have you developed to support you in this process?

## BECOMING A PROACTIVE LEARNER

Have you learned how to be a proactive learner? The proactive learner seeks experiences to add knowledge, skills, and abilities to her or his expertise. Carter, Bishop, and Kravitz (2002) describe techniques for becoming a lifelong learner. They note that knowledge in every field is doubling every 2 to 3 years. This certainly is true in nursing! Thus, lifelong learning is essential. One must become self-directed, resourceful, and a critical thinker. Carter et al. also describe the "strategic learner," one who puts herself/himself into new learning situations to help toward one's identified goals.

### ▶ Thinking Critically

Assess your study skills and resources. Identify those you possess and those you need to develop to support yourself in the ADN program. Are you a strategic learner? What can you do to develop yourself in this area? (Save this information for use in designing your PEP.)

## DEVELOPING MENTORS

In addition to study skills and resource materials, developing mentors and participating in study groups are strategies that increase your chances of success. Vance and Olson (1998) discuss the "mentor connection" in nursing:

> We believe that mentoring is essential to our full development as human beings and as professionals. It is possible, of course, to have a productive career without a significant mentor, but mentoring promotes career success faster and easier. Mentor relationships have a profound impact on self and career development. Mentor relationships shape and nourish us. They have the capacity to transform the path of our human journey. (p. 3)

A mentor is someone with whom you can consult, who will give you advice, and who will counsel, guide, and help you in the learning process. More advanced students, program graduates, instructional aides, and learning resource specialists are examples of people who may be appropriate mentors for you.

Much has been written in recent years about the value of mentoring, especially in today's world where information changes rapidly and job turnover often occurs every 2 to 3 years. Fletcher (2000) has defined mentoring:

> Mentoring is the potential of a one-to-one professional relationship that can simultaneously empower and enhance practice. Mentoring means guiding and supporting trainees to ease them through difficult transitions; it is about soothing the way, enabling, reassuring as well as directing, managing, and instructing. It should unlock the ways to change by building self-confidence, self-esteem and a readiness to act as well as to engage in ongoing constructive interpersonal relationships. (p. 1)

When choosing a mentor, you must decide on qualities in prospective mentors that will enhance your success based on your individual learning style and personality. An individual who is a good mentor for one student may be a poor one for another. For example, do you want a mentor who will challenge you with prodding questions about program content or one who will act as a sounding board for your ideas? Do you want a mentor who will be nurturing and offer words of encouragement or one who will challenge you and assist you in disciplining yourself to study? What role(s) do you want your mentor to play?

Choosing a mentor is another area in which you need to be proactive. Duff (1999) emphasizes the importance of

1. women mentoring women as career professionals with job and personal lives;
2. not "waiting" for a mentor to appear, but rather taking the initiative to seek a mentor;
3. overcoming the fear of appearing demanding, needy, or weak or of being rejected; and
4. choosing a mentor you admire, respect, can confide in, and whose values are those with which you feel comfortable.

## STUDY GROUPS

Likewise, forming or joining a study group can greatly enhance thinking, problem-solving, and decision-making skills. However, selecting or forming a study group must take into account your preference for learning. The ground rules for the study group must be clear. For example, does each member read all material and then discuss it with the group, or does each member take a portion of the assignment and then present or teach it to the others? Will the purpose of the study group be to meet frequently and discuss all the content or to meet infrequently bringing only answered questions or problems to the group? What will be the format of the sessions? How small or large will it be? These questions must be addressed.

> ### Thinking Critically
>
> Think about the type of learning required in an ADN program and your strengths and growth needed to achieve this learning level. On a piece of paper, make a large box with four quadrants. Label each of the four quadrants as follows: mentor characteristics, mentor role, study group characteristics, study group role. Fill in each box, and examine your results. Do you know anyone who will meet your needs to be your mentor? Do you know classmates with whom you might work well in a study group? (Save this information for use in designing your PEP.)

## Time Management

A last important area to examine in assessing your preparedness for the student role is the area of time management. Often the LPN/LVN entering an ADN program must balance a number of roles, such as spouse, parent, student, worker, and community citizen. The nursing program can be demanding at times. As discussed in Chapter 1, preparing for the student role involves such time management success strategies as balancing personal, career, and student roles; reassessing commitments to committees, boards, and service groups; and enlisting the support of significant others through the use of win/win agreements.

> ### Thinking Critically
>
> On a sheet of paper, identify your roles, group commitments, and significant others. Write an action plan for time management that takes into account these three items and the win/win agreements you developed in Chapter 1. (Save this action plan for use in designing your PEP.)

## Assessing Learning Style

The second step in individualizing a plan for transition from the LPN/LVN to the ADN level is to assess your learning style. In Chapter 1, you learned that we each have different ways in which we learn best. Chapter 5 discusses characteristics of adult learners. Some people are visual learners, whereas others are auditory learners. Some learn best through teaching strategies in which the learner uses manipulative skills or body kinetic (motion) or kinesthetic (sensory) approaches to learn course content. Take a moment and review the four styles of learners presented in Chapter 1 and the characteristics of adult learners discussed in Chapter 5.

> ### Thinking Critically
>
> Based on material learned and exercises completed in Chapter 1 and reflecting on learning activities that have been the most helpful to you in the past, assess and write in your own words a description of your learning style. Give examples of learning activities that fit your learning style. (Save this information for use in designing your PEP.)

# The Reflective Process: Assessing Adult Learner Uniqueness

The third step in individualizing a plan for role transition is to identify your unique characteristics as an adult learner. In Chapter 5, you learned about the characteristics of adult learners and driving forces that motivate such learners in the educational setting. Adult learners bring with them to the educational setting a variety of personal and professional life experiences. Each adult learner has developed values, biases, and fears; each is motivated by her or his own unique driving forces. Each has identified personal and career goals that guide her or him in the learning process. Wymard (1999) conducted numerous interviews with successful women to gain their insights. One trend she found is the importance of being able to see one's self in a lead role to actually assume one. As you begin your transition from the LPN/LVN role to the RN role, how do you view yourself? Can you see yourself in the lead role?

### ▶ Thinking Critically

Reflect on yourself as an adult learner. Take a moment to write down specific areas of nursing expertise you feel you have developed in the practice of nursing, things that motivate you to learn in classroom and clinical settings, and personal goals you hope to achieve by participating in the ADN program. (Save this information for use in designing your PEP.)

# Assessing Prior Learning: Standardized and Nonstandardized Tests

The fourth step in individualizing a plan for role transition from the LPN/LVN to the ADN level is to assess your prior learning. You acquire knowledge, skills, and abilities in the cognitive, affective, and psychomotor domains through formal education and experiential learning processes. (For a discussion of the three learning domains, refer to Chapter 5.)

In addition to a review of transcripts for course work completed, assessment tests are available to assist you in assessing your knowledge base and to guide you as you pursue a career as an RN. Many standardized tests are available for individual use, and many nursing schools use standardized or nonstandardized tests for assessment and selection purposes. A standardized test has undergone numerous validity and reliability research studies to ensure that content is valid and unbiased and that test takers would provide the same answers if the same test were administered again or by a different test administrator. It also has been administered to several populations, resulting in available normative data (information on the norms from various populations of test takers). Standardized tests are often published by formal organizations and are usually copyrighted. In contrast, nonstandardized tests are locally prepared (often by a teacher or school) and may contain regional questions.

## Assessment Tests for General Education

Many standardized tests are available to assess reading, writing, and mathematical computation skills. Most 2-year colleges require some form of general education assessment in their college admission process.

## Subject Area Assessment Tests for Nursing and Support Curricula

Assessment tests are available to assist LPN/LVNs in assessing knowledge in specific nursing curricular areas. Test areas include nursing fundamentals, medical–surgical nursing, obstetric nursing, pediatric nursing, nutrition, pharmacology, anatomy and physiology, microbiology, and the behavioral sciences. Your nursing school may require some of these, but you also may want to take some of these on your own. Professional organizations (e.g., the National League for Nursing) and the private sector (e.g., American College Testing and the College-Level Examination Program) have assessment tests for specific subject areas in the discipline of nursing.

## Integrated Nursing Assessment Tests

Many books have been written on test-taking strategies. Nugent and Vitale (2000) provide excellent suggestions for nursing students on how to take multiple choice tests. Because many tests you will take during your ADN education (and ultimately the NCLEX-RN) are in this format, it may help you to examine your skill in this area. The author's suggestions include how to read questions well, understand the intent of the question, and eliminate answer choices as a result, in order to select the correct answer.

## Nursing Review Tests

An additional self-evaluation technique LPN/LVNs have found useful in assessing their prior learning in preparation for role transition to the ADN level is published review texts. Subject-specific and integrated nursing review texts are available, providing you with the opportunity not only to assess strong and weak areas in your knowledge base, but also to practice answering multiple choice test questions in preparation for the nursing program and the NCLEX-RN, which you will take after you complete the ADN program.

> ▶ **Thinking Critically**

Examine the course work in the ADN program for which you will receive challenge or equivalency credit (or beyond which you will be advance placed). Reflecting on your own learning needs, identify in writing the methods or tests you would like to use and those required by your nursing program to assess your prior learning in nursing. Contact your school's nursing department, counseling office, bookstore, or testing center to determine the process for accessing the assessment tests you have identified. (Save this information for use in designing your PEP.)

## The Instructor–Student Partnership

Throughout this chapter, you have worked through several Thinking Critically exercises for self-assessment. In preparing to design a PEP, you have assessed your preparedness for the student role, learning style, adult learner uniqueness, and prior learning. As you use this information to design your plan, another area to consider will be the instructor–student partnership.

The goal of the instructor–student partnership is the growth and success of the student. The more the instructor understands your learning style, strengths, areas for growth, and individual uniqueness, the more the partnership will be able to meet your learning needs. Lofmark and Wikblad (2001, p. 43) studied nursing students to determine from their view which factors facilitated and which obstructed learning in clinical practice and reported the following results:

> The students emphasized responsibility and independence, opportunities to practice different tasks, and receiving feedback as facilitating factors. Others perceived promoting factors included perceptions of control of the situation and understanding of the "total picture." Examples of obstructing factors were the nurses as supervisors not relying on the students, supervision that lacked continuity and lack of opportunities to practice. Perception of their own insufficiency and low self-reliance were drawbacks for some students. (p. 43)

Do you share some of these same perceptions?

Sharing your PEP, including information about how you learn best, your goals, barriers to overcome, accommodations needed, clinical experiences needed, and methods of feedback that are most helpful to you, will maximize the ability of your partnership with the instructor to reach its goal: your success.

## Designing Your Personal Education Plan

Now that you have completed the Thinking Critically sections of this chapter, you are ready to design your PEP (**Display 6-1**). Gather all exercises you have completed throughout the text for entry into your PEP.

*(text continues on page 133)*

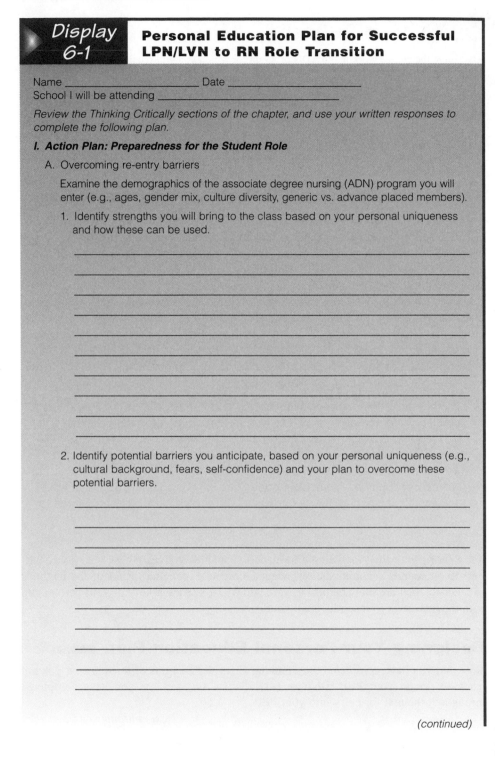

**Display 6-1**

**Personal Education Plan for Successful LPN/LVN to RN Role Transition**

Name _____ Date _____
School I will be attending _____

*Review the Thinking Critically sections of the chapter, and use your written responses to complete the following plan.*

**I. Action Plan: Preparedness for the Student Role**

A. Overcoming re-entry barriers

   Examine the demographics of the associate degree nursing (ADN) program you will enter (e.g., ages, gender mix, culture diversity, generic vs. advance placed members).

   1. Identify strengths you will bring to the class based on your personal uniqueness and how these can be used.

   _____

   _____

   _____

   _____

   _____

   _____

   _____

   _____

   _____

   2. Identify potential barriers you anticipate, based on your personal uniqueness (e.g., cultural background, fears, self-confidence) and your plan to overcome these potential barriers.

   _____

   _____

   _____

   _____

   _____

   _____

   _____

   _____

   _____

*(continued)*

B. Preparing for the school setting

1. List below the areas with which you need to locate and familiarize yourself on campus. Obtain a campus map, and plot a self-guided tour.

_____

_____

_____

_____

_____

_____

_____

_____

2. Write below the campus processes or systems with which you need to familiarize yourself and who you need to see or where you need to go to obtain information.

_____

_____

_____

_____

_____

_____

_____

_____

_____

| Process/System | Who or Where |
| --- | --- |
|  |  |
|  |  |
|  |  |
|  |  |
|  |  |
|  |  |
|  |  |
|  |  |

(continued)

3. Write below the library and research skills you need to acquire to become oriented to the library and to use it effectively.

_____

_____

_____

_____

_____

_____

_____

_____

_____

C. Developing student success strategies

1. Write below the texts and other resources you will need to buy or borrow to prepare for the nursing program.

_____

_____

_____

_____

_____

_____

_____

_____

2. Write below the traits (characteristics) and roles of mentors and study groups that will enhance your success at the ADN level.

_____

_____

_____

_____

_____

_____

_____

_____

*(continued)*

| Mentor Traits | Mentor Roles |
|---|---|
|  |  |
|  |  |
|  |  |
|  |  |
|  |  |
|  |  |
|  |  |
|  |  |

| Study Group Traits | Study Group Roles |
|---|---|
|  |  |
|  |  |
|  |  |
|  |  |
|  |  |
|  |  |

D. Time management

Write below your action plan for effective time management as you transition to the student role. Include elements of the win/win agreements you established with significant others.

_____

_____

_____

_____

_____

_____

_____

_____

_____

*(continued)*

## II. Action Plan for Needed Course Work

List below all course work needed to complete ADN requirements and college graduation requirements. Note course work completed or in progress. If course work was completed at another school or if you received equivalency or advance standing credit, indicate course(s) or experience for which you were granted that status. For course work needed, indicate the term and year you plan to take each course.

| Nursing and Graduation Requirements | Course Work Course Work Needed | Completed |
|---|---|---|
| At This School (Term/Year) (IP = In-Progress) | Another School Equivalency (Course, School) | Term/Year Planned |
| | | |
| | | |
| | | |
| | | |
| | | |
| | | |
| | | |
| | | |
| | | |
| | | |
| | | |
| | | |
| | | |
| | | |
| | | |
| | | |
| | | |
| | | |
| | | |
| | | |
| | | |
| | | |
| | | |
| | | |
| | | |
| | | |
| | | |
| | | |
| | | |
| | | |
| | | |
| | | |

## References

Carter, C., Bishop, J., & Kravitz, S. L. (2002). *Keys to college studying: Becoming a lifelong learner.* Upper Saddle River, NJ: Prentice Hall.

Duff, C. S. (1999). *Learning from other women: How to benefit from the knowledge, wisdom, and experience of female mentors.* New York: AMACOM, American Management Association.

Fletcher, S. (2000). *Mentoring in schools: A handbook of good practice.* London: Kogan Page.

Lofmark, N. J., & Wikblad, K. (2001). Facilitating and obstructing factors for development of learning in clinical practice: A student perspective. *Journal of Advanced Nursing, 34*(1), 43–50.

Nugent, P. M., & Vitale, B. A. (2000). *Test success: Test-taking techniques for beginning nursing students* (3rd ed.). Philadelphia: FA Davis.

Vance, C., & Olson, R. K. (Eds.). (1998). *The mentor connection in nursing.* New York: Springer.

Wymard, E. (1999). *Conversations with uncommon women: Insights from women who've risen above life's challenges to achieve extraordinary success.* New York: AMACOM, American Management Association.

## Suggested Reading

Brown, H., & Edelmann, R. (2000). Project 2000: A study of expected and experienced stressors and support reported by students and qualified nurses. *Journal of Advanced Nursing, 31*(4), 857–864.

Palmer, P. J. (1998). *The courage to teach: Exploring the inner landscape of a teacher's life.* San Francisco: Jossey-Bass.

*On the Web* • • • • • • • • • • • • • • • • • • • • • • • • • • • • • • • • • • • • • • • •

*www.daytracker.com*: This is a good site for organizational calendars.

*www.efn.org/~nurses/*: This student-oriented site includes study tips and sample math calculations/sample exams.

*www.aamn.org*: This is the website for the American Association for Men in Nursing.

*www.back2college.com/*: This is an excellent source for information on this topic with links to tutoring sites.

# Core Competencies for Professional Nursing Practice

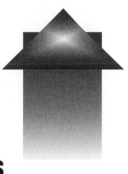

# CHAPTER 7

# Practicing Within Regulatory Frameworks

## LEARNING OBJECTIVES

*By the end of this chapter, the student will be able to:*

1. Relate the differences between regulations, policies, and standards of practice in nursing.
2. Identify boundaries and restrictions of practice of the licensed practical/vocational nurse (LPN/LVN).
3. Describe the differences between LPN/LVN and registered nurse (RN) scopes of practice.
4. Discuss the meaning of and need for regulation language in nurse practice acts.
5. Write a statement that reflects the scope of practice of the RN in the United States, after examining the nurse practice acts.
6. Differentiate among directed, autonomous, and collaborative nursing practices.
7. Analyze sample situations to determine directed, autonomous, and collaborative nursing practices in action.
8. Describe mechanisms for identifying differences in the knowledge and roles of LPN/LVNs and RNs.
9. Differentiate between the National Council test plans for LPN/LVNs and RNs.
10. Differentiate between the roles of the LPN/LVNs and RNs in the nursing process.
11. Contrast the differences between core competencies for the LPN/LVN and those for the RN.

## KEY TERMS

affective learning
American Nurses
   Association
autonomous nursing
   practice
cognitive learning
collaborative nursing
   practice
competency
directed nursing
   practice

evidence-based
   practice
learning domains
National League for
   Nursing
NCLEX-PN
NCLEX-RN
nurse practice act
nursing diagnosis
nursing process

permissive language
policy
psychomotor learning
regulation
restrictive language
scope of practice
standards of practice
state board of nursing

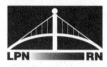

### VIGNETTE

Lori Ann Dietz, LPN, is discussing entering an ADN program with another LPN-to-RN student. The discussion has centered on validation for clinical practice.

**Lori Ann:** I have been a licensed practical nurse for 20 years. In that time I have done multiple catheterizations, charted on hundreds of clients, monitored rhythm disturbances by telemetry, and passed medications effectively and safely. Why do I have to do this entirely over again? Why do I have to demonstrate performance in skills I have already mastered as an LPN?

As you enter the RN program, you are embarking on a whole new scope of practice level. Perhaps you have felt like the LPN in the vignette provided. As an LPN/LVN, you have practiced under the direction of the RN or physician to whom you have reported. Your role has been a directed role, for the most part restricted by state law to performing certain nursing procedures, administering medications (depending on the state), and perhaps even (with additional certification) performing some intravenous therapy procedures.

To answer the question of this nursing student, your scope of practice as an RN will not only be broader in the types and complexity of procedures you perform, but also will require additional knowledge and independent thinking and problem-solving skills. More and more, you will be expected to use research to maintain and upgrade your nursing practice. This is called evidence-based practice. You will acquire the ability to collaborate with other healthcare team members to design plans for comprehensive care to patients and clients and to foster prevention and self-care among these consumers of healthcare.

## Regulations, Policies, and Standards

Regulations, policies, and standards all play a role in defining the practice of the RN. A thorough understanding of each of these is essential as you embark on an RN educational program.

# Regulations

According to the National Council of State Boards of Nursing (NCSBN, 2001), nursing regulation is the "governmental oversight provided for nursing practice in each state" (p. 1). Such laws are written to protect the consumer from someone who is incompetent or not prepared to practice. Because of this, health professions are heavily laden with regulations. State and federal regulations exist to govern various aspects of the healthcare industry and healthcare professionals.

Regulations at the state level define the scope of practice, requirements for licensure and relicensing, certification and continuing education requirements, and disciplinary consequences for healthcare practitioners. Regulations that define the practice of individuals licensed in a particular area are called practice acts. Nursing practice acts are laws established in a state or province to regulate the practice of nursing. Although practice acts may differ from state to state or province to province, much similarity and support of reciprocity are increasingly evident as states attempt to meet the needs of consumers, healthcare workers, and the healthcare industry. Extensive use of the National Council Licensure Examination for Registered Nurses (NCLEX-RN) throughout the states is an example of this effort. In many states, a single nurse practice act defines the practice of RNs and LPN/LVNs. Some states have two separate practice acts for these two levels of practitioners.

Regulations, especially those with the purpose of defining the scope of practice of various healthcare professionals, can be written with either restrictive or permissive language. Restrictive language restricts the practitioner to performing only the functions and procedures outlined in the regulation. LPN/LVN practice acts are often written in this manner.

Permissive language in regulations allows practitioners to use judgment and make decisions to serve their purpose in performing their roles. **Display 7-1** contrasts restrictive and permissive language in LPN/LVN and RN practice acts in the state of Kansas. Permissive language is used for the more autonomous practice of the RN. Similar restrictive and permissive language for LPN/LVN and RN practice acts, respectively, exists in many other states.

## ▶ Thinking Critically

Differentiate between restrictive and permissive language in other rules you have encountered in your life and describe the difference in your ability to think and act independently in each.

# Policies

To implement and enforce regulations, governing bodies (often in the form of appointed boards) are established to develop policies. A policy is a "plan or course of action, as of a government, political party or business, designed to influence actions" (*Webster's II New College Dictionary*, 2001, p. 854).

**Display
7-1**

# Restrictive and Permissive Language in Practical/Vocational and Registered Nurse Practice Acts in the State of Kansas

▶ **RESTRICTIVE LANGUAGE FOR THE PRACTICAL NURSE**

"The practice of nursing as a licensed practical nurse means the performance for compensation or gratuitously,...of tasks and responsibilities...based on acceptable educational preparation within the framework of supportive and restorative care under the direction of a registered professional nurse, a person licensed to practice medicine and surgery or a person licensed to practice dentistry" (p. 9).

▶ **PERMISSIVE LANGUAGE FOR THE REGISTERED NURSE**

"The practice of professional nursing as performed by a registered professional nurse for compensation or gratuitously,...means the process in which substantial specialized knowledge derived from the biological, physical, and behavioral sciences is applied to: the care, diagnosis, treatment, counsel and health teaching of persons who are experiencing changes in the normal health processes or who require assistance in the maintenance of health or the prevention or management of illness, injury or infirmity; administration, supervision or teaching of the process as defined in this section; and the execution of the medical regimen as prescribed by a person licensed to practice medicine and surgery or a person licensed to practice dentistry" (p. 9).

Kansas State Board of Nursing. (2002). *Nurse Practice Act.* Topeka, KS: Author.

In nursing, each state establishes a state board of nursing to develop guidelines for interpreting regulations. The state boards of nursing also ensure implementation of regulations with continuity. State boards of nursing include the lay public on their boards of directors to ensure consumer protection as regulations are implemented. With only a few exceptions (California, Georgia, Louisiana, Texas, and West Virginia), most states have a single state board of nursing for governing the practice of the LPN/LVN and the RN.

An example of a regulation and a corresponding policy by the California State Board of Nursing for implementing the regulation are shown in **Display 7-2**. The policy is a guide for nursing schools to ensure that the regulation is implemented with continuity throughout the state.

## ▶ Thinking Critically

Describe the difference between a rule (regulation) and an interpretation (policy) related to one or more rules that you have seen in an organization, service club, charity group, or social organization. What confusion or differing interpretations of the rule led to the need for the policy to be developed?

# Standards

Regulations and policies denote only minimal requirements for licensed nurses. Professional organizations play a key role in further defining the discipline of nursing, identifying entry-level competencies, and establishing standards of practice for the discipline.

**Display 7-2** | **Sample Regulation and Corresponding Interpretation (Policy for Implementation): California (2001)**

▶ STATE OF CALIFORNIA BOARD OF REGISTERED NURSING FACULTY QUALIFICATIONS AND CHANGES INTERPRETATION OF RULES AND REGULATIONS, 1425

| Regulation | Interpretation |
|---|---|
| (b) The registered nurse director of the program shall have:<br>(1) A master's or higher degree from an accredited college or university, which includes coursework in nursing, education, or administration; | 1. Master's or higher degree in nursing, education, or administration |
| (2) A minimum of 1 year's experience in an administrative position; | 1. Administrative position is defined as a director or assistant director who has direct responsibility for the administrative decision-making process of the educational program: budgeting, employing, delegating assignments, planning, and allocating resources.<br>2. Administrative responsibility in a professional program in nursing education includes diploma, associate and baccalaureate degree registered nursing programs, director of nursing or in-service education program, postlicensure baccalaureate programs.<br>3. An academic year of two semesters or three quarters will be regarded as equivalent to 1 year's administrative experience. |
| (3) A minimum of 2 years' experience teaching in prelicensure or postlicensure nursing programs; | 1. An academic year is defined as two semesters of three quarters.<br>2. Full-time teaching experience preferred.<br>3. Prelicensure or postlicensure nursing program includes diploma, associate, or baccalaureate degree registered nursing programs. |
| (4) At least 1 year's experience as registered nurse providing direct patient care; or<br>(5) equivalent experience and/or education as determined by the Board. | 1. One year's continuous full-time experience as a registered nurse providing direct patient care. |
| (c) The registered nurse assistant director shall meet the education requirements set forth in subsection (b)(1) above and the experience requirements set forth in subsections (b)(3) and (b)(4) above or such experience as the Board determines to be equivalent. | 1. Master's degree, which includes course work in nursing, education, or administration.<br>2. Two years' teaching experience in prelicensure or postlicensure program—diploma, associate, or baccalaureate degree registered nursing program.<br>3. One year's continuous experience as a registered nurse providing direct patient care. |

*(continued)*

▶ STATE OF CALIFORNIA BOARD OF REGISTERED NURSING FACULTY QUALIFICATIONS
AND CHANGES INTERPRETATION OF RULES AND REGULATIONS, 1425 *(Continued)*

| Regulation | Interpretation |
|---|---|
| (d) An instructor shall meet the following requirements: (1) Those set forth in subsections (b)(1) and (b)(4) above and | 1. Master's or higher degree, which includes course work in nursing, education, or administration. 2. The equivalent of 1 year's full-time experience as a registered nurse providing direct patient care within the last 5 years. (Clinical teaching applies toward direct patient care.) |
| (2) Completion of at least 1 year's experience teaching courses related to nursing or a course that includes practice in teaching nursing. | 1. One academic year's experience teaching nursing courses in diploma, associate, or baccalaureate degree registered nursing program or as in-service educator. 2. Course in practice teaching is defined as a course given by an accredited college or nursing school, which includes teaching strategies, course outline, and lesson plan development, practice teaching, and evaluation. 3. Clinically competent as defined in 1420(c) means that a nursing program faculty member possesses and exercises the degree of learning, skill, care, and experience ordinarily possessed and exercised by staff-level registered nurses of the clinical unit to which the instructor is assigned. |
| (e) An assistant instructor shall have: (1) A baccalaureate degree from an accredited college, which shall include courses in nursing or in natural, behavioral, or social sciences relevant to nursing practice. | 1. Baccalaureate degree must be in nursing or related fields. 2. May teach in classroom but may not take full responsibility for the course. 3. May not serve as content expert. |
| (2) At least 1 year's continuous, full-time experience in direct patient care practice as a registered nurse. | 1. Must demonstrate clinical competency. 2. One year's experience in the requested clinical area of nursing. |
| (f) A clinical teaching assistant shall have had at least 1 year's experience within the previous 5 years as a registered nurse providing direct patient care. | 1. May not have any responsibility for classroom instruction. 2. Must work under the direction of the instructor who has the final responsibility for the students and the clinical area. 3. Instructor is not required to be physically present. |

A standard is a measurement that denotes the degree or worth of an action. "The purpose of the standards of clinical nursing practice is to describe the responsibilities for which nurses are accountable" (Kozier, Erb, Berman, & Burke, 2000, p. 10).

The American Nurses Association (ANA) and the National League for Nursing (NLN) are two professional organizations that establish standards of practice for the discipline of nursing. Other specialty organizations, such as the American Association of Critical Care Nurses (AACN), have standards that are based on the general standards but are more specific for nurses who work in a specialty area, for example, in the critical care units. Many states have a state chapter of each organization (e.g., the California Nursing Association and the California League for Nursing). One of the most notable publications by the ANA (1980a) is its *Nursing: A Social Policy Statement*. An excerpt from this document is shown in **Display 7-3**. This ground-breaking statement provided clarity on the definition of nursing as a discipline, identifying it as an entity discrete from medicine, with its own unique purpose and autonomous practice. This social policy statement was updated and expanded in 1995.

Both the ANA and the NLN, each of which is composed of nurses who pay dues as members of the discipline, continue to set standards and publish documents that identify nursing's role in the healthcare industry, entry-level competencies of practitioners in the discipline of nursing, and professional accrediting standards for nursing education programs.

### ▶ Thinking Critically

Visit the American Nurses Association website (site address provided at the end of this chapter). Choose a position statement from the "readroom." What does this policy statement say about nursing? What does it say about protecting the public?

## Nurse Practice Acts ▬▬▬▬▬

Nurse practice acts exist in each state as part of the state's regulations (laws). Nurse practice acts vary in length, from a simple document only several pages in length (such as the act for Louisiana) to complex documents more than 30 pages in length for each of the practice levels (such as the LVN and RN practice acts in California). States provide additional clarity and interpretation of the practice of nursing through policies established by the state boards of nursing.

Changing regulations (laws) requires a lengthy political process. The choice of the extent to which specifics of nursing practice are incorporated into law is at the discretion of the state and may or may not be desirable, depending on the state's desire for flexibility and ease of change of such language. However, policies can be changed by the state's board of nursing as needed. Because the role of nurse practice acts and sub-

### ▶ Display 7-3    Nursing: A Social Policy Statement

Nursing is the diagnosis and treatment of human responses to actual or potential health problems.

American Nurses Association. (1980). *Nursing: A social policy statement* (p. 1). Kansas City, MO: Author.

---

### NCLEX–RN Might Ask 7-1   ❓❓❓

An RN is explaining to a family about how the scope of his/her practice is governed by the state nursing practice acts. These acts are considered

    A. regulations.
    B. policies.
    C. permissive language.
    D. standards of care.

• *See Appendix A for correct answer and rationale.*

---

sequent policies by the state board of nursing for implementing and enforcing such laws is to protect the consumer, public hearings are often held when major regulation or policy changes are proposed.

Since the 1950s, the ANA has played a key role in shaping nurse practice acts and providing guidance to states in restructuring nurse practice act language. In *The Nursing Practice Act: Suggested State Legislation*, the ANA (1980b) outlines standards considered essential in structuring legislative language related to the practice of nursing (**Display 7-4**). More recently, the National Council of State Boards of Nursing (NCSBN) has developed the *Model Nursing Practice Act* and *Model Nursing Administrative Rules* (August, 2001). These models and the current nurse practice acts of states can be viewed at the NCSBN's website.

## Directed, Autonomous, and Collaborative ▬▬▬▬ Nursing Practice

A key factor differentiating the scopes of practice of LPN/LVNs and RNs is the extent of independence legislated by nurse practice act language.

### Directed Nursing Practice

The restrictive language used in outlining the scope of practice of the LPN/LVN delimits this nurse's practice to a directed role. *Directed*, as defined by *Webster's II New College Dictionary* (2001), means "to supervise the performance of " (p. 321). Although many LPN/LVNs have achieved a great deal of independence in their practice, particularly as it relates to caring for patients with common disorders or dysfunctions, their practice remains by law a directed nursing practice. Practical/vocational nursing has been defined by the ANA (1980b) as:

> The practice of practical nursing means the performance for compensation of technical services requiring basic knowledge of the biological, physical, behavioral, psychological, and sociological sciences and of nursing procedures. These services are performed under the supervision of a registered nurse and utilize standardized procedures leading to predictable outcomes in the observation and care of the ill, injured and infirm; in the maintenance of health, in action

## Display 7-4 — American Nurses Association's Standards for Nurse Practice Acts

▶ **THE NURSING PRACTICE: SUGGESTED STATE LEGISLATION**

1. The primary purpose of a licensing law for the regulation of the practice of nursing is to protect the public health and welfare by establishing legal qualifications for the practice of nursing. Such legal standards are determined adequate to provide safe and effective nursing practices.
2. All people practicing or offering to practice nursing or practical nursing should be licensed. Protection of the public is accomplished only if all who practice or offer to practice nursing are licensed. The public should not be expected to differentiate between incompetent and competent practitioners.
3. Because nursing is one occupational field, there should be one nursing practice act that licenses both registered nurses and licensed practical nurses. The public and the practitioners may be confused when there is more than one law regulating the practice of nursing and the practice of practical nursing.
4. The enactment of one nursing practice act necessitates only one licensing board for nursing in a state. The board of nursing should be composed of nurses whose practice is regulated by the licensure law and by a representative or representatives of the public.
5. Candidates for licensure should complete an educational program approved by the board and pass the licensing examination before a license to practice is granted.
6. The nursing practice act should provide for the legal regulation of nursing without reference to a specialized area of practice. It is the function of the professional association to establish the scope and desirable qualifications required for each area of practice and to certify individuals as competent to engage in specific areas of nursing practice. It also is the function of the professional association to upgrade practice above the minimum standards set by law. The law should not provide for identifying clinical specialists in nursing or require certification or other recognition for practice beyond the minimum qualifications established for the legal regulation of nursing.

American Nurses Association. (1980). *The nursing practice act: Suggested state legislation* (pp 2-3).

to safeguard life and health; and in the administration of medications and treatment prescribed by any person authorized by state law to prescribe. (p. 6)

Inherent in this definition is the standard that the educational preparation of the LPN/LVN provides this practitioner with the basic knowledge for practice in a directed role. It also allows the LPN/LVN to use standardized procedures within that directed role.

Consistent with the ANA's definition of nursing is the NLN's 1989 *Entry-Level Competencies of Graduates of Educational Programs in Practical Nursing*, which defines the role of the practical/vocational nursing program graduate.

The graduate of the practical/vocational nursing programs is eligible to apply for licensure. Licensed practical/vocational nurses practice under the guidance of a registered nurse or licensed physician/dentist. The primary role of the licensed practical/vocational nurse is to provide nursing care for clients experiencing common, well-defined health problems in structured health care settings. In their roles as members of the discipline of nursing, practical/vocational nurses actively participate in and subscribe to legal and ethical tenets of the discipline. (p. 1)

## Autonomous Nursing Practice

*Webster's II New College Dictionary* (2001) defines autonomous as "independent, self-contained or independent of the laws of another state or government" (p. 77). Autonomous nursing practice is engaging in the practice of nursing independently, without external supervision. The ANA (1980b) contrasts the practice of nursing (i.e., registered nursing) with the practice of practical nursing.

> The practice of nursing [i.e., registered nursing], means the performance for compensation of professional services requiring substantial specialized knowledge of the biological, physical, behavioral, psychological, and sociological sciences and of nursing theory as the basis for assessment, diagnosis, planning, intervention, and evaluation in the promotion and maintenance of health; the case finding and management of illness, injury, or infirmity; the restoration of optimum function; or the achievement of a dignified death. Nursing practice [i.e., registered nursing], includes but is not limited to administration, teaching, counseling, supervision, delegation, and evaluation of practice and execution of the medical regimen, including the administration of medications and treatments prescribed by any person authorized by state law to prescribe. Each RN is directly accountable and responsible to the consumer for the quality of nursing care rendered. (p. 6)

The substantial specialized knowledge enables the RN to exercise judgment, design, and implement plans of care, and engage in a variety of independent functions.

> ### ▶ Thinking Critically
>
> Compare and contrast the areas in your personal life in which you perform in a directed role versus an autonomous role. What additional specialized knowledge enables you to exercise judgment and perform independently when in the autonomous role?

## Collaborative Nursing Practice

Collaboration among healthcare providers is essential for meeting an array of client needs and fostering health in a holistic manner. As defined by *Webster's II New College Dictionary* (2001), to *collaborate* is to "work together, especially in a joint intellectual effort" (p. 219). Collaborative nursing practice, also called *interdependent nursing practice*, is working jointly with others (often physicians) in performing nursing roles within the legislated scope of practice.

The nurse and the physician practice autonomously in making nursing diagnoses and medical diagnoses, respectively. However, collaboration improves comprehensiveness, efficiency, and consistency in fostering health in clients. Many states have created practice act language to allow for the development of standardized procedures, developed jointly by physicians and nurses. Standardized procedures enhance the nurse's ability to function independently. Standardized procedures are developed for use in organized healthcare systems (e.g., hospitals, clinics, home health agencies, community health services, physicians' offices). **Display 7-5** depicts a sample of standardized procedure guidelines from the California Nursing Practice Act (2002).

| *Display* 7-5 | **California Nurse Practice Act (2002) Standardized Procedure Guidelines** |
| --- | --- |

**▶ 1470. PURPOSE.**

The Board of Registered Nursing in conjunction with the Medical Board of California (see regulations of the Medical Board of California, Article 9.5, Chapter 13, Title 16 of the California Code of Regulations) intends, by adopting the regulations contained in the article, to jointly promulgate guidelines for the development of standardized procedures to be used in organized health care systems which are subject to this rule. The purpose of these guidelines is:

(a) To protect consumers by providing evidence that the nurse meets all requirements to practice safely.
(b) To provide uniformity in development of standardized procedures.

**▶ 1474: STANDARDIZED PROCEDURE GUIDELINES.**

Following are the standardized procedure guidelines jointly promulgated by the Medical Board of California and by the Board of Registered Nursing:

(a) Standardized procedures shall include a written description of the method used in developing and approving them and any revision thereof.
(b) Each standardized procedure shall:
  (1) Be in writing, dated, and signed by the organized healthcare system personnel authorized to approve it.
  (2) Specify which standardized procedure functions registered nurses may perform and under what circumstances.
  (3) State any specific requirements that are to be followed by registered nurses in performing particular standardized procedure functions.
  (4) Specify any experience, training, or education requirements for performance of standardized procedure functions.
  (5) Establish a method for initial and continuing evaluation of the competence of registered nurses authorized to perform standardized procedure functions.
  (6) Provide for a method of maintaining a written record of people authorized to perform standardized procedure functions.
  (7) Specify the scope of supervision required for performance of standardized procedure functions, for example, immediate supervision by a physician
  (8) Set forth any specialized circumstances under which the registered nurse is to immediately communicate with a patient's physician concerning the patient's condition.
  (9) State the limitations on settings, if any, in which standardized procedure functions may be performed.
  (10) Specify patient record keeping requirements.
  (11) Provide for a method of periodic review of the standardized procedures (p. 65).

California Office of Administrative Law. (2002). Title 16: California code of regulations. Division 14: Board of registered nursing. California Nurse Practice Act. Sacramento, CA: Author.

---

## NCLEX–RN Might Ask 7-2 ❓❓❓

In working with clients, the nurse uses the resources of many other healthcare workers to achieve acceptable outcomes in client care. In this role, the nurse is working

    A. independently.
    B. as an advocate.
    C. autonomously.
    D. collaboratively.

• *See Appendix A for correct answer and rationale.*

---

# Mechanisms for Identifying Differences ▬▬▬ in Knowledge and Roles

Although there is a common core of knowledge and competencies in the practice of LPN/LVNs and RNs, the knowledge base and practice roles differ between these two licensed healthcare providers. How does an individual, organization, council, or licensing board determine the knowledge and roles of a specific practitioner? How do the knowledge and roles of the LPN/LVN differ from those of the RN? What expectations should an employer have of these two levels of practitioners? What additional knowledge and role abilities should the LPN/LVN expect to gain by participating in and completing an associate degree nursing educational program? What knowledge, skills, and abilities should be tested under the governance of the state boards of nursing to ensure the public that individuals are competent to be licensed to practice within the scope of practice outlined in state law? These questions are addressed in this chapter as the knowledge and roles of the LPN/LVN and the RN are explored, explained, compared, and contrasted. Several mechanisms are used to identify such differences in knowledge and roles.

## Job Analysis Studies

An important mechanism for determining the knowledge needed and the roles played by a particular licensed healthcare provider is to survey those already in the work setting who are licensed to practice at that level. Such job analysis studies have been conducted for LPN/LVNs and RNs.

Kane and Colton (1988) conducted the initial job analysis of newly licensed LPN/LVNs to examine the entry-level practices of such nurses. Activities these respondents cited were analyzed in relation to the frequency of their performance, their impact on maintaining client safety, the various settings in which they were performed, and the age ranges of clients. A framework for entry-level performance was established, incorporating the nursing process, specific client age and needs, and the practice setting. This job analysis was updated in 1997 by Yocom (1997). The framework continues to be used by the NCSBN in designing the National Council Licensure Examination for Practical Nurses (NCLEX-PN).

Chornick, Yocom, and Jacobson (1993) conducted a similar job analysis study of entry-level performance of RNs. This work was updated by Hertz, Yocom, and Gawel in 2000. Survey results in these studies were similarly analyzed, resulting in a framework for entry-level performance that incorporated the nursing process and specific client needs. The NCSBN is using the framework from this recent study to design the NCLEX-RN.

## Licensure Examination Test Plans

As described previously, job analysis studies play a key role in the design of licensure examination test plans. It is critical that such test plans identify the knowledge and roles of practitioners at the designated licensure level. Thus, in addition to job analysis studies, the NCSBN examines the scope of practice for that licensure level by its member jurisdictions and uses item writers (nurses and nurse educators) to operationalize the test plan for actual test construction. The NCLEX-PN differs from the NCLEX-RN in relation to the results of the respective job analyses, the scopes of practice as defined by member jurisdictions, and the levels of knowledge, skills, and abilities tested.

## Licensure Requirements and Nurse Practice Acts

Nurse practice acts in each state outline eligibility and requirements for licensure within that state. Although not required, most states use the NCLEX-PN and NCLEX-RN to determine eligibility for licensure. Minimum examination scores needed for licensure eligibility are determined according to the nurse practice act language in each state.

Nurse practice acts in each state also delineate the nursing education program content and clinical experience needed for the program to be accredited by the state board of nursing and for the program graduate to be eligible for licensure. Any additional knowledge or course work required for licensure beyond that in the LPN/LVN or RN program also is outlined in the nurse practice act. In addition to behavioral and biological sciences and core nursing content, some states specify a certain number of hours of education in such areas as communication skills, communicable diseases, pharmacology, child and elder abuse, and substance abuse. Nurse practice acts also may designate specific roles for LPN/LVNs and RNs related to such areas as medication administration, intravenous therapy, blood administration or withdrawal, and chemotherapy.

## Professional Organization Standards

Although job analysis studies identify activities being performed by newly licensed LPN/LVNs and RNs and state boards of nursing establish licensure eligibility, these represent only minimal competencies for licensed practice. An additional mechanism

## NCLEX–RN Might Ask 7-3

An LVN is asking an RN about the NCLEX-RN test. The LVN is correct when he/she states to the RN that passing NCLEX-RN demonstrates

   A. specialty competency.
   B. excellence in practice.
   C. average competency.
   D. minimal competency.

• *See Appendix A for correct answer and rationale.*

for identifying differences in the knowledge and roles of LPN/LVNs and RNs are the standards set by professional organizations.

The NLN's (1999) *Entry-Level Competencies of Graduates of Educational Programs in Practical Nursing* describes the role and competencies that should be expected from the graduate LPN/LVN. Likewise, the NLN's (2000) *Educational Outcomes of Associate Degree Nursing Programs: Roles and Competencies* defines three interrelated roles and eight core competencies of the associate degree nurse. Knowledge critical to each role and the expected competencies of graduates are outlined in the document. **Display 7-6** provides an overview of the roles and competencies.

# National Council Licensure Examinations

## Practical/Vocational Nursing Test Plan

The *Test Plan for the NCLEX®* Examination for Practical Nurses (NCSBN, 1998) provides a concise summary of the content and scope of the NCLEX-PN examination and

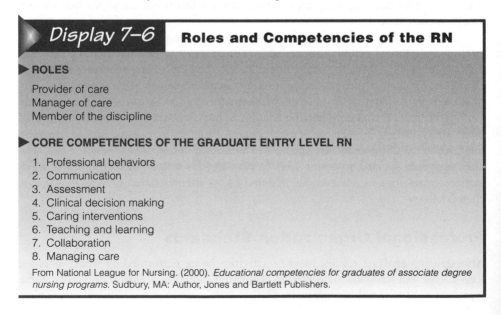

### Display 7-6   Roles and Competencies of the RN

▶**ROLES**

Provider of care
Manager of care
Member of the discipline

▶**CORE COMPETENCIES OF THE GRADUATE ENTRY LEVEL RN**

1. Professional behaviors
2. Communication
3. Assessment
4. Clinical decision making
5. Caring interventions
6. Teaching and learning
7. Collaboration
8. Managing care

From National League for Nursing. (2000). *Educational competencies for graduates of associate degree nursing programs.* Sudbury, MA: Author, Jones and Bartlett Publishers.

serves as a guide for candidates preparing to write the examination and for those individuals involved in developing it. The test plan provides the foundation for the development of each licensure examination so that each NCLEX-PN examination reflects the knowledge, skills, and abilities essential for the application of the phases of the nursing process to meet the needs of clients with commonly occurring health problems having predictable outcomes.

As indicated, the test plan designed by the NCSBN (1998) is based on the job analysis study by Yocom (1997). The NCLEX-PN examination includes test items at the cognitive levels of knowledge, comprehension, and application, with most items at the comprehension and application levels.

The test plan notes that the LPN functions in a directed role, contributing to care planning and participating in the nursing process. The NCSBN (1998) states:

> The entry-level practical/vocational nurse, under appropriate supervision, provides competent care for the clients with commonly occurring health problems having predictable outcomes. The practical/vocational nurse uses the nursing process to collect and organize relevant health care data to assist in the identification of health care needs/problems of clients throughout the clients' life span and a variety of settings. (p. 3)

The NCSBN (1998) test plan details client needs that can be addressed by the LPN/LVN and emphasizes that this level practitioner requires "basic" knowledge of nursing in four major categories: safe, effective care; health promotion and maintenance; psychosocial integrity; and physiologic integrity. The following elements are integrated throughout the NCLEX-PN: caring, communication, cultural awareness, documentation, nursing process, self-care, and teaching/learning.

## Registered Nursing Test Plan

The *Test Plan for the NCLEX® Examination for Registered Nurses* (2000), similar to that for practical nursing, serves as a guide for those preparing to take the NCLEX-RN examination and for item writers in their development of the exam. The test plan was developed based on the job analysis study by Hertz et al. (2000). In contrast with the test plan for the NCLEX-PN, test items for the NCLEX-RN are at the cognitive levels of knowledge, comprehension, application, and analysis, with most items at the application and analysis levels.

The test plan for registered nursing delineates this practitioner's role in nursing process, noting (in contrast with that of practical nursing) autonomous functions, such as assessment, nursing diagnosis, plan development, and evaluation; and collaborative functions, such as planning with other health team members, delegating, and providing referrals. Similar to the test plan for practical nursing, the test plan for registered nursing outlines the knowledge, skills, and abilities needed to address client needs. However, unlike the practical nursing test plan, the test plan for registered nursing calls for a more in-depth knowledge base and skills in teaching, communication, and management. **Table 7-1** compares several elements of the test plan of the NCLEX-PN with that of the NCLEX-RN.

**TABLE 7-1**
TEST PLANS FOR NCLEX-RN AND NCLEX-PN

| Test Plan Element | NCLEX-PN | NCLEX-RN |
|---|---|---|
| 1. Levels of cognitive ability | Knowledge<br>Comprehension<br>Application<br>Analysis (fewer) | Knowledge (fewer)<br>Comprehension<br>Application<br>Analysis |
| 2. Safe, effective care environment | Coordinated care:<br>Collaborates with other health care team members to facilitate effective client care | Management of care:<br>Providing integrated, cost-effective care to clients by coordinating, supervising, and/or collaborating with members of the multidisciplinary health care team |
| 3. Health promotion and maintenance | Assists the client and significant others in the normal expected stages of growth and development from conception to advanced old age | Provides and directs care that incorporates the knowledge of expected growth and development principles and the prevention and/or early detection of health problems |
| 4. Psychosocial integrity | Promotes the client's ability to cope, adapt, and/or solve situations related to illnesses or stressful events | Provides and directs nursing care that promotes and supports the emotional, mental, and social well-being of the client and significant others |
| 5. Physiological integrity | Provides comfort and assistance in the performance of ADLs | Promotes physical health and well-being by providing care and comfort, reducing client risk potential, and managing the client's health alterations |

*From National Council State Board of Nursing NCLEX-PN and NCLEX-RN Test Plans.

# Practical/Vocational Nursing Roles and Competencies

## Practical/Vocational Nursing Roles

The NLN (1999) defines the roles of the LPN/LVN as follows:

> The primary role of the licensed practical/vocational nurse is to provide nursing care for clients who are experiencing common, well defined health problems in structured health care settings. In their roles as members of the discipline of nursing, practical/vocational nurses actively participate in and subscribe to the legal and ethical tenets of the discipline. (p. 1)

This definition clearly designates two roles for the LPN/LVN: care provider and member of the discipline of nursing.

## Competencies in the Care Provider Role

Within the care provider role, the NLN (1999) outlines competencies of the LPN/LVN in each of the four phases of the nursing process: assessment, planning, implementation, and evaluation.

### ASSESSMENT

In the assessment phase, the LPN/LVN assesses basic needs of clients by collecting data and identifying deviations from normal. She or he documents these data and communicates findings.

### PLANNING

In the planning phase, the LPN/LVN contributes to the development of nursing care plans, determines client care need priorities, and assists in revising such care plans. She or he uses established nursing diagnoses in this planning process for clients with common, well-defined health problems.

### IMPLEMENTATION

In the implementation phase, the LPN/LVN provides care using effective communication, collaborating with other health team members, and instructing clients regarding health maintenance. She or he uses accepted standards of practice and records and reports implementation activities. The LPN/LVN also maintains the privacy and dignity of clients.

### EVALUATION

In the evaluation phase, the LPN/LVN seeks guidance and continues collaboration with others in modifying nursing approaches and revising nursing care plans.

## Competencies in the Member of the Discipline Role

As a member of the discipline of nursing, the LPN/LVN, as delineated by the NLN (1999), describes her or his role in the healthcare delivery system and complies with the state's nurse practice act. She or he identifies personal strengths, weaknesses, and potential, using educational opportunities; she or he not only adheres to nursing's code of ethics, but also functions as a healthcare consumer advocate.

# Associate Degree Nursing Roles and ▬▬▬ Competencies

## Associate Degree Nursing Roles

In 1990, the NLN identified three interrelated roles of the associate degree nurse: provider of care, manager of care, and member within the discipline of nursing. With the 2000 document, the NLN Council of Associate Degree Competencies Task Force thought that the role expectancies would be simpler and duplication would be avoided by organizing expected competencies into eight core components that crossed the traditional boundaries of the three roles of provider of care, manager of care, and member within the discipline of nursing. The three roles and eight core components depicted in Display 7-6 provide an organizing framework for expected RN entry-level competencies, and therefore the educational outcomes for graduates of associate degree nursing programs.

# Competencies in the Care Provider Role

The associate degree nurse uses the nursing process when engaging in the care provider role.

## ASSESSMENT

In addition to competencies specified at the practical nursing level, the associate degree nurse conducts a more extensive data collection process, using a variety of resources. She or he contributes this information to a database and is able to identify changes in the client's health status.

## DIAGNOSIS

Unlike the practical nurse, the associate degree nurse has the educational preparation to analyze and interpret data, identifying actual or potential healthcare needs and selecting nursing diagnoses.

## PLANNING

In addition to competencies at the practical nursing level, the associate degree nurse establishes client-centered goals, develops client-specific care plans, and develops individualized teaching plans in collaboration with other healthcare workers.

## IMPLEMENTATION

In addition to competencies at the practical nursing level, the associate degree nurse initiates nursing interventions, implementing care plans according to priorities of goals and making adjustments as client situations change. The associate degree nurse also fosters a health-supportive environment, promoting rehabilitation potential, providing for physical and psychological safety, and using communication techniques that assist clients with coping and problem solving. Individualized, client-centered care management and teaching plans are implemented, providing continuity of care, and referrals are provided as needed.

## EVALUATION

The associate degree nurse evaluates the client's progress toward goals and the effects of interventions, revising care plans as needed.

## Other Core Competencies

The NLN task force identified 68 expected competencies of the entry-level RN, including the nursing process steps described above, inherent in the care provider, manager, and member of the discipline roles. The task force organized these competencies under eight core component headings: professional behaviors, communication, assessment, clinical decision making, caring interventions, teaching and learning, collaboration, and managing care (Display 7-6). Specific competencies in each of these eight components can be found in the NLN publication (NLN, 2000).

## Licensed Practical/Vocational Versus ▬▬▬▬ Registered Nurse Knowledge, Skills, and Abilities

The knowledge, skills, and abilities of those in the nursing profession progress along a continuum, with increasing complexity at each practice level. The educational curricula for the LPN/LVN, the RN, and the baccalaureate and higher degree nurse prepare these healthcare providers to perform within the scope of the practice prescribed by law and in the roles identified by professional organizations, such as the NLN.

As discussed in Chapter 5, in the mid-1900s Benjamin Bloom and others identified three learning domains that provided a basis for the development of educational curricula for decades to follow. These learning domains include cognitive (knowledge), affective (values), and psychomotor (manipulative skills) learning abilities. Within the cognitive learning domain, six increasingly complex learning achievement levels are identified: knowledge, comprehension, application, analysis, synthesis, and evaluation.

Nursing process, nursing diagnosis, and nursing care plan design require abilities in all six of the cognitive learning levels and in the affective and psychomotor domains. Related to these abilities in the three learning domains, LPN/LVNs and RNs demonstrate different competencies within their roles. As cited, the *Test Plan for the NCLEX®* *Examination for Practical Nurses* (NCSBN, 1998) includes test items at the knowledge, comprehension, and application levels; subsequent editions include some analysis questions. The *Test Plan for the NCLEX® Examination for Registered Nurses* (NCSBN, 2001) includes test items at the knowledge, but mostly, comprehension, application, and analysis levels. More emphasis is now being placed on the higher analysis level. This reflects the increased complexity inherent in the scope of practice and job analysis study for registered nursing. Chapter 5 describes associate degree nursing curricular content and learning activities in each of the three learning domains and in the six achievement levels of the cognitive domain.

## Conclusion ▬▬▬▬▬▬▬▬▬▬▬▬▬▬▬▬▬▬▬▬▬▬▬▬▬▬▬▬▬▬▬▬

This chapter examines the scopes of practice of the LPN/LVN and the RN. A differentiation among regulations, polices, and standards of practice in nursing is provided, along with discussion of restrictive and permissive language. Directed practice, autonomous practice, and collaborative practice are described, and sample language from states' nurse practice acts illustrates the difference in scopes of practice of the LPN/LVN and the RN.

This chapter also compares and contrasts the knowledge and roles of LPN/LVNs and RNs. Four mechanisms for identifying the knowledge and roles of these two practitioners are described: job analysis studies, licensure examination test plans, licensure requirements and nurse practice acts, and professional organization standards. The NCSBN's test plans for practical and registered nurses are compared and contrasted. Associate degree nursing and LPN/LVN roles are discussed, including competencies and each practitioner's role in the nursing process.

## ▌ Student Exercise

1. Review the LPN/LVN and RN nurse practice acts from your state.
2. Outline several RN activities that fall within each of the three practice functions: directed, autonomous, and collaborative practice.
3. Write in your own words a broad definition of the scope of practice of the RN in the United States.
4. Develop a chart comparing and contrasting the care provider role competencies in each phase of the nursing process for the LPN/LVN and the associate degree nurse.

## References

American Nurses Association (ANA). (1980a). *Nursing: A social policy statement*. Kansas City, MO: Author.

American Nurses Association (ANA). (1980b). *The nursing practice act: Suggested state legislation*. Kansas City, MO: Author.

American Nurses Association (ANA). (1995). *Nursing's social policy statement*. Washington , D.C.: Author.

California Office of Administrative . (2002). *Title 16: California code of regulations*. Division 14: Board of registered nursing. California Nurse Practice Act. Sacramento, CA: Author. *www.rn.ca.gov/practact\title16.htm*.

Chornick, N., Yocom, C., & Jacobson, J. (1993). *1993–94 job analysis study of newly licensed entry-level registered nurses*. Chicago: National Council of State Boards of Nursing.

Hertz, J., Yocom, C., & Gawel, S. (2000). *Linking the NCLEX-RN examination to practice: 1999 practice analysis of newly licensed registered nurses in the U.S.* Chicago: National Council of State Boards of Nursing, Inc.

Kane, M., & Colton, D. (1988). *Job analysis of newly licensed practical/vocational nurses: 1986–87*. Chicago: National Council of State Boards of Nursing.

Kansas State Board of Nursing. (2002). *Nurse practice act*. Topeka, KS: Author.

Kozier, B., Erb, G., Berman, A., & Burke, K. (2000). *Fundamentals of nursing: Concepts, process and practice* (6th ed.). Upper Saddle River, NJ: Prentice Hall Health.

National Council of State Boards of Nursing (NCSBN). (1998). *Test plan for the NCLEX® examination for practical nurses*. Chicago: Author.

National Council of State Boards of Nursing (NCSBN). (2000). *Test plan for the NCLEX® examination for registered nurses*. Chicago: Author.

National Council of State Boards of Nursing (NCSBN). (2002). *Model nursing practice act and nursing administrative rules*. Chicago: Author.

National League for Nursing (NLN): Council of Associate Degree Programs. (2000). *Educational outcomes of associate degree nursing programs: Roles and competencies.* New York: Author.

National League for Nursing (NLN): Council of Practical Nursing Programs. (1999). *Entry-level competencies of graduates of educational programs in practical nursing.* New York: Author

*Webster's II new college dictionary.* (2001). Boston: Houghton Mifflin Company.

Yocom, C. (1997). *1997 job analysis study of newly licensed entry-level practical/vocational nurses.* Chicago: National Council of State Boards of Nursing.

## Suggested Reading

Bloom, B. S. (Ed.). (1956). *Taxonomy of educational objectives: The classification of educational goals.* New York: David McKay.

Bloom, B. S. (Ed.). (1974). *The taxonomy of educational objectives: Affective and cognitive domains.* New York: David McKay.

Bylone, M., & Ritchie, K. (2001). Should staffing ratios be legislated by state governments. *Advances for Nurses, 3,* 5, 7.

Clarke, H., & Wearing, J. (2001). Regulation of registered nursing: The Canadian perspective. *Reflections on Nursing Leadership, 27*(4), 26–27, 35.

Crawford, L. (2001). Regulation of registered nursing: The American perspective, *Reflections on Nursing Leadership, 27*(4), 28–29, 34.

*On the Web* • • • • • • • • • • • • • • • • • • • • • • • • • • • • • • • • • • • • • • • •

*www.nln.org:* National League for Nursing

*www.ncsbn.org:* National Council of State Boards of Nursing

*www.nursingworld.org:* American Nurses Association

*www.rn.ca.gov/practact\title16.htm*: California Nurse Practice Act

*www.nlnac.org:* National League for Nursing Accrediting Commission

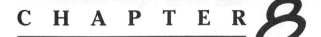

# Critical Thinking and Clinical Judgment in Nursing

*By the end of this chapter, the student will be able to:*

1   Describe the importance of critical thinking in today's society and in registered nursing practice.
2   Describe the role of clinical judgment in the profession of nursing.
3   Describe the major contributions throughout the 1900s to the evolving definition of critical thinking.
4   Compose a definition of critical thinking.
5   Describe the role played by context in critical thinking.
6   Differentiate between critical thinking and feeling.
7   Identify critical thinking abilities and dispositions.
8   Describe the importance of critical thinking abilities, dispositions, and judgment.
9   Differentiate between critical and creative thinking.
10  Describe the role of critical thinking in nursing process.
11  Analyze client situations using a variety of critical thinking modes.

## K E Y   T E R M S

analysis
background
  assumptions
belief
clinical judgment
context
creative thinking
critical thinking

critical thinking
  abilities
critical thinking
  dispositions
deductive reasoning
inductive reasoning
inference
informal logic
judgment

metacognition
nursing process
reasoning
reflective practitioner
reflective skepticism
self-regulation
synthesis
world view

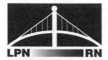

**VIGNETTE**
Sally Caruthers is a first semester LVN returning to school. Tim DeMot is a second-year student.

**Sally:** Critical thinking, critical thinking, critical thinking. What is it? We have a quiz every week, a test every month, and now the instructor says we have to take this critical thinking test. How do I prepare for this?

**Tim:** Boy, I know it sounds like a lot, but you'll be able to do it! This test is not high up there on the ones you need to be concerned about. This critical thinking test is taken in the first semester and again before you graduate. You don't really get the results, but they are critical to the faculty. They told me that they use the information for the National League for Nursing to show if students have developed these skills within the program.

**Sally:** You mean we take this test, but we don't even get the results? How are we to learn from that?

**Tim:** Through the teaching learning process and the assignments given like group projects, case studies, computer-assisted learning tools, and many others. The faculty needs the information to make necessary changes within the program curriculum.

**Sally:** OK, if you say I don't have to worry, I won't.

**Tim:** The tools the instructors use are trying to help us be prepared to do the complex thinking, problem solving, analysis, and creative thinking required of a nurse. So you see, even though we don't get graded or learn how we did on the test, it's all part of the big picture that is needed to prepare us professionally. However, the class content on critical thinking will be coming up for you with the nursing care planning process in about 2 weeks if I remember correctly. Do you want to go over my notes from last year? It may help you understand more about what is going on.

**Sally:** Not right now. I have to study for a psychology class. But can we have lunch together in the student center this afternoon? You've stimulated my curiosity. It helps me to know the big picture in my learning.

**Tim:** Now you've got it. See you soon. 'Bye now.

# The Need for Critical Thinking

"Being in favor of critical thinking is like being in favor of freedom, justice, or a clean environment" (McPeck, 1981, p. 1).

What is critical thinking? When is thinking critical rather than just thinking? Why is there such a need for critical thinking in today's world?

Stephen Brookfield (1987) emphasizes the worth of critical thinking in maintaining a healthy democracy. Smith (1990) describes the role critical thinking plays in shaping and reframing values and cultural beliefs:

Why do some cultures elevate the role of women and others demean it? Why do different groups take differing views on abortion, sex, child labor, material wealth, education, and respect for all people, for all animals, for the entire world? Economics or power may have been at the beginning of some or all of these attitudes, but they are perpetuated by stories. They are believed, and held to be natural and right, simply because they make sense to people; it is what they think.

The great problems of the world today—political, environmental, social, and economic—are not due to lack of facts, and probably not to lack of thought either. They reflect the values of people and governments, the stories they believe. There will be no solutions if we constantly wait for new skills and knowledge; what is required is an ability to recognize and understand the stories that are currently being played out, their consequences, and how they might be changed, in ourselves and others. (p. 132)

As the structure and concept of church, family, community, and civic responsibility undergo rapid, extensive change, the importance of critical thinking is intensified. Brookfield (1987) states, "Making sense of, and trying to feel some sense of control over [such] changes is central to becoming critically thoughtful" (p. 51). He also notes the societal expectation that adults be able to reflect critically on the truth of general rules taught to them in childhood. Paul (1992) further emphasizes, "An open society requires open minds. Collectively reinforced egocentric and sociocentric thought, conjoined with massive technical knowledge and power, are not the foundations for a genuine democracy" (p. 180).

The need for critical thinking "is particularly acute today when our culture's output of information far exceeds our ability to think critically about that information," (Meyers, 1986, p. xi). Creasia and Parker (2001) emphasize the need for conceptual foundations and critical thinking by professionals in nursing to meet the challenges of today's world. Norris (1985) notes the following:

Critical thinking is not just another educational option. Rather it is an indispensable part of education, because being able to think critically is a necessary condition for being educated, and because teaching with the spirit of critical thinking is the only way to satisfy the moral injunction of respect for individuals which must apply to students as well as to anyone else. According to this reasoning, students have a moral right to teaching that embodies the spirit of critical thinking and a moral right to be taught how to think critically. Thus, to abide by the moral principle of respect for person, teachers must recognize the student's right to question, to challenge, and to demand reasons and justifications for what is being taught (Siegel, 1980, p.14).. ...In addition, there is a responsibility to teach them to do these things well, because in the end students must choose for themselves: there is no escaping this truth. (p. 40)

In *Playgrounds of Our Minds*, Barell (1990) writes that we must create an environment where children can "play" in their minds. Through imagination, creativity, and novelty, new realities emerge, and background assumptions are reshaped. The notion of what is and what can be can thereby be dynamic and continually evolving. This also applies to the adult learner. Munnich (1990) notes that current curricula in schools are relativistic and based on the "tradition" of white, male Western dominance. She advocates including the "different voice" (described by Gilligan, 1982) of women and various cultures and races in structuring curricula, writing texts, and designing learning activities. Critical thinking during the creating and reshaping of background assumptions can take place only in an environment of such "alternative traditions."

## Thinking Critically

Can you think of any learning activities in which you were involved in which the teacher's assignment or exercise caused you to see things differently? What techniques were used that assisted you in seeing things through a new lens? What were your reactions to the exercise?

Failure to develop thinking skills impedes the ability to continue to learn as adult workers (Wurman, 1989). According to Adams and Hamm (1990), "Critical thinking involves the ability to raise powerful questions about what's being read, viewed or listened to" (p. 39). They stress the need for critical thinking and collaboration in a democratic society to balance reason, individualism, and community. The lifelong tasks of thinking and learning are especially critical in the global positioning of countries in an era of international competition and continuous, rapid technologic and sociologic change.

Catterall (1988) describes the importance of noting societal economic trends. The shift away from manufacturing to focus on information and services means that society is decreasing its dependence on the human hand and increasing its dependence on the human brain. Tucker (1988) expresses the need for increasing students' capacity for higher order thinking to assimilate complex information, solve problems, and engage in lifelong learning.

McTighe and Schollenberger (1985) emphasize the importance of fostering critical thinking skills in students who will join an Information Age work force. They describe the extraordinary rate of emerging knowledge and the brief time in which such information becomes obsolete.

## Thinking Critically

Recall a time in your nursing experience when you were able to solve a problem, answer a question, or work through a situation for which you had not been taught the information. How were you able to do this? What thinking tools had you learned that you were able to modify or adapt and use in this new situation?

# Critical Thinking in Nursing

The need for critical thinking in nursing has never been greater. As we embark on healthcare reform and changes in the healthcare industry, encounter rapid technologic change, experience great demographic shifts, and confront difficult ethical dilemmas, registered nurses (RNs) must bring with them the critical thinking skills to make wise decisions and collaborate on change that will have a positive impact on future generations. Also, as the opening vignette shows, many schools have opted to test critical thinking skills before entry and exit of the program. So, licensed practical/vocational nurses (LPN/LVNs) who are returning to school need to know more about critical thinking. Bandman and Bandman (1988) describe the need for critical thinking in graduates entering registered nursing practice at this time of tension in the discipline:

> By defining the conditions under which sound and valid conclusions are drawn, critical thinking facilitates the use of the nursing process. Critical thinking is a liberating force in all human thoughtful activity, but especially to nurses. . . . Nursing is in a state of change; activity in defining its theory, practice and social mandate and critical toward its current status. The nursing profession is experiencing distress and pressure from within and without regarding its purposes, educational preparation, practice, roles, theory, research, and in its relation to medicine. This is, therefore, an auspicious time in which to use cannons of critical thinking and logic to inquire openly into the assumptions, beliefs, goals, and values that characterize nursing. (pp. 1–2)

This is still true today. Wilkinson (1996; 2001) notes the challenges for nursing brought about by scientific and technological advances in a rapidly changing care environment.

LeStorti et al. (1999) describe the evolving role of the professional nurse from the traditional role of being task oriented (such as reporting and recording and executing physician's orders) to one of being role oriented, including being a problem solver, decision maker, educator, and change agent.

In its most recent review of the practice of professional nursing, the National League for Nursing (NLN, 2000) identified clinical decision making as one of eight core components of nursing practice for entry-level registered nurses. In addition, the NLN (2000, p. 13) delineated 51 assumptions about the future environment in which the registered nurse educated in an associate degree nursing program will practice. One of these assumptions was that "critical thinking skills will be essential."

# Critical Thinking Defined

Critical thinking has been defined a number of ways. In the early 1900s, critical thinking was viewed as problem solving, creative thinking, or what Dewey (1933) termed "reflective thinking." He used this term to refer to "the kind of thinking that consists in turning a subject over in the mind and giving it serious consecutive consideration" (p. 3). He also used such terms as "suspended judgment" and "healthy skepticism" when speaking of what we now call critical thinking.

In the mid-1900s, attempts were made to define critical thinking in a more concrete way. Ennis (1962) developed what he believed to be a comprehensive yet simple approach to the concept. He defined critical thinking as "the correct assessing of statements" (p. 83) and outlined 12 aspects of critical thinking, including grasping the meaning of statements and making judgments about them.

Lists of critical thinking skills (also termed *proficiencies* or *abilities*) appeared during the next 2 decades with the following frequently appearing: "identifying assumptions, both stated and unstated, both one's own and others; clarifying, focusing, and staying relevant to the topic; understanding logic (including inference, deduction, and induction); and judging sources, their reliability and credibility" (Idol & Jones, 1991, p. 14). Snook (1974) took exception to this approach, stating, "To imagine that thinking can be broken down into its component parts which are then programmed is to misunderstand the nature of thinking" (p. 154).

The third quarter of the century brought about contributions from the disciplines of mathematics, science, and engineering, with "problem solving" receiving much attention. Polya (1971) outlined a four-stage approach: understanding the problem, devising a plan, carrying out the plan, and looking back. Woods, Wright, Hoffman, Swartmen, and Doig (1975) described an adaptation of Polya's approach, adding a "think about it" step before planning for their engineering students.

Continued research in the areas of reasoning and problem solving by scientists, psychologists, and philosophers provided multiple facets to the evolving concept of critical thinking. Guilford (1967) described "creative problem-solving," in an attempt to merge the two concepts. In a manner similar to Woods et al., Guilford incorporated the step of "incubation" into Polya's method to allow for what he called "intuitive leaps."

The 1960s saw an intense focus on feelings, challenging beliefs, and using drugs to escape reality and to refute mores of "the establishment." It was a time to "do your own thing" and "go your own way." Ruggiero (1984) notes, "The result of that extremism was the neglect of thinking" (p. xiii). However, an important contribution was made to the development of the concept of critical thinking. Creativity, challenging background assumptions, and exploring alternatives became important elements in the discussion of critical thinking during the following decade. Such discussion also gave rise to the importance of dispositions of the thinker. To think critically, one must not only possess the skills and abilities to reason, problem solve, and explore alternatives, but one also must be inclined to do so and have the desire to engage in such activity.

The 1980s witnessed a renewed fervor of discussion about critical thinking. More fuel was added to the fire in the debate regarding whether or not critical thinking skills could be learned out of context (i.e., on their own, separate from a specific discipline of subject matter). In addition, an emphasis on metacognition (thinking about thinking) emerged, as authors examined the thinking process and how one assesses and regulates one's thinking process.

Current literature explores the relationships among the concepts of problem solving, reasoning, critical thinking, creative thinking, and metacognition and how we teach these. Does critical thinking incorporate the others? Are they distinct but interrelated concepts? Can they be taught, and if so, how can they be taught in and out of context? Do our current teaching methods teach them?

Katz, Carter, Bishop, and Kravits (2001) describe critical thinking for nurses as important thinking that requires essential questioning. They note, "Using critical thinking, you question established ideas, create new ideas, turn information into tools to solve problems and make decisions, and take the long-term view as well as the day-to-day view" (p. 114).

Raingruber and Haffer (2001) also emphasize the power of questioning for nurses: Learning to ask "What else?" and "What if?" They define critical thinking as

> a multi-faceted process that includes logical, rhetorical, and humanistic skills and attitudes that promote the ability to determine what one should believe and do. Critical thinking requires one to actively process and evaluate information, to validate existing knowledge, and to create new knowledge. It involves reflective thinking. (p. 3)

# Critical Thinking Versus Feeling

When developing critical thinking skills and abilities, and when thinking critically in context, we cannot avoid confronting issues through our own "lenses." We each bring with us our own "world view," which is composed of our age and gender-related, cultural, ethnic, religious, and sociologic viewpoints. We rely on feelings, intuitions, and experiential knowledge when posing and selecting solutions for new problems and when confronting issues that arise.

Bar-Levav (1988) writes,

> We hold on to our rationalizations tenaciously, since our view of ourselves as rational beings depends on their validity . . . Man still tends to hide even from himself the fact that many of his life's most important choices and decisions are made on the basis of feelings, not rationally. (p. 343)

He further notes:

> Feelings commonly camouflage themselves as thoughts . . . But much thinking is circular and ruminative and leads to conclusions already arrived at by our feelings. . . . Learning to really think requires first that we make room for it by diminishing the domain of feelings. . . . Notions from our infantile past in the form of feelings commonly persist as guideposts in adult living. (p. 34)

O'Neill (1985) stresses that the major concept in critical thinking is the ability to distinguish bias from reason and fact from opinion. This is difficult, at best, as Brookfield (1987) describes, because critical thinking is not seen as a wholly rational, mechanized activity. It involves such emotive aspects as feelings, intuition, and sensing. As Bar-Levav (1988) points out, "Feelings are the residues of our lifelong individual experiences. . . . Rather than reflecting current reality, feelings express our expectations based on what we already know from before. They are therefore totally unreliable as a guide to actions in the present" (p. 116).

## NCLEX–RN Might Ask 8-1

The nursing instructor is explaining critical thinking to a new LVN student. The instructor knows the student needs further clarification when the student incorrectly states:

A. "Critical thinking is acting on my feelings."
B. "Critical thinking is looking at all possible options."
C. "Critical thinking involves using new technologies to solve problems."
D. "Part of critical thinking involves looking at how age, culture, and backgrounds influence how nurses think."

• *See Appendix A for correct answer and rationale.*

When transitioning to the RN role, the practical/vocational nurse, to practice independently, is challenged daily to identify feelings and to discriminate between fact and opinion. She or he, when thinking critically, notes personal beliefs and "brackets" (or sets aside) these feelings and background assumptions to confront issues and approach and solve problems in an unbiased, nonjudgmental manner.

## Thinking Critically

Can you remember some occasions when your own beliefs and background assumptions have prevented you from seeing alternative solutions to problems or additional facets of some issues?

The NLN (2000) has described the need for critical thinking in entry-level registered nurses in order to make decisions and exercise clinical judgment. The group states:

> Clinical decision making encompasses the performance of accurate assessments, the use of multiple methods to access information, and the analysis and integration of knowledge and information to formulate clinical judgments. Effective clinical decision making results in finding solutions, individualizing care, and assuring the delivery of accurate, safe care that moves the client and support person(s) toward positive outcomes. Evidence based practice and the use of critical thinking provide the foundation for appropriate clinical decision making. (p. 8)

## Critical Thinking and Creative Thinking

Although controversy exists regarding the relationship of creative thinking to critical thinking (namely whether or not one encompasses the other or if they are distinct, discrete forms of thinking), there is agreement that they work synergistically to produce "good thinkers."

Dale noted the need for creativity in society, stating that imitating the past yields death. Only a creative society can survive. Dale (1972) states, "To be creative is to be thoughtfully involved, to be a concerned and active participant, not a disengaged spectator" (p. 76). Perkins (1984) points out that the ultimate criterion of creativity is output. He describes creative thinking as

> thinking patterned in a way that tends to lead to creative results. . . . We call a person creative when that person consistently gets creative results, meaning, roughly speaking, original and otherwise appropriate results by the criteria of the domain in question. (pp. 18–19)

As in descriptions of critical thinking, a common theme is the emphasis on attitudes or dispositions of the thinker. Ruggiero (1988) suggests, "Creative ideas often come from associating things not commonly associated or from actively bringing together antithetical elements" (pp. 24–25). He also attributes the "disposition to be curious, to wonder, to inquire" as the "trigger mechanism for creative thinking" and notes that the "production of ideas is stimulated by deferring judgments" (pp. 25–26).

The interrelatedness of critical thinking and creative thinking is readily apparent. As Marzano (1991) points out, "Creative thinking is closely related to critical thinking, however, the emphasis is more on the generation of new and unique ways of conceiving information than on the thoughtful analysis of information" (p. 427). He says the following dispositions, taken from his list of thinking dispositions, form the basics for creative thought:

- Engaging intensely in tasks even when answers or solutions are not immediately apparent;
- Pushing the limits of one's knowledge and abilities to keep improving one's knowledge and skills;
- Generating, trusting, and maintaining one's own standards of evaluation; and
- Generating new ways of viewing a situation outside the boundaries of standard conventions (p. 426)

Egan (1986) and Brookfield (1987) also note the presence of risk taking as a characteristic of creative thinkers, along with such characteristics as "optimism, confidence, acceptance of ambiguity and uncertainty, a wide range of interests, flexibility, tolerance of complexity, curiosity, persistence, and independence" (Brookfield, 1987, p. 115). Brookfield further notes commonalities among creative thinkers.

- Creative thinkers reject standardized formats for problem solving.
- They have interests in a wide range of related and divergent fields.
- They can take multiple perspectives on a problem.
- They view the world as relative and contextual, rather than universal and absolute.
- They frequently use trial-and-error methods in their experimentation with alternative approaches.
- They have a future orientation; change is embraced optimistically as a valuable developmental possibility.
- They have self-confidence and trust in their own judgment. (pp. 115–116)

Brookfield summarizes that "developing these capacities is a major task of those helping adults to think critically" (p. 116).

> ### ▶ Thinking Critically
>
> Do any of these lists of creative thinking dispositions sound familiar? Which dispositions describe you? What implication does this have for you as you transition to the RN role?

Smith (1990) provides a detailed account of the concept of creative thinking:

> Most people who talk about creative thinking want something more than imaginativeness. There are usually three other requirements: the thinking (or, rather, its observable consequence) must reach *high standards*, it must be *original*, and it must be the result of *intention* [italics added] rather than chance. (p. 13)

# Modes of Critical Thinking

After reading and thinking about the nature of critical thinking, you should have not only a greater understanding of the concept, but also a greater appreciation of the need for critical thinking in nursing. You may be wondering if, given the need for critical thinking at the RN level, the associate degree nursing educational program will be different from your prior education at the practical/vocational nursing level.

As discussed, the higher order thinking skills of analysis, synthesis, and evaluation are integral to the practice of registered nursing and beyond what is required of the practical/vocational nurse. As Billings (2002) notes, although the NCLEX-RN test plan includes questions to test knowledge, comprehension, application, and analysis, most of the questions test at the levels of application and analysis. These higher order thinking skills are included in the associate degree nursing curriculum and are developed through four modes of critical thinking: problem-solving (using the nursing process); reasoning and informal logic; reflection, challenging beliefs, and imagining alternatives; and metacognition and self-regulation. The following sections explore each of these four modes of critical thinking and learning activities within each mode that foster critical thinking.

## Problem Solving

Problem solving as a mode of critical thinking has received a great deal of attention throughout the years in the areas of science and mathematics. In 1971, Polya outlined a four-stage approach to problem solving: understand the problem, devise a plan, carry out the plan, and look back. In an effort to incorporate more reasoning and reflection, Guilford (1967) included an incubation step, and Woods et al. (1975) added a "think about it" step before planning. Bransford and Stein's (1984) IDEAL problem-solving method was a further adaptation: **I**dentify the problem, **D**efine the problem, **E**xplore alternative approaches, **A**ct on a plan, and **L**ook at the effects.

Nursing as a science-based discipline also embraced a problem-solving method. The American Nurses Association (ANA, 1973) adopted into their *Standards of Nursing Practice* a five-step nursing process model of assessment, analysis, planning, implementation, and evaluation. This model has evolved during the last 2 decades, and especially during the last decade, with the incorporation of nursing diagnosis as a core concept in the model. The use of nursing diagnosis reflects the increased independent and interdependent (collaborative) nature of registered nursing practice. At its roots, nursing process as a science-based problem-solving model is a linear model. Higher order thinking skills (such as analysis, synthesis, and evaluation) are incorporated, and reasoning and informal logic can be applied.

LeStorti et al. (1999) combined the concepts of problem solving and creative thinking to formulate "creative problem solving." They define this as "thinking directed toward the achievement of a goal be means of a novel and appropriate idea of product" (p 63). Nursing today requires creative problem solving in new roles such as patient advocacy and case management. In addition, as noted by Silverman and Casazza (2000), some of us think and learn in a linear analytical manner, whereas others use a more holistic, visual approach.

Registered nursing programs use nursing process extensively for developing thinking skills in students. A study by Harrington (1992) of nursing faculty in 70 associate degree nursing programs in the state of California revealed that 40% of respondents defined critical thinking as problem solving and the use of nursing process. An additional 25% described critical thinking as using analysis, synthesis, and evaluation. Nearly all schools (98%) reported using case studies involving problem solving and nursing process as a learning activity and found them highly effective in fostering critical thinking skills in students.

## Reasoning and Informal Logic

Reasoning and informal logic as modes for critical thinking also have received a great deal of attention. Focusing on reasoning as a description of critical thinking, Glasman, Koff, and Spiers (1984) outline four areas of activity:

1. The ability to identify and formulate problems, as well as the ability to propose and evaluate ways to solve them;
2. The ability to recognize and use inductive and deductive reasoning and to recognize fallacies in reasoning;
3. The ability to draw reasonable conclusions from information found in various sources (written, spoken, tables, graphs), and to defend one's conclusions rationally; and
4. The ability to distinguish between fact and opinion. (p. 467)

Authors often equate critical thinking with reasoning and informal logic. In the discipline of nursing, an important contribution was made by Bandman and Bandman (1988), who stress the need for reasoning and informal logic in registered nursing practice. The purpose of their text *Critical Thinking in Nursing* was "to identify and strengthen the critical thinking skills of nurses by demonstrating the role of scientific reasoning, logic, and philosophy in increasing the effectiveness of the nursing process, and every-day nursing decisions" (p. xi).

Such learning activities as inductive and deductive reasoning exercises and formal debates foster reasoning skills. In the Harrington (1992) study, inductive and deductive reasoning activities were used widely, whereas formal debates had been used by only 19% of those surveyed.

## Reflecting, Challenging Beliefs, and Imagining Alternatives

Many authors have cited limitations to the informal logic and problem-solving approaches to critical thinking. Subject matter knowledge, the role played by background assumptions, and the need to take an active role in modifying beliefs have emerged as important elements of critical thinking. Meyers (1986) notes serious limitations to the general logic and problem-solving approaches, including concern that skills taught separate from subject matter have shown little carry over to the disciplines and that these approaches do not support "a central element in critical thinking [which] is the ability to raise relevant questions and critique solutions without necessarily posing alternatives" (p. 5).

Consistent with the writings of McPeck, Brookfield (1987) writes that thinking critically is "reflecting on the assumptions underlying our and others' ideas and actions, and contemplating alternative ways of thinking and living" (p. x). He further states that critical thinking "involves calling into question the assumptions underlying our customary, habitual ways of thinking and acting and then being ready to think and act differently on the basis of this critical questioning" (p. 1).

Brookfield (1987) also notes nine important critical thinking themes. Five of these deal with *recognizing* critical thinking:

1. Critical thinking is a productive and positive activity.
2. Critical thinking is a process, not an outcome.
3. Manifestations of critical thinking vary according to the contexts in which it occurs.
4. Critical thinking is triggered by positive and negative events.
5. Critical thinking is emotive as well as rational (p. 5).

Four Brookfield identified as *components* of critical thinking:

1. Identifying and challenging assumptions is central to critical thinking.
2. Challenging the importance of context is crucial to critical thinking.
3. Critical thinkers try to imagine and explore alternatives.
4. Imagining and exploring alternatives lead to reflective skepticism (p. 5).

The role played by background assumptions in impeding critical thinking and the necessity for the critical thinker to modify these as needed also was addressed by experts in the 1980s. Drawing on the work of psychologist Jean Piaget (1976), Meyers (1986) writes, "If we view mental structures as components of larger disciplinary perspectives for problem solving and analysis, we can say that when we teach students to think critically, we are helping them alter or replace their mental structures" (p. 13).

Brookfield (1987) emphasizes that although critical thinking involves identifying and challenging assumptions and exploring and imagining alternatives, it is not a passive process. Rather, it is a "praxis of alternating analysis and action" (p. 23) as you refute new ideas or integrate them, modifying current beliefs. Paul's (1992) strong sense definition of critical thinking, in which multilogical issues are examined from a variety of perspectives, challenging values and beliefs, is consistent with Brookfield's notion of "critical thinking praxis." As Brookfield notes, the ability to imagine alternatives to one's current ways of thinking and living is one that often entails a deliberate break with rational modes of thought in order to prompt forward leaps in 'creativity'" (p. 12).

It is often difficult to set aside our biases and challenge our beliefs. It is only through reflection and empathic listening that we can imagine alternatives. In registered nursing practice, making accurate nursing diagnoses and designing a plan of care with a client demand that such multiple perspectives be used. Learning activities in the affective domain and case studies in which problems arise and the nurse is confronted with multifaceted issues foster critical thinking skills in this mode.

Raingruber and Haffer (2001) suggest four critical thinking approaches that nurses can use: reading and reflecting on narratives, asking questions consistent with Stephen Brookfield's critical thinking processes, using "mind maps," and using a reflective journal.

## Metacognition and Self-regulation

Most authors who have written in the area of critical thinking have discussed the importance of thinking about thinking, or metacognition. Beyer (1987) and others emphasize the synergy among critical thinking skills, dispositions, and metacognition. Beyer describes the importance of "helping students become independent thinkers, proficient at self-initiated and self-directed thinking. . . . The teaching of thinking consists of teaching students to think about their own thinking, consciously and deliberately, while engaged in thinking for functional purposes" (p. 191). Some authors include the concept of metacognition as part of the critical thinking process, whereas others clearly distinguish it as a discrete thinking process but one that is essential to being a critical thinker.

Beyer (1987) concurred with the concept of self-regulation, delineating three major metacognitive operations: planning, monitoring, and assessing. He notes that "although these operations may appear to be sequential, in practice they are not strictly linear but recursive" (p. 192) and that these metacognitive operations (in addition to thinking skills and dispositions) are vital to effective thinking or critical thinking.

Burton (2000) describes the necessity of "reflective practice" in today's nursing profession. Such self-regulation is important to the nurse's ability to think critically, considering unique patient/client needs. Reflection allows the nurse to check her/his own background assumptions and biases to be more objective in individualizing care.

Costa (1984) defines metacognition as the

ability to know what we know and what we don't know . . . to plan a strategy for producing what information is needed, to be conscious of our own steps and strategies during the act of problem solving, and to reflect on and evaluate the productivity of our own thinking. (p. 57)

He differentiates this from mere "inner language," which begins in most children around the age of 5 years, noting that metacognition, a formal thought operation, does not develop until about 11 years. He further states, "Probably the major component of metacognition is developing a plan of action and then maintaining that plan in mind over time" (p. 58).

Marzano (1991) equates metacognition with self-regulation. He adds that metacognition, like critical and creative thinking, is dispositionally based, noting that an "individual is behaving in a self-regulated, metacognitive manner when he or she plans, is sensitive to feedback, evaluates progress, and uses available resources" (p. 427).

In nursing school, your ability to think about your thinking, why you developed a nursing care plan a certain way, or why you took specific actions in caring for a client will be valuable to your learning. Raingruber and Haffer (2001) suggest using mind maps or a journal to "track" your thinking process. This is an example of metacognition.

Appearing more recently in the literature is an emerging redefinition of the concept of metacognition to include aspects of motivation and initiative in the learner. Idol, Jones, and Mayer (1991) write that metacognition refers to two dimensions of learning: self-appraisal and self-regulation. They comment on metacognition's newly defined relation to motivation, stating, "In the past, metacognition was defined largely as an individual behavior and was not initially linked to motivation. Now, it is defined as shared behavior (thinking aloud), and it includes the learner's beliefs, judgments, attitudes, motivation, and self-concept" (p. 73).

As you embark on the associate degree nursing program, you may encounter learning activities that cause you to think about your thinking patterns and process. You may be asked to keep a journal, record verbatim communications you have had in the clinical area, or draw cognitive maps (mind maps) representing your thinking process. Teacher role modeling of thinking patterns and processes also assists students in understanding metacognition and self-regulation.

---

## NCLEX–RN Might Ask 8-2

A senior nursing student is being evaluated on critical thinking during client care. Which of the following statements by the student would show the need for additional education on the subject?

    A. "It is important to find out if the client if telling me the truth."
    B. "It is important to verify evidence to support what the client is saying."
    C. "I have a feeling that this is the right thing to do."
    D. "I am making this decision based on all of the facts I have found."

• See Appendix A for correct answer and rationale.

# Critical Thinking and the ▬▬▬▬
# Teaching–Learning Process

Meyers (1986) states,

> Despite a growing body of literature on the subject, college teachers have found few suggestions for ways to improve the critical thinking of their students. Most of this literature has been highly theoretical, far removed from the practical concerns that constantly confront teachers and their students. (p. xi)

He adds that what makes this even more difficult is that the methods for critical thinking vary from discipline to discipline.

Several authors have described techniques that are discussed in the context of a particular discipline but could be used across disciplines. Raths, Wassermann, Jonas, and Rothstein (1986) state, "Thinking activities . . . are open-ended, in that no single, 'correct' answers are being sought. . . . Many answers are acceptable and appropriate. Each activity calls for the exercise of one or more higher-order mental functions" (p. 47). Dale (1972) suggests that the role of the teacher is to give the student just enough help to avoid frustration but not too much, or the student becomes dependent and is robbed of the joys and risks of independent thinking. He describes that the teacher's role is not to provide knowledge on which the student makes choices, but rather to stimulate the student to think independently about choices and their consequences and to develop values: "To be creative is to be thoughtfully involved, to be a concerned and active participant, not a disengaged spectator" (p. 76). See **Display 8-1** for more ideas for promoting critical thinking.

Teaching strategies for critical thinking often involve reading and writing techniques. Paul (1992) describes the important role of critical reading:

> *Critical reading is an active, intellectually engaged process* [italics added] in which the reader participates in an inner dialogue with the writer. Most people read uncritically and so miss some part of what is expressed while distorting other parts. A critical reader realizes the way in which reading, by its very nature,

---

▶ *Display 8-1* **Fostering Critical Thinking**

Group work
Noting patterns
Building outlines or models
Bringing dissimilar ideas or opposing views together
Modeling
Mind mapping
Case studies
Position papers
Computerized instructive scenarios

means entering into a point of view other than our own, the point of view of the writer. A critical reader actively looks for assumptions, key concepts and ideas, reasons and justifications, key concepts and experiences, implications and consequences, and any other structural features of the written text, to interpret and assess it accurately and fairly. (p. 642)

Paul also provides a discussion of critical writing:

"To express oneself in language requires that one arrange ideas in some relationship to each other. When accuracy and truth are at issue, then we must understand what our thesis is, how we can support it, how we can elaborate it to make it intelligible to others, what objections can be raised to it from other points of view, what the limitations are to point of view, and so forth. *Disciplined writing requires disciplined thinking; disciplined thinking is achieved through disciplined writing* [italics added]. (pp. 643–644)

Jones, Tinzmann, Friedman, and Walker (1987) use the term "strategic teaching," meaning the use of teaching strategies to decrease teacher direction so students take responsibility for their own learning. The teacher must assist the learner in constructing meaning so that the "learner is strategic, working actively to link the new information to prior knowledge and drawing on a repertoire of thinking strategies" (p. 10). They note that learning is recursive and nonlinear, with the learner returning to earlier thoughts for revision as new information is understood and assimilated.

Teaching strategies whereby students assimilate and group information, note patterns, or build models are useful in fostering critical thinking. Jones et al. (1987) suggest students use organizational patterns and graphic outlining or mapping. Dale (1972) recommends building outlines, models, and paradigms to classify ideas and to use mental scanning to bring dissimilar ideas together. In addition, he adds that the student must think about thinking through systematic critique. This includes reading between the lines for implications and reading beyond the lines for application. Ruggiero (1988) concurs with this, suggesting that faculty encourage students to be curious and ask questions, such as "How will it be when applied?" and "How will different people react to it?"

There is increasing support in the literature for modeling and the use of exemplars. Critical thinking is an abstract concept that is difficult to describe and operationally define. Often, the learner can best learn its use through modeling and effective use of exemplars. Meyers (1986) states that "by modeling reflective thought in lectures and discussion, teachers can do much to encourage this frame of mind in their students" (p. 47). Paul (1985) stresses that the teacher must raise opposing views, explore background assumptions, and examine inconsistencies. To facilitate this process in students, the teacher must be able to model these behaviors.

Grant (1988) advocates the use of models, metaphors, and images as modeling techniques. Adams and Hamm (1990) advocate the use of collaborative teaching strategies, citing debates, role play, composition of letters to newspapers and the media, and other collaborative processes as means for developing critical thinking skills. Interdisciplinary small group projects also are effective teaching strategies in the cooperative learning approach. Adams and Hamm also advocate the use of computers to stimulate interaction, thinking, and collaboration

Heyman and Daly (1992) suggest a number of teaching strategies for occupational programs, including visualization techniques, literature, case studies and oral communications, and problem solving and models. Marzano and Evy (1989) stress the need for programs to emphasize self-management skills (setting goals, planning, adjusting, and evaluating), knowledge extension skills (composing, problem solving, decision making, and inquiry), and enabling skills (comparing, classifying, deducing, analyzing, supporting, and abstracting).

Miller and Malcolm (1990) advocate critical thinking in nursing, stating,

> Changes could be made whereby students could engage in more problem-solving activities, case study analysis, more discussion and reflection, and position papers rather than passively listening to lectures. . . . Nursing educators can foster critical thinking in students by reinforcing the spirit of inquiry and independent critical thought. (p. 73)

Miller and Malcolm also stress the need for nurse educators to consider not only the students' cognitive levels, but also their learning styles. Klaassens (1988) provides the following as teaching strategies that apply to higher educational settings and nursing education in particular: use of reflective responses, analysis, free writing, brainstorming, journal writing, case studies, and computer simulations. Harrington (1992) provides numerous examples of teaching strategies used in associate degree nursing programs to foster critical thinking in students.

Teaching strategies to foster critical thinking in clinical practice proposed by Persaud, Leedom, and Land (1986) include the use of feedback lectures, with students divided into groups and given problems to solve; clinical simulations using a decision-making model; computer-assisted video instruction; and case studies integrating medical–surgical and maternal–child content areas. Chau (2001) advocates the use of videotaped vignettes to enhance students' critical thinking abilities. Kirkpatrick, Ford, and Castelloe (1997) note the role of storytelling by nurses as a means for thinking critically about the actual experiences of others. Benner, Tanner, and Chesla (1996) concur, noting the need for nurse "experts" to serve as role models for those who are at a novice level. Gambrill (1990) suggests that clinical practitioners strive to improve their accuracy of judgments and decisions about clients by learning more about sources of error. Teaching strategies such as role modeling and critiquing case studies allow for such learning, especially among students who have experience at a novice level in clinical practice.

As you participate in the associate degree nursing program, you may encounter a number of the mentioned teaching strategies and learning activities to foster critical thinking. View these as an opportunity for growth as you transition to the more autonomous practice of the RN.

## Student Exercise

1. Set a timer for 10 minutes. Write as many words or phrases as you can that come to mind when you hear the words "critical thinking."

2. Using the words or phrases you listed, compose your own definition of critical thinking. Describe a situation in nursing when you took inappropriate or incomplete actions. What aspect of critical thinking could you have used to strengthen or correct your actions? (Suggestions: Bracketing feelings or background assumptions; using reasoning and judgment skills; using analysis, synthesis, and evaluation better; challenging assumptions or exploring alternatives; applying metacognitive or self-regulatory processes.)

## References

Adams, D. M., & Hamm, M. E. (1990). *Cooperative learning: Critical thinking and collaboration across the curriculum.* Springfield, IL: Charles C. Thomas.

American Nurses Association (ANA). (1973). *Standards of nursing practice.* Kansas City, MO: Author.

Bandman, E. L., & Bandman, B. (1988). *Critical thinking in nursing.* Norwalk, CT: Appleton and Lange.

Bar-Levav, R. (1988). *Thinking in the shadow of feelings.* New York: Simon and Schuster.

Barell, J. (1990). *Playgrounds of our minds.* New York: Teachers College Press (Teachers College, Columbia University).

Benner, P., Tanner, C., & Chesla, C. (1996). *Expertise in nursing practice: Caring, clinical judgment, and ethics.* New York: Springer.

Beyer, B. K. (1987). *Practical strategies for the teaching of thinking.* Boston: Allyn and Bacon.

Billings, D. M. (2002). *Lippincott's review for NCLEX-RN* (7th ed.). Philadelphia: Lippincott Williams & Wilkins.

Bransford, J., & Stein, B. S. (1984). *The IDEAL problem solver: A guide for improving thinking, learning, and creativity.* New York: WH Freeman.

Brookfield, S. D. (1987). *Developing critical thinkers: Challenging adults to explore alternative ways of thinking and acting.* San Francisco: Jossey-Bass.

Burton, A. J. (2000). Reflection: Nursing's practice and education panacea? *Journal of Advanced Nursing, 31*(5), 1009–1017.

Catterall, J. (1988, March). *Tomorrow's workforce: Overcredentialed and under-prepared?* Paper presented at the conference Can California Be Competitive and Caring? Sponsored by the Institute of Industrial Relations, University of California at Los Angeles.

Chau, J. P. C. (2001). Effects of using videotaped vignettes on enhancing students' critical thinking abilities in a baccalaureate nursing program. *Journal of Advanced Nursing, 36*(1), 112–119.

Costa, A. L. (1984). Mediating the metacognitive. *Educational Leadership, 4*(3), 57–62.

Creasia, J. L., & Parker, B. (2001). *Conceptual foundations of professional nursing practice: The bridge to professional nursing practice* (3rd ed.). St. Louis: Mosby.

Dale, E. (1972). *Building a learning environment.* Bloomington, IN: Phi Delta Kappa.

Dewey, J. (1933). *How we think.* Boston: DC Health.

Egan, G. (1986). *The skilled helper: A systematic approach to effective helping.* Monterey, CA: Brooks and Cole.

Ennis, R. H. (1962). A concept of critical thinking. *Harvard Educational Review, 32*(1).

Gambrill, E. (1990). *Critical thinking in clinical practice: Improving the accuracy of judgments and decisions about clients.* San Francisco: Jossey-Bass.

Gilligan, C. (1982). *In a different voice.* Cambridge: Harvard University Press.

Glasman, N., Koff, R., & Spiers, H. (1984). Preface. *Review of Educational Research, 54,* 461–471.

Grant, G. E. (1988). *Teaching critical thinking.* New York: Praeger.

Guilford, J. P. (1967). Problem solving and creative production. In J. P. Guilford (Ed.), *The nature of human intelligence*. New York: McGraw-Hill.

Harrington, N. (1992). *A survey of teaching strategies used in California community college nursing programs to foster critical thinking*. Unpublished doctoral dissertation, University of San Diego, California.

Heyman, G. A., & Daly, E. R. (1992). Teaching critical thinking in vocational–technical and occupational classes. In C. A. Barnes (Ed.), *Critical thinking: Educational imperative, new directions for community colleges* (No. 77). San Francisco: Jossey-Bass.

Idol, L., & Jones, B. F. (Eds.). (1991). *Educational values and cognitive instruction: Implications for reform*. Hillsdale, NJ: Erlbaum.

Idol, L., Jones, B. F., & Mayer, R. E. (1991). Classroom instruction: The teaching of thinking. In L. Idol & B. F. Jones (Eds.), *Educational values and cognitive instruction: Implications for reform*. Hillsdale, NJ: Erlbaum.

Jones, B. F., Tinzmann, M. B., Friedman, L. B., & Walker, B. B. (1987). *Teaching thinking skills: English/language arts*. Washington, DC: National Education Association of the United States.

Katz, J. R., Carter, C., Bishop, J., & Kravits, S. L. (2001). *Keys to nursing success*. Upper Saddle River, NJ: Prentice Hall.

Kirkpatrick, M. K., Ford, S., & Castelloe, B. P. (1997). Storytelling: An approach to client-centered care. *Nurse Educator, 22*(2), 38–40.

Klaassens, E. L. (1988). Improving teaching for thinking. *Nurse Educator, 13*(6), 15–19.

LeStorti, A. J., et al (1999). Creative thinking in nursing education: Preparing for tomorrow's challenge. *Nursing Outlook, 47*(2), 62–66.

McPeck, J. E. (1981). *Critical thinking and education*. Oxford: Martin Robertson & Company.

McTighe, J., & Schollenberger, J. (1985). Why teach thinking: A statement of rationale. In A. L. Costa (Ed.), *Developing minds: A resource book for teaching thinking* (pp. 3–6). Roseville, CA: Association for Supervision and Curriculum Development.

Marzano, R. J. (1991). Creating an educational paradigm centered on learning through teacher-directed, naturalistic inquiry. In L. Idol & B. F. Jones (Eds.), *Educational values and cognitive instruction: Implications for reform* (pp. 411–442). Hillsdale, NJ: Erlbaum.

Marzano, R. J., & Evy, R. W. (1989). Thinking for tomorrow. *Vocational Education Journal, 64*(5), 28–29.

Meyers, C. (1986). *Teaching students to think critically: A guide for faculty in all disciplines*. San Francisco: Jossey-Bass.

Miller, M. A., & Malcolm, N. S. (1990). Critical thinking in the nursing curriculum. *Nursing and Health Care, 11*(2), 67–73.

Munnich, E. K. (1990). *Transforming knowledge*. Philadelphia: Temple University Press.

National League for Nursing (NLN). (2000). *Educational competencies for graduates of associate degree nursing programs*. Sudbury, MA: Jones and Bartlett Publishers.

O'Neill, T. (1985). *Censorship-opposing views*. St. Paul, MN: Greenhaven Press.

Paul, R. W. (1985). Bloom's taxonomy and critical thinking instruction. *Educational Leadership, 43*(2), 36–45.

Paul, R. W. (1992). *Critical thinking: What every person needs to survive in a rapidly changing world*. Rohnert Park, CA: Center for Critical Thinking and Moral Critique, Sonoma State University.

Perkins, D. N. (1984). Creativity by design. *Educational Leadership, 42*, 18–25.

Persaud, D., Leedom, C., & Land, L. (1986). Facilitating critical thinking in clinical practice. In Thinking across the disciplines, *Proceedings of the Fifteenth Annual Conference of the International Society for Individualized Instruction* (pp. 1–10). Atlanta, GA.

Piaget, J. (1976). *Psychology of intelligence*. Totowa, NJ: Littlefield Adams.

Polya, G. (1971). *How to solve it*. Princeton, NJ: Princeton University Press.

Raingruber, B., & Haffer, A. (2001). *Using your head to land on your feet: A beginning nurse's guide to critical thinking*. Philadelphia: FA Davis

Raths, L. E., Wassermann, S., Jonas, A., & Rothstein, A. (1986). *Teaching for thinking: Theory, strategies, and activities for the classroom*. New York: Teachers College Press.

Ruggiero, V. R. (1984). *Beyond feelings: A guide to critical thinking* (2nd ed.). Mountain View, CA: Mayfield.

Ruggiero, V. R. (1988). *The art of thinking: A guide to critical and creative thought* (2nd ed.). New York: Harper and Row.

Siegel, H. (1980). Critical thinking as an educational ideal. *Educational Forum, 45*(1), 7–23.

Silverman, S. L., & Casazza, M. E. (2000). *Learning and development: Making connections to enhance teaching.* San Francisco: Jossey-Bass.

Smith, F. (1990). *To think.* New York: Teachers College Press.

Snook, I. A. (1974). Teaching pupils to think. *Studies in Philosophy and Education, 8*(3), 154–155.

Tucker, M. S. (1988). Peter Drucker, knowledge, work, and the structure of schools. *Educational Leadership, 45*(5), 44–46.

Wilkinson, J. M. (1996). *Nursing process: A critical thinking approach.* Menlo Park, CA: Addison-Wesley.

Wilkinson, J. M. (2001). *Nursing process and critical thinking* (3rd ed.). Upper Saddle River, NJ: Prentice-Hall.

Woods, D. R., Wright, J. D., Hoffman, T. W., Swartmen, R. K., & Doig, I. D. (1975). Teaching problem-solving skills. *Engineering Education, 66*(3), 238–243.

Wurman, R. S. (1989). *Information anxiety.* New York: Doubleday.

## Suggested Reading

Adams, B. L. (1999). Nursing education for critical thinking: An integrative review. *Journal of Nursing Education, 38,* 111–119.

Alfaro-LeFevre, R. (2002). *Applying nursing process: Promoting collaborative care.* (5th ed.). Philadelphia: Lippincott Williams & Wilkins.

Alfaro-LeFevre, R. (1998). *Critical thinking in nursing* (2nd ed.). Philadelphia: WB Saunders

Argyris, C. (1982). *Reasoning, learning, and action.* San Francisco: Jossey-Bass.

Arons, A. B. (1985). Critical thinking and the baccalaureate curriculum. *Liberal Education, 71*(2), 141–157.

Benner, P. (1984). *From novice to expert: Excellence and power in clinical nursing practice.* Menlo Park, CA: Addison-Wesley.

Beyer, B. K. (1985). Critical thinking: What is it? *Social Education*, April, 270–276.

Bloom, B. S. (Ed.). (1974). *The taxonomy of educational objectives: Affective and cognitive domains.* New York: David McKay.

Burns, S., & Bulman, C. (2000). *Reflective practice in nursing: The growth of the professional practitioner* (2nd ed.). London: Blackwell Science.

Carper, B. (1978). Fundamental patterns of knowing in nursing. *Advances in Nursing Science, 31*(5), 1009–1017.

Carr, E. C. J. (1996). Reflecting on clinical practice: Hectoring talk or reality? *Journal of Clinical Nursing, 5,* 289–298.

Clarke, J. H. (1990). *Patterns of thinking: Integrating learning skills in content thinking.* Boston: Allyn and Bacon.

Cohen, J. (1971). *Thinking.* Chicago: Rand McNally.

Ennis, R. H. (1981). Rational thinking and educational practice. In J. F. Soltis (Ed.), *Philosophy and education, Eightieth yearbook of the National Society for the Study of Education* (Part I). Chicago: University of Chicago Press.

Ennis, R. H. (1987). Critical thinking and the curriculum. In M. Heiman & J. Slomianko (Eds.), *Thinking skills instruction: Concepts and techniques.* Washington, DC: National Education Association.

Ennis, R. H. (1987). A taxonomy of critical thinking dispositions and abilities. In J. B. Baron & R. J. Sternberg (Eds.), *Teaching thinking skills: Theory and practice* (pp. 9–26). New York: Freeman.

Ennis, R. H. (1989). Critical thinking and subject specificity: Clarification and needed research. *Educational Researcher, 18*(3), 4–10.

Green, C. (2000). *Critical thinking in nursing: Case studies across the curriculum.* Upper Saddle River, NJ: Prentice-Hall.

Halpern, D. F. (1984). *Thought and knowledge: An introduction to critical thinking.* Hillsdale, NJ: Erlbaum.

Hyde, A. A., & Bizar, M. (1989). *Thinking in context: Teaching cognitive processes across the elementary school curriculum.* New York: Longman.

Kennedy, M., Fisher, M. B., & Ennis, R. H. (1991). Critical thinking: Literature review and needed research. In L. Idol & B. F. Jones (Eds.), *Educational values and cognitive instruction: Implications for reform* (pp. 11–40). Hillsdale, NJ: Erlbaum.

Long, G. A. (1989). Cooperative learning. A new approach. *Journal of Agricultural Education, 30*(2), 2–9.

McPeck, J. E. (1990). *Teaching critical thinking.* New York: Routledge, Chapman, and Hall.

Manlove, C. (1989). *Critical thinking: A guide to interpreting literary tests.* New York: St. Martin's Press.

Mezirow, J. (1983). *Transformations in adult learning.* Paper presented at the Annual Conference of the American Association for Adult and Continuing Education, Philadelphia, November 29, 1983.

Michenbaum, P. (1985). Teaching thinking: A cognitive-behavioral perspective. In S. F. Chipman, J. W. Segal, & R. Glaser (Eds.), *Thinking and learning skills: Vol. 2. Research and open questions* (pp. 407–426). Hillsdale, NJ: Erlbaum.

Nickerson, R. S. (1987). Why teach thinking? In J. B. Baron & R. J. Sternberg (Eds.), *Teaching thinking skills: Theory and practice* (pp. 27–37). New York: Freeman.

Norris, S. P. (1985). Synthesis of research on critical thinking. *Educational Leadership, 42*(8), 40–45.

O'Flahavan, J. F., & Tierney, R. J. (1991). Reading, writing, and critical thinking. In L. Idol & B. F. Jones (Eds.), *Educational values and cognitive instruction: Implications for reform* (pp. 41–64). Hillsdale, NJ: Erlbaum.

Paul, R. W. (1984). Critical thinking: Fundamental for education in a free society. *Educational Leadership, 42*, 4–14.

Perkins, D. N. (1990). The nature and nurture of creativity. In B. F. Jones & L. Idol (Eds.), *Dimensions of thinking and cognitive instruction* (pp. 415–444). Hillsdale, NJ: Erlbaum.

Rubenfeld, M., & Scheffer, B. (1999). *Critical thinking in nursing: An interactive approach* (2nd ed.). Philadelphia: Lippincott Williams & Wilkins.

Rubinstein, M. F., & Firstenberg, I. R. (1987). Tools for thinking. In J. E. Stice (Ed.), *New directions for teaching and learning: Developing critical thinking and problem-solving abilities.* San Francisco: Jossey-Bass.

Ruggiero, V. R. (1986). *Teaching thinking across the curriculum.* New York: Harper and Row.

Schein, E. H. (1985). *Organizational culture and leadership: A dynamic view.* San Francisco: Jossey-Bass.

Siegel, H. (1988). *Educating reason: Rationality, critical thinking, and education.* New York: Routledge.

Sternberg, R. J. (1987). Questions and answers about the nature and teaching of thinking skills. In J. B. Baron & R. J. Sternberg (Eds.), *Teaching thinking skills: Theory and practice* (pp. 251–259). New York: Freeman.

Sternberg, R. J., & Baron, J. B. (1985). A statewide approach to measuring critical thinking skills. *Educational Leadership, 43*(7), 40–43.

Sternglass, M. S. (1988). The presence of thought: Introspective accounts of reading and writing. In *Advances in Discourse Processes, 34.* Norwood, NJ: Ablex.

Vanetzian, E. V. (2001). *Critical thinking: An interactive tool for learning medical–surgical nursing.* Philadelphia: FA Davis.

## On the Web  . . . . . . . . . . . . . . . . . . . . . . . . . . . . . . . . . . . . . .

*www.ncsbe.org*: National Council of State Boards of Nursing

*www.nln.org*: National League for Nursing

*www.nursingworld.org*: American Nursing Association website for online resources

*www.findarticles.com*: website for articles on any topic. Suggestions: (1) critical thinking and nursing; (2) nursing and clinical judgment.

# Role Concepts Essential for RN Practice

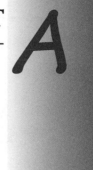

P A R T

# A

# Provider of Care

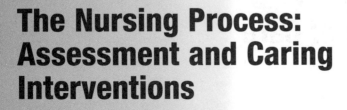

# The Nursing Process: Assessment and Caring Interventions

*By the end of this chapter, the student will be able to:*

1 Discuss the historical development of the nursing process.
2 Explain the reasons the nursing process was developed.
3 Discuss the importance of the nursing process in guiding nursing practice.
4 Describe the five components of the nursing process.
5 Formulate an actual nursing diagnostic statement using the PES format.
6 Write a measurable nursing goal with expected outcomes using a case study.
7 Describe the difference between goals, expected outcomes, and interventions.
8 Discuss the significance of evaluating the nursing goal.

## KEY TERMS

analysis
American Nurses
  Association
assessment
collaborative problem
cues
data
diagnosis
evaluation

focused assessment
goals/expected outcomes
holistic approach
implementation
measurable
need
North American Nursing
  Diagnosis Association
  (NANDA)

National Council of State
  Boards of Nursing (NCSBN)
nursing diagnosis
nursing process
objective data
outcome criteria

planning
primary source
problem
secondary source
subjective data
validation

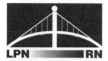

### VIGNETTE

Jane Smith, LPN, and Enrique Martinez, RN, are having a coffee break together at Paterno Medical Center. Jane is a first semester student at State Community College and yesterday had her first classroom lesson in planning nursing care.

**Jane:** Boy, we just had a really difficult class on the nursing process.

**Enrique:** Oh, yes. I remember the days in school where we had to do those monster 20-page care plans.

**Jane:** Well, we don't have to do that this semester. We have a care plan due in a week on our clients. It sure is a time-consuming process to do the research and to follow the plan through.

**Enrique:** Yes, and although the hospital doesn't require care plans like you do them in school, we use the nursing process in a hospital to guide our patient care. Care plans become very useful when there is a change from the usual things that you do for the client. That is something that needs to be communicated to everyone. If it weren't for care plans, everything I know about a client would be here! [He points to his head.]

**Jane:** I know. Our instructor says it's a way to learn a disciplined approach so I don't overlook anything. She also says that care plans are a way to communicate the client's many complex problems. But you are right; care plans are also a learning tool to help me think critically. And besides...I need all the help I can get learning how to put it all in here! [She points to her head, giggles and laughs.]

## From Licensed Practical Nurse to ▬▬▬▬ Professional Nursing Practice

Jane Smith and Enrique Martinez are discussing learning and using the nursing process in clinical practice. If you had licensed practical nurse (LPN) training during the past decade, you probably learned about the nursing process and are using it at work to assess and evaluate client care. However, if you were trained more than 10 years ago, you may have not learned the nursing diagnosis piece of the nursing process.

Practicing LPNs continue to perform and have input into many vital functions in the nursing process. As a professional nurse, you will be designing, implementing, and evaluating the entire process. You will be involved in the process from beginning to end and thus, as Jane stated, will be using a disciplined approach to think critically and solve complex problems.

# An Historical Overview of the Nursing Process

Nursing as a profession is in its infancy as far as other professions go. Although nursing in various forms has existed throughout history, it wasn't until the profession defined what nurses were and what nursing did that the nursing process was first established. Many of the interventions that nurses did in the past were based on trial-and-error, intuitive problem solving and scientific methods. Although Hall first used the term *nursing process* in 1955, it wasn't until 1967 that Yura and Walsh first published what they described as the steps in the nursing process. At that time, the steps of the nursing process were assessment, planning, intervention and evaluation. In 1974, Gebbie and Lavin established nursing diagnosis as a step in the process.

In 1973, the first national conference on nursing diagnosis was held and, in 1982, the North American Nursing Diagnosis Association (NANDA) was born. Every 2 years, NANDA meets to contribute to growing knowledge and to revise nursing diagnosis terminology. This provides a common language for all nurses.

Many nursing organizations have espoused the nursing process as the organizer of nursing care. The American Nurses Association (ANA, 1998) addresses the steps of the nursing process in their Standards of Clinical Nursing Practice, and the National League for Nurses (NLN) requires that all educational programs incorporate the steps of the nursing process into the curriculum. The National Council of State Boards of Nursing (NCSBN) has rewritten the *National Council Licensure Examination for Registered Nurses* (NCLEX-RN) in terms of the nursing process.

Other healthcare organizations also use the nursing process. The Joint Commission on Accreditation of Healthcare Organizations (JCAHO) mandates that documentation must be according to the nursing process. So you see, the nursing process is used widely throughout nursing and other health care arenas. So what is the nursing process?

# The Nursing Process: Overview and Steps

The nursing process is a systematic problem-solving method that guides nurses in giving client-centered, goal-oriented care in an effective and efficient manner. The process is systematic in that it consists of sequential steps or phases similar to the steps of the scientific method used in laboratory studies and the general problem-solving process. **Table 9-1** shows a comparison of these three processes.

The nursing process is dynamic and flexible, with a great deal of interaction and overlap, as depicted in **Figure 9-1**. In uncomplicated situations, the nursing process can be followed sequentially, with each step relying on the accuracy of the one preceding it and influencing the one that follows it. In complicated situations, all five phases may

**T A B L E   9 - 1**
COMPARISON OF THE SCIENTIFIC METHOD, PROBLEM-SOLVING PROCESS, AND NURSING PROCESS

| Scientific Method | Problem-Solving Method | Nursing Process |
|---|---|---|
| 1. Define problem. | 1. Encounter problem. | 1. Assess |
| 2. Collect data. | 2. Collect data. | 2. Diagnose |
| 3. Formulate hypothesis. | 3. Analyze data to specify problem. | 3. Plan |
| 4. Design plan to test hypothesis. | 4. Determine plan of action to resolve problem. | 4. Implement |
| 5. Test hypothesis. | 5. Execute action plan. | 5. Evaluate |
| 6. Interpret results. | 6. Evaluate plan for effectiveness in problem resolution. | |
| 7. Evaluate for study conclusion or revision. | | |

occur simultaneously. In any event, the various elements of the process enable the nurse to do the following:

Systemically collect client data
Critically think about the data
Identify client strengths and needs or problems
Establish priorities and goals
Develop an individualized plan of care
Provide client-centered individual care
Evaluate the effectiveness of care and attainment of client goals

**Table 9-2** shows the steps and activities of the nursing process.

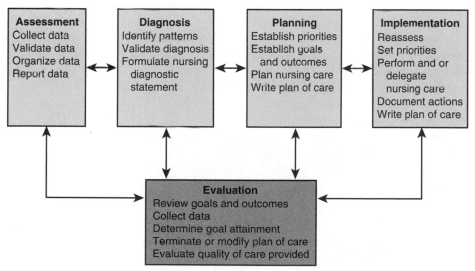

**FIGURE 9–1** ▼ Steps and activities of the Nursing Process.

**TABLE   9-2**
STEPS AND ACTIVITIES OF THE NURSING PROCESS

| Assessment | Diagnosis | Planning | Implementation | Evaluation |
|---|---|---|---|---|
| Collect data | Identify patterns | Establish priorities | Reassess | Review goals and outcomes |
| Validate data | Validate diagnosis | Establish goals and outcomes | Set priorities | Collect data |
| Organize data | Formulate nursing diagnostic statement | Plan nursing care | Perform or delegate nursing care | Determine goal attainment |
| Report data | | Write plan of care | Document actions | Terminate or modify plan of care Evaluate quality of care provided |

The nursing process is recognized as client centered because it involves the nurse and client interacting in each phase to ensure that an individualized plan is produced. The plan focuses on client strengths and specifies the client's desired goals and the nursing actions needed to meet those goals. If the client is unable to participate in the process because of age or condition, a family member or support person participates in the process. Although the primary purpose of the nursing process is to help the nurse manage client care, as mentioned in the beginning of the chapter, the process has gained acceptance in use for documenting client care, writing nursing care plans, defining professional standards of clinical practice, and testing nursing knowledge and abilities for licensure. In nursing education programs and healthcare organizations and institutions, the nursing process also provides a means for conducting research to improve the quality of care. This research is called evidenced-based research.

Reviewing client outcomes and evaluating the extent to which a client has achieved goals can help to identify factors that positively or negatively influence goal achievement. Identification of nursing actions that affect goal attainment can guide self-improvement (e.g., better handwashing in an individual nurse's practice) and nursing in-service programs. Recognition of needed system changes, such as a more timely medication delivery system, can lead to development of more efficient institutional practices, policies, and procedures.

The nursing process consists of five essential steps or phases: assessment, diagnosis, planning, implementation, and evaluation (ADPIE) (see Figure 9-1). Following these steps helps the nurse to identify and handle a client's problems in an orderly and systematic way.

## Assessment

The first phase of the nursing process, assessment, is the continuous and systematic collection, validation, and communication of client data. During the assessment phase, the nurse establishes and develops a comprehensive database by observing, interviewing, and exam-

## NCLEX–RN Might Ask 9-1

The primary nurse is providing orientation to a new nurse. Together they are reviewing the nursing plan of care for an elderly client. The primary nurse knows that the new nurse needs additional help with the nursing process when the new nurse states the nursing process is

    A. an extension of the medical plan.
    B. developed with the client.
    C. comprehensive.
    D. a systematic problem-solving method.

• *See Appendix A for correct answer and rationale.*

ining the client with the goal of gaining insight and information about the client's condition and situation. As an LPN, you probably have been asked to help with data collection, such as obtaining vital signs or weight. The registered nurse (RN) then used that information to make sound clinical nursing judgments in the diagnostic and planning phases.

Assessment activities that are necessary for greater understanding of the client's situation are:

**Collect data:** Gather client information.
**Validate data:** Determine accuracy of information.
**Organize data:** Cluster information into related groups that show illness or
    health patterns.
**Report data:** Document and report findings.

## COLLECTING DATA

Because nursing is a holistic profession, data collection involves gathering information about the client, family, or even the community. Information is gathered about physiologic, psychosocial, cultural, developmental, spiritual, and environmental aspects of the client.

When it comes to an individual client, data collection involves making general observations, obtaining a health history, reviewing diagnostic studies, and performing a physical examination. Additional information can be gained from secondary sources, such as reviewing client records and consulting with the client's family members and other healthcare professionals.

The focus of a nursing assessment is getting to know the person. Nurses should attempt to gain as much information as possible directly from the client. The client is considered the primary source of information. Secondary sources, such as records, family members, and other healthcare providers, are useful for supplementing and validating the information obtained from the client. Good interviewing skills are essential to obtaining the required client data and communicating concern for the client (see Chapter 10). The physical examination should be accomplished in a thorough and organized way using a consistent and systematic approach, such as head-to-toe or body systems. As an RN student nurse, you will be learning to conduct a more in-depth physical assessment and will be adding to that skill throughout your nursing career. The history/database and physical assessment should be obtained as soon as possible after a client presents for care (hospital admission, home health visit, or clinic appointment).

The nursing assessment should be comprehensive and include data concerning all aspects of the client's health. Most healthcare facilities and nursing schools have developed assessment tools (forms) to collect and report assessment data (**Display 9-1**). These tools follow an organizing framework, such as body systems, Gordon's (1994) functional health patterns, NANDA's human response patterns, or a conceptual model of nursing, such as Orem's self-care model. Use of an assessment tool helps prevent omissions in data collection and improves data analysis in the diagnostic phase.

Regardless of the model used, a comprehensive database should include subjective (client's and family verbal information) and objective (observable, measurable data) information about the client (**Display 9-2**).

The depth and breadth of data collected in assessment depend on the purpose for the assessment as determined by the client's developmental stage and nursing care needs. Once the nurse establishes a comprehensive database and determines priorities for ongoing assessment, a more focused assessment can be used to update and evaluate specific problems or needs that have been identified. A focused assessment is done to concentrate on one area, specifically the patient's primary problem, and gather as much

---

> **Display 9-2**    **Body Systems Assessment Tool (Quick Physical Assessment Tool)**

| *Appearance* *Overall* | *Head/Neck* | *Thorax/Lungs* | *Heart/Vascular* |
|---|---|---|---|
| Skin color | Eyes | Respiratory pattern | Heart sounds |
| Respiratory pattern | Nasal flaring | Tracheal midline | Pulses |
| Response to nurse | Mouth/lips | Breath sounds | JVD |
|  | (dry, moist/color) | Retractions |  |
|  |  |  | *Equipment/* |
| *VS/TPR* | *Skin* | *Abdomen* | *Invasive Lines* |
| T: _____ | Color | Configuration | IV type, drip rate |
| P: _____ | Temperature | Bowel sounds | $O_2$ type, flow |
| R: _____ | Texture | Percussion | Foley catheter |
| BP: _____ | Turgor | Palpation | Drainage tubes |
| $SaO_2$ _____ | Pressure ulcers | Pulsations | Dressings |
| *Neurologic* | *Extremities* | *Safety* | *Psychosocial* |
| Orientation | Strength | Bed position | Strengths |
| GCS | Capillary refilling | Call bell | Needs |
| Speech pattern | Positioning | Bed rails | Family |
| Follows commands | Edema | Bed check | Religion |
| Cranial nerve check |  | Assistance | Coping skills |
| Pupils/direct/ |  | OOB order | Education level |
| consensual |  | Level of activity |  |

*Abbreviated terms:* JVD: jugular venous distension. VS/TPR: vital signs/temperature, pulse, respirations. BP: blood pressure. $SaO_2$: peripheral oxygenation. $O_2$: oxygen. GCS: Glasgow Coma Scale. OOB: out of bed.

| Display 9-2 | Objective and Subjective Data* |
| --- | --- |

- Personal demographics: name, age, sex, race, culture, language, occupation, and education
- Developmental stage and ability to meet developmental tasks
- Values, beliefs, and perceptions concerning health and illness
- Health habits and patterns contributing to health and illness
- Physical and emotional responses to illness and health
- Internal (coping abilities) and external resources (support systems, finances, environmental factors) for dealing with illness and health
- Family history
- Past and current physical and emotional state
- Expectations and preferences for treatment and care

*Objective data are what the nurse observes; subjective data are what the client says.

information as possible in this area. A comprehensive assessment is obtained during initial contact with the client (admission to hospital, home health, or clinic). To strengthen and update the information, an ongoing focused assessment of the client's problem areas is conducted during each client–nurse contact.

## VALIDATING DATA

Incomplete or inaccurate assessment data might lead to false assumptions. Data should be validated always with the client or another source. Validation ensures that information is accurate and complete. The nurse must confirm subjective data by asking more questions, eliciting confirmation from a secondary source, or confirming the data with objective information. For example, a nurse might infer that a child is not hungry because he did not eat the pork chop and squash served at dinner. However, seeking validation of the observed behavior by asking, "You did not eat very much. Aren't you hungry tonight?" can lead the nurse to discover that the child did not like the food but would eat ravenously if given an alternative choice. Inconsistency in a client's behavior and verbal responses should always be double-checked to avoid misunderstandings or incorrect inferences. Using inaccurate or incomplete information can result in errors of problem identification in the diagnostic phase of the nursing process. Validating data prevents missing information, misunderstanding situations, jumping to conclusions, and focusing in the wrong direction (Alfaro-LeFevre, 1997).

## ORGANIZING DATA

It is necessary to organize collected data to identify problems and formulate nursing diagnoses. Use of an assessment tool facilitates some organization of the data during collection, but it does not always give the full picture by bringing related information together for a more holistic view of the client. Clustering data into established categories for interpretation can produce a better clinical picture of the client's strengths and problems. A nursing model is more effective for establishing nursing diagnoses because it reveals the functional health or human response patterns that nursing interventions are most effective in managing.

## REPORTING DATA

The final activity in the assessment phase is reporting abnormalities to expedite treatment and documenting all collected data in a clear, concise, and timely manner to facilitate continuity of care by other members of the healthcare team. Record specific objective observations of client status and avoid use of nonspecific terms, such as good, average, normal, and poor, that are subject to interpretation. Documented information should be written legibly and according to legal and professional standards.

Read the following case study. Then look at **Display 9-3**. The client data on Bill Akins is organized according to Gordon's (1994) functional health patterns. We will be asking questions throughout this chapter about the story of Bill and Roy Akins and their nurse, Gloria Linquist.

### CASE STUDY OF BILL AKINS

Roy Akins, age 35 years, enters his father's room at Seaview Medical Center to visit for the first time since Bill Akins, age 69 years, was admitted after experiencing a heart attack 3 days earlier. Gloria Linquist, RN, is standing at the bedside talking to Bill about the heart medications he had just taken for the first time. As Roy quickly and briefly touches his father's outstretched hand, he looks nervously at the intravenous bottles, monitors, and oxygen tubing attached to his father's nose.

*Roy:* How's it going, Dad?

*Bill:* Not too well. They say I've had a heart attack.

Gloria notices Roy's pale color, shaky voice, and trembling hands and offers him a chair.

*Gloria:* Your father has had a heart attack, and his condition is stabilizing.

*Roy:* How long does he have to stay here? I'd like to take him home as soon as possible.

*Gloria:* A few days. As soon as we get his medications regulated and his condition remains stable.

*Bill:* Could you help me get comfortable in this bed, Gloria? This is the hardest mattress I've ever laid on. I could use some fresh air and something to drink.

*Gloria:* Sure thing.

Gloria assists Bill to turn, arranges the pillow more comfortably under his head and shoulders, opens the window, and retrieves some juice from the unit kitchen.

*Gloria:* You two relax and visit for a while. I'll go see about getting a foam mattress pad for your bed. We'll go for a short walk in about an hour, Bill. Ring if you need anything.

Later, Roy comes to the nurses' station to speak with Gloria.

*Roy:* I'd like to leave the phone number of my motel so that you can get in touch with me if necessary. I'm glad my Dad's OK. I sure was scared when my sister called and told me he had a heart attack. I wasn't sure I could come visit him.

## Display 9-3   Data Organization According to Gordon's Functional Health Patterns

▶ **CLIENT DATA: BILL AKINS**

1. 69-year-old male
2. Widowed 2 years: two children
3. Occupation: retired economics professor
4. Religion: Baptist
5. Ht: 5 ft 11 in; weight: 170 lb
6. T: 98°F; P: 62, irregular; R: 16
7. BP: 112/64
8. Alert and oriented
9. Swims 4 days a week at college pool
10. Walks a 3-mile course 3 days a week
11. Smoked cigars and pipe for 30 years; quit 8 years ago
12. Lungs clear
13. Episodic mild-moderate chest pain with activity controlled with nitroglycerin SL
14. Voiding clear urine; 250-300 mL every 3-4 h
15. No bowel movement in 3 days
16. Son states hospitals terrify him.
17. Son asks lots of questions about father's condition.
18. Son and daughter visit frequently.
19. Allergic to ampicillin
20. Patient states he likes to take care of himself; doesn't want to be a burden to children.
21. Awakens frequently during night
22. Wants to know what kind of activity restrictions he will have
23. Likes to barbecue and picnic in summer with family members
24. Intermittent headaches relieved with Tylenol
25. Abdominal cramping; passing gas
26. Bedrest

▶ **DATA ORGANIZATION BY FUNCTIONAL HEALTH PATTERNS**

Health perception–health management pattern: 9, 10, 20
Nutritional metabolic pattern: 5, 6, 7, 11, 12, 14, 15, 19, 23, 25
Elimination pattern: 14, 15, 24, 25, 26
Activity–exercise pattern: 9, 10, 13, 22, 23
Cognitive–perceptual pattern: 8
Sleep–rest pattern: 13, 21, 24
Self-perception–self-concept pattern: 20
Role-relationship pattern: 1, 2, 3, 4, 17, 18
Sexuality–reproductive pattern: 2
Coping–stress tolerance pattern: 11, 13, 22, 24
Value–belief pattern: 4, 20

## ▶ Thinking Critically

1. List the subjective data the nurse would obtain from Bill and Roy.

2. What objective data would Gloria be collecting about Bill and Roy?

# Diagnosis

When the nurse has completed the collection, validation, and organization of client data, it is time to begin the second phase of the nursing process to analyze and synthesize the data to determine what the client needs. The purpose of the second phase is to determine the actual problems, the human response condition for which the client is at risk.

The use of the nursing diagnosis to describe what nurses can do for clients experiencing a human response to injury or illness is still somewhat controversial and inconsistently applied in clinical nursing practice. Resistance may arise from reluctance to devote the time it takes to develop a nursing diagnosis, confusion about the difference between nursing and medical diagnoses, or confusion about the changing terminology proposed by NANDA.

## NURSING DIAGNOSIS DEFINED

As defined by NANDA, the nursing diagnosis is a clinical judgment about individual, family, or community responses to actual or potential health problems or life process. Nursing diagnoses provide the basis for the selection of nursing interventions to achieve outcomes for which the nurse is accountable (NANDA, 2001).

The activities in the diagnostic phase include:

1. Identifying patterns or clustering data;
2. Validating diagnosis; and
3. Formulating diagnostic statements.

## IDENTIFYING PATTERNS

The interrelationship of the assessment phase and the diagnosis phase occurs when the nurse organizes data and identifies patterns to determine the client's nursing diagnosis.

The ability to cluster data intuitively and to identify problems develops with experience (Benner, 2001). Nursing students and beginning practitioners should expect to follow guides and use resources to accomplish this diagnostic activity. Caution should be taken to avoid making decisions about client strengths and problems with insufficient, inaccurate, or inconsistent information. If cues do not match or seem inadequate for the category, additional information should be gathered (focused assessment) to validate the diagnosis. **Display 9-4** provides an example of data analysis for the clinical example of Bill Akins.

## VALIDATING DIAGNOSIS

When the client's information has been analyzed and a nursing diagnosis selected, it needs to be validated with the client. Validation with the client provides an opportunity to examine the client's perception of the problem and determine if there is a willingness to participate in its resolution. Through validation, the client's motivation and desires regarding care can be realized. Some clients are not ready or motivated to resolve problems that are clearly evident to healthcare providers. Use of client validation allows the client to be an informed and willing participant in his or her care.

## Display 9-4   Data Analysis for Clinical Example of Bill Akins

Gloria has a concern about Bill Akins' level of rest and reviews the clustered cues for his sleep-rest pattern category:

1. Episodic mild–moderate chest pain with activity; controlled with nitroglycerin SL
2. Awakens frequently during night
3. Intermittent headaches relieved with Tylenol

Before drawing any conclusions about Bill's inability to achieve a restful sleep at night, Gloria questions the completeness and accuracy of the existing information and conducts a focused assessment. Although she knows that he awakens frequently during the night, no information indicates the reason for this. Gloria further evaluates the physiologic, psychological, and environmental factors that might be contributing to Bill's inability to get a good night's rest.

Gloria's focused assessment includes the following:

1. Frequency of voidings secondary to increases in diuretics
2. His tolerance for unit noise, lights, and presence of staff in the room; noise and activities concerning other patients in the unit
3. Bill's concern over his condition, fear of dying, and lifestyle changes after discharge
4. Bill's level of comfort and frequency of chest pain during the night
5. Bill's ability to obtain rest during other periods during the day

## FORMULATING DIAGNOSTIC STATEMENTS

When you have completed the assessment phase and have clustered the data, it is time to determine if the client's situation is normal, altered, or at risk for altered functioning and to name the problem by using the NANDA label that most closely matches your patient's cues. Patients can have four types of nursing problems: actual, risk for, possible, and wellness diagnoses (**Display 9-5**).

If the client is acutely ill, you will be formulating an actual nursing diagnostic statement. Such a statement has three parts. Because it is an actual problem, this is the *only* nursing diagnostic statement that has all three parts. A list of problem descriptions (title/labels and definitions) has been developed by NANDA for clinical use and testing. These are sometimes called the NANDA stems because they need to be selected from a standardized list that comes from NANDA (see Appendix C). The list is reviewed and updated every 2 years. Each NANDA stem (a problem statement) is accompanied by a list of defining characteristics (a cluster of signs and symptoms commonly associated with the diagnosis) and related causes or etiologies (factors that cause or contribute to the problem).

## Display 9-5   Types of Nursing Diagnostic Statements

**Actual:** Three-part nursing diagnostic statement
**Risk for:** Two-part nursing statement
**Possible:** Two-part nursing statement
**Wellness:** Two-part nursing statement

> **Display 9-6**

# The PES Format for Writing Actual Nursing Diagnostic Statements

P = problem statement (NANDA stem)
E = Etiology or causes/risk factors
S = Signs/symptoms: defining characteristics

When writing diagnostic statements, use the proper components of the PES format (P = problem; E = etiology or cause; and S = sign/symptoms supporting the problem), as outlined in **Display 9-6**.

Link the NANDA stem (problem) and etiology (cause) with the words "related to" (RT), and state the signs/symptoms (defining characteristics) that support the diagnosis with the phrase "as evidenced by" (AEB).

Here are more examples of actual nursing diagnostic statements.

- Constipation related to bed rest and lack of exercise, as evidenced by decreased frequency of bowel movements, headache, and abdominal cramping.
- Ineffective airway clearance related to excessive, tenacious secretions and inability to cough, as evidenced by copious amounts of thick gray sputum and weak coughing.

**Risk Diagnosis** ▼ The client's database shows evidence of related risk factors but no evidence of defining characteristics. The following are examples.

- Risk for infection related (RT) to break in integument
- Risk for injury RT diminished visual acuity
- Risk for ineffective coping RT complex self-care regimen

**Possible Diagnosis** ▼ A possible diagnosis is formulated when the nurse has insufficient data on defining characteristics and related risk factors to make a definitive diag-

---

# NCLEX–RN Might Ask 9-2   ? ? ?

The nurse is formulating a nursing diagnostic statement for a client with an actual health care problem. Which of the following statements is *correct* regarding an actual nursing problem?

    A. Ineffective airway clearance RT thick sputum
    B. Risk for fall RT weakness and orthostatic hypotension
    C. Sleep pattern disturbance RT death of spouse AEB inability to get to sleep and excess sleepiness during the day
    D. Decreased cardiac output RT ineffective heart pumping and death of myocardial tissue

- *See Appendix A for correct answer and rationale.*

nosis. In this situation, the nurse selects the problem that appears to be most probable, and the diagnostic statement is written like an actual diagnosis, except the etiology is stated as "unknown cause" or "unknown etiology." The following are examples.

- Possible interrupted family processes related to unknown cause
- Possible disturbed sleep pattern related to unknown etiology

**Wellness Diagnosis ▼** A wellness diagnosis is formulated when a healthy client wants to attain a higher level of function in a specific area. Wellness diagnoses are written as one-part statements using the phrase "potential for enhanced" followed by the listed problem label. The following are examples.

- Potential for enhanced community coping
- Potential for enhanced therapeutic regimen management

---

## ▶ Thinking Critically

Review the database for Bill Akins in Display 9-3, and write actual, possible, and potential (risk) nursing diagnoses using the PES format.

### 1. Actual Nursing Diagnosis

NANDA stem: _____

Etiology (RT): _____

Signs/symptoms (AEB):

### 2. Possible Nursing Diagnosis

NANDA stem: _____

Etiology (RT): _____

### 3. Potential Nursing Diagnosis

NANDA stem (risk for): _____

Etiology (RT): _____

- *See Appendix B for answers.*

---

## MEDICAL VERSUS NURSING DIAGNOSES

Medical diagnoses and nursing diagnoses differ in several ways. Medical diagnoses identify disease and organ dysfunctions, whereas nursing diagnoses describe the client's response to actual or potential health problems or conditions. A second major difference is that medical diagnoses do not change as long as the disease is present, whereas nursing diagnoses can change from day to day as the client's response to illness changes. Most significantly, medical diagnoses require medical intervention and

**TABLE 9-3**
COMPARISON OF NURSING VERSUS MEDICAL DIAGNOSIS

| Medical Diagnosis | Nursing Diagnosis |
|---|---|
| Strep throat | Ineffective thermoregulation |
| Cerebral vascular incident (stroke) | Risk for injury |
| Chemical burn | Impaired skin integrity |
| Alzheimer's disease | Wandering |

treatment, whereas nursing diagnoses are within the legal scope of independent nursing practice. The use of medical diagnoses in nursing diagnostic statements should be avoided when possible (**Table 9-3**).

## COLLABORATIVE PROBLEMS

When interventions require medical and nursing treatment, a collaborative health problem exists. A collaborative problem is an actual or potential physiological complication to a disease, injury, treatment, or diagnostic study for which the nurse shares accountability for treating with the physician. Nursing care for a collaborative problem is directed toward detecting and reporting actual and potential complications that require medical intervention, implementing medical interventions, and initiating nursing interventions to manage the problem.

Because the focus of a collaborative problem is a potential complication(s) of a problem, the statement begins with PC (for "potential complication"), followed by a colon, and a list of the complications that might occur. For clarity, the potential complication and the collaborative problem are linked with "related to." The following examples depict the format to use when writing collaborative problems:

**PC:** Dysrhythmia related to myocardial infarction
**PC:** Infection related to intravenous therapy

# Planning

The planning phase of the nursing process involves developing strategies to resolve the client's identified problems and help the client achieve an optimal level of functioning. When possible, client strengths identified in the diagnostic phase should be used to resolve problems. Planning and implementation activities often occur concurrently in simple or complex situations. The written plan of care is a major outcome for this step in the nursing process. Planning phase activities include the following:

Establishing priorities
Establishing client goals and outcomes
Planning nursing interventions
Writing an individualized plan of care

| Display 9-7 | Establishing Priorities for Nursing Diagnoses: Questions the RN Should Ask |
|---|---|

1. Does it involve the ABC of emergency care?
2. Can you use Maslow's hierarchy of needs?
3. How many symptoms does the client exhibit?
4. What priority does the client place on the problem?

## ESTABLISHING PRIORITIES

The initial step in developing a nursing care plan is to examine the identified needs and set priorities. The ABCs of CPR can be used when setting priorities because they allow quick and easy screening for problems that require immediate attention (suctioning an airway, breathing, circulation, etc). Maslow's (1968) hierarchy of needs may be used with problems that are not life threatening (positioning, pain, nutrition), need referral to others (diet consultation), or require ongoing attention (wound care, counseling). Priorities are set by considering the severity of the situation (life-threatening conditions take priority over personal enrichment) and recognizing the differences between clients. A plan is tailored to meet the client's individualized needs. One client may be ready and willing to perform his or her own dressing change after watching the nurse one or two times, whereas another may need a supportive family member to do it. **Display 9-7** shows a few suggestions on how to establish priorities for client nursing diagnoses.

## ESTABLISHING EXPECTED OUTCOMES

The terms *goals*, *objectives*, and *expected outcomes* are often used interchangeably in practice, references, and educational situations. Generally, a patient goal or objective is a general description or broad statement about the state of the client, whereas an outcome is more specific. Most often, a goal or objective is a reflection of the problem.

**Problem:** Self-concept disturbance
**Goal:** Positive self-concept

---

### NCLEX–RN Might Ask 9-3   ❓❓❓

The nurse has identified the following problems list for a client who has been admitted to a long-term care facility. Which of the following would be a top priority nursing diagnosis?

   A. Constipation
   B. Activity intolerance
   C. Risk for decreased cardiac output
   D. Ineffective airway clearance

• *See Appendix A for correct answer and rationale.*

Client expected outcomes are written statements of specific, measurable, realistic, and timed statements of goal attainment. They restate the goal and present information that facilitates evaluation. Expected outcomes help all the nurses involved in a client's care to know specifically what the planned care is trying to accomplish.

> **Problem:** Risk for self-esteem disturbance related to perceived effects on sexuality
> **Goals:** Client will communicate feelings about hysterectomy before the surgery.

Client will acknowledge changes in body structure and function.

The ANA's *Standards for Clinical Practice* (1998) specifically states that expected outcomes need to be individually tailored to clients. The standards address six criteria that planning outcomes must achieve. **Display 9-8** lists the ANA's criteria for measurable outcomes.

Alfaro-LeFevre (2002) recommends a five-part outcome statement: subject (client), a verb (will walk), condition (with walker), criteria (50 ft), and specific time (three times a day). If the subject is assumed to be the client for whom the nursing care plan is written, the outcome statement begins with the verb. The following are examples.

1. *Nursing problem:* Imbalanced nutrition: less than body requirements. *Goal:* Improved nutritional status. *Expected outcome:* (Client and family members) will gain 5 pounds by the end of 5 weeks.
2. *Nursing problem:* Acute pain. *Goal:* Decrease pain. *Expected outcome:* (Client) will rate pain as 0 to 1 on a 1 to 10 scale within 4 hours.

Verbs used in outcome statements should be behavioral, measurable, and specific. Choose action verbs that measure success. Verbs such as *know*, *understand*, *think*, *accept*, and *feel* should be avoided.

Goals may be short or long term, depending on the specific problem being addressed. Short-term goals can be achieved in a few hours, a day, or a week. Long-term goals require more time, perhaps several weeks or months. Care should be taken to sequence large objectives into smaller increments to prevent discouragement and

---

**Display 9-8    Measurable Outcome Criteria According to the ANA**

1. Expected outcomes must be related to the nursing diagnosis.
2. When appropriate, expected outcomes must be formulated with the target population (i.e., patient, family, community).
3. Expected outcomes must address current and potential capabilities of the client and be culturally sensitive.
4. Expected outcomes need to take into consideration the resources available to the client.
5. Expected outcomes need to provide continuity of care.
6. Expected outcomes must be documented as measurable goals.

## NCLEX–RN Might Ask 9-4   ❓❓❓

The nurse is designing expected outcomes for a client with the nursing diagnosis of excess fluid volume related to (RT) excess oral fluid intake as evidenced by (AEB) S3 heart sounds and crackles in the lungs. Which of the following would be a properly written expected outcome for this client?

A. The client will list foods high in cholesterol.
B. The client will have an output greater than intake within the next 4 hours.
C. The client will lose 5 pounds within the next week.
D. The client will have his/her lung sounds assessed every 4 hours.

• *See Appendix A for correct answer and rationale.*

ensure compliance with the care plan. For example, a client who wishes to lose 150 pounds may become discouraged when facing a weight reduction goal of such magnitude. A more realistic approach may be a goal of 5 pounds per month.

### ▶ Thinking Critically

Write goal or client outcome statements for the nursing diagnoses you developed for Bill Akins in the previous Thinking Critically activity.

• *See Appendix B for answers.*

## PLANNING NURSING INTERVENTIONS

In the planning phase, it is important to identify specific nursing measures that can resolve the issues and problems identified in the diagnostic phase. Nursing interventions are activities performed by the nurse in the implementation phase. They consist of any nursing treatment that a nurse performs for a client, including ongoing assessing for possible complications, teaching, counseling, consulting, giving referrals, and performing direct client care tasks, such as bathing, dressing, toileting, and ambulating. Sometimes this may be referred to as the "AMT method." **Display 9-9** gives the components of the AMT method of writing nursing interventions.

Nurses use their clinical judgment and experience to determine which nursing actions and activities will best achieve established client-centered goals and out-

### *Display 9-9*   **Nursing Interventions: The AMT Method**

A = Assessments: What ongoing assessments do I need to perform?
M = Measures: What nursing interventions do I need to do?
T = Teaching: What kinds of teaching do I need to do with this client?

comes. Standardized planning guides are usually available in nursing schools and clinical practice settings to make the work of planning care easier. However, these plans are guides that need to be adapted and individualized to each client situation. In using standard plans, such as standards of care, standard care plans, and critical pathways, it is important to screen the material and apply only information that applies to a particular client. Not all the information given in a standard plan is applicable to every client. In addition, the nurse must use scientific rationale for the selected interventions and be creative and willing to add alternative activities and actions so that nothing is missed. When used correctly by nursing students and clinical nurses, standard plans can provide valuable direction for developing an individualized nursing care plan. If used incorrectly, they can block professional growth and may bring harm to a client.

## WRITTEN PLAN OF CARE

Once the interventions are identified, it is time to write a nursing care plan (nursing orders) so that all nursing personnel involved in the client's care have clear direction for implementing the plan of care. The written plan needs to include the nursing orders, which clearly reflect the four dimensions of any nursing action: assessing,

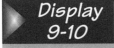

## Display 9-10   Sample Individualization of Standard Nursing Care Plan

**Nursing Diagnosis:** Risk of ineffective thermoregulation related to limited metabolic compensatory regulation secondary to age (neonate)

**Client-centered goals/outcomes:**
1. Infant will maintain temperature between 36.4° and 37°C. (target date)
2. Parents will explain and demonstrate techniques that keep infant's temperature stable/normal. (target date)

| Standardized Care Plan | Individualized Care Plan |
| --- | --- |
| 1. Monitor infant's temperature. | 1. Assess axillary temperature every hour until stable after birth; check once per shift thereafter. |
| 2. Teach parents how to protect infant from hypothermia and hyperthermia. | 2. Show parents how to dress and bundle infant for home and outings and how to conserve heat during bathing. Explain how to protect infant from drafts and heat loss in the environment. |
| 3. Reduce/eliminate sources of heat loss; prevent hyperthermia. | 3. Wrap infant in one or two blankets; use that and booties if appropriate to keep temperature between 37.4° and 37°C; protect from dampness, drafts, and cold surfaces. Keep room temperature at 70°F. Place infant in crib away from windows, doors, and walls. |
| 4. Make referrals to community resources for infant care. | 4. Offer free public health/neonatal nursing home visit(s) after discharge. Give name, address, telephone number, or appointment to well-baby clinic or pediatrician. |

doing and teaching. Note in **Display 9-10** that nursing orders include these dimensions.

Written nursing orders should be specific, clear, and always contain the date the order was written, the action to be performed, who is to do it, and a descriptive phrase that includes all the specifics needed for the activity (how, when, where, how much, how long). For example, 4/2/95: Assist Kate to walk to the end of hall with walker 10 AM, 1 PM, 4 PM, and 7 PM daily. M. Wilson, RN.

Written nursing care plans come in a variety of designs, including portable cards, Kardexes, multiple-page forms, or computer-generated documents. Despite the differences in forms, the basic components for written care plans are inclusion of the nursing diagnosis, client-centered outcomes, and specific nursing interventions. Nurses and nursing students need to become competent in the use of whatever type is required in their own clinical practice or educational program settings to implement and document a client's care properly.

## ▶ Thinking Critically

Write nursing orders for the outcome criteria you developed for Bill Akins in the previous Thinking Critically activity. Be sure to include interventions appropriate for reassessing, doing, and teaching activities of nursing care.

• *See Appendix B for answers.*

# Implementation

Implementation is the action phase of the nursing process. During this phase, the written nursing care plan is followed, and the nursing orders are executed to move the client toward achievement of his or her established goals. Implementation activities include the following.

- Reassess
- Set priorities
- Perform or delegate nursing interventions
- Document actions

## REASSESSING

Implementation requires more that just doing; it requires revisiting some of the activities used in previous phases to ensure that new events and changes in the client's situation are constantly being identified and incorporated into the client's care. In each client encounter, the nurse gathers information on the client's condition to identify changing problems. The data obtained are used to document the client's condition and evaluate if nursing interventions are effective and if client outcomes are being met.

## SETTING PRIORITIES

Just as priorities were established during the diagnostic phase, priorities need to be re-established on a daily and sometimes hourly basis to ensure that the client's immediate needs are met.

## PERFORMING OR DELEGATING NURSING INTERVENTIONS

The RN carries the primary authority and responsibility for directing client care in institutional and community settings. When implementing the plan, the nurse either performs the interventions personally or delegates them to another member of the nursing team (nursing assistant or LPN). When a group of clients is under the care of a nurse, the nurse is responsible for assessing and reviewing the plan of care with each client and communicating the needs and schedule of planned interventions with the other members of the nursing care team. The nurse generally reserves direct performance of nursing interventions for educating, communicating, and providing complex technical skills and procedures.

# Evaluation

Evaluation is the final step in the nursing process. It is recognized as a separate, distinct phase and an ongoing process (Alfaro-LeFevre, 2002). Evaluation might be described as using nursing process within nursing process. Activities include reassessment, rediagnosis, replanning, and in some situations, reimplementation. The goal, not each intervention, should be evaluated (**Display 9-11**). When possible, the client and family should participate in the evaluation of goal attainment.

Nurses begin evaluation by reviewing client goals/expected outcomes to determine if they were measurable, realistic, and appropriate for resolving the client's problems. It is then necessary to collect data about the client's condition, being alert for changes and unknown factors that have positively or negatively influenced goal achievement.

Barriers and facilitators to goal achievement may be unknown factors, such as client reactions, worsening condition, cultural beliefs, moral values, and religious beliefs of the family. Reviewing how the nursing team applied the interventions is equally important when developing a comprehensive database on which to make a judgment about goal attainment.

After collecting subjective and objective data, the nurse analyzes the information to formulate a conclusion about the client's behavioral responses to the nursing interventions used. Some nursing diagnoses will be resolved, whereas others will be completely or partially unmet. It also is possible for new problems and new diagnoses to

---

> *Display 9-11*   **Evaluation of the Goal**

Goals/expected outcomes are evaluated.
Interventions are not evaluated.

develop simultaneously. If the nursing diagnosis is resolved, it can be eliminated from the plan. Partially met nursing diagnoses should be additionally assessed, and necessary modifications should be made to the plan of care. If new problems have developed, new nursing diagnoses should be identified and a new plan of treatment written.

## Conclusion

The nurse uses the nursing process in a variety of settings with clients of all ages to identify actual and potential health issues and problems and to design strategies for resolving them.

This chapter has provided a brief review of the five basic steps of the process and has explored its application in meeting the goals/expected outcomes of nursing care. By providing individualized care through a combination of independent and collaborative actions, nurses are valued contributors to the healthcare system in providing holistic, comprehensive care.

## References

Alfaro-LeFevre, R. (2002). *Applying nursing process: A step-by-step guide* (5th ed.). Philadelphia: Lippincott Williams and Wilkins.

American Nurses Association (ANA). (1998). *Standards of clinical nursing practice* (2nd ed.) Washington, DC: Author.

Benner, P. (2001). *From nurse to expert: Excellence and power in clinical nursing practice.* Upper Saddle River, NJ: Prentice-Hall Health.

Gebbie, K., & Lavin, M. A. (1974). Classifying nursing diagnoses. *American Journal of Nursing, 74*(2), 250–252.

Gordon, M. (1994). *Nursing diagnosis: Process and application.* St. Louis: Mosby Yearbook.

Hall, L. E. (1995). Quality of nursing care. *Public Health News, June.*

Maslow, A. (1968). Toward a psychology of being (2nd ed.). New York: Van Nostrand Reinhold.

North American Nursing Diagnosis Association (NANDA). (2001). *Nursing diagnosis: Definitions and classification, 2001–2002.* Philadelphia: Author.

Yura, H., & Walsh, M. B. (1988). *The nursing process: Assessing, planning, implementing, evaluating* (5th ed.). Norwalk, CT: Appleton-Century-Crofts.

## Suggested Reading

Ackley, B. & Ladwig, G. (2002). *Nursing diagnosis handbook: A guide to planning care* (5th ed.). St. Louis: Mosby.

Craven, R. F., & Hirnle, C. J. (2001). *Fundamentals of nursing: Human health and function.* Philadelphia: Lippincott Williams & Wilkins.

Carpenito, L. (2002). *Nursing diagnosis: Application to clinical practice* (9th ed.). Philadelphia: Lippincott Williams & Wilkins.

Murray, M., & Atkinson, L. (2000). *Understanding the nursing process in a changing care environment.* New York: McGraw-Hill.

Rubenfeld, M. G., & Scheffer, B. K. (1995). *Critical thinking in nursing: An interactive approach.* Philadelphia: JB Lippincott.

Taylor, C., Lillis, C., & LeMone P. (2001). *Fundamentals of nursing: The art and science of nursing care* (4th ed.). Philadelphia: Lippincott Williams & Wilkins.

Wilkinson, J. M. (2001). *Nursing process and critical thinking* (3rd ed.). Upper Saddle River, NJ: Prentice-Hall.

**On the Web** ✦ . . . . . . . . . . . . . . . . . . . . . . . . . . . . . . . . . . . . .

*www.careplans.com*: Gives sample care plans.

*www.NANDA.org*: Address for NANDA for the latest discussions on what's new in the nursing diagnosis world.

*www.ncsbn.org*: Home website for the National Council of State Boards of Nursing. This site offers educational programs, NCLEX-RN style questions, and information on the latest in NCLEX-RN testing styles. The organization constantly seeks RNs for item reviewers and item writers for the NCLEX-RN.

*www.rncentral.com*: Contains a lot of information on care plans and nursing.

# The Nurse as Communicator

*By the end of this chapter, the student will be able to:*

1  Describe the importance of effective communication to quality nursing care.
2  Distinguish between therapeutic and social relationships.
3  Describe the characteristics of effective therapeutic, caring nurses
4  Discuss the two types (forms) of communication.
5  Identify factors promoting effective communication.
6  Describe blocks to communication
7  Discuss the effective communication techniques used in therapeutic communication.
8  Evaluate therapeutic communications by using a checklist or process recording
9  Describe effective communication techniques applicable across the life span.
10  Evaluate a communication scenario with clients for effective communication techniques.

## KEY TERMS

| | | |
|---|---|---|
| active listening | empower | paralanguage |
| blocks to communication | encoding | problem solving |
| caring behaviors | false assurance | process recording |
| clarification | feedback | reflection |
| cultural sensitivity | general leads | silence |
| decoding | goal oriented | social relationships |
| empathy | nonverbal communication | summarization |
| | | sympathy |

therapeutic          therapeutic humor          verbal communication
   communication          trust                              blocks

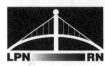

LPN ████████ RN

## VIGNETTE

James Clancy, a 48-year-old retired Irish–American firefighter, has severe bilateral arterial occlusive disease. Treatment for his disease at a rehabilitation center has failed, and tomorrow he will be sent to the hospital for bilateral above-the-knee amputations. Charles Seymour, RN, and student nurse Marie Laurent are entering Mr. Clancy's room for his morning assessment.

Today, Mr. Clancy is very disheveled, hasn't shaved, and has puffy eyes. He is very difficult to wake up.

**Marie:** Hello, Mr. Clancy. My name is Marie Laurent. I am a student nurse and will be doing your care today.

**Mr. Clancy:** Why do you always have to be doing something with me? Leave me alone. I just want to sleep.

**Marie:** Mr. Clancy, you look tired. Did you sleep well last night?

Mr. Clancy's legs are twisted together; he moves them back and forth in an agitated manner. He states in a much louder voice, "What do you think? I'm losing my legs tomorrow. Why don't you just let me die? I'm no good to anyone this way."

Marie looks at Charles with a helpless look on her face and backs away from Mr. Clancy. She remains silent but sad and thoughtful looking.

**Charles:** Was it pain in your legs that caused you to lose sleep last night, or worrying about what is going to happen?

**Mr. Clancy:** Both. What do you think! You are always doing things with me. Don't you understand how much pain I'm in. Now I hear I need to go for more tests today. I'm in agony when I get onto that stretcher.

**Charles:** (Moves closer to Mr. Clancy, leans over his bed, pauses, and looks directly at him.) I can give you something stronger for the pain and I can also ask if we can transport you for your test in your bed.

**Mr. Clancy:** All I'm asking is that someone meet me half-way. I really don't want to have this surgery, and I'm in more pain when I'm moved.

**Charles:** I feel this is a very difficult decision for you, am I wrong? (Charles pauses, stays close to Mr. Clancy, has a look of genuine concern on his face, and remains silent.)

**Mr. Clancy:** I don't want this. What will I do with the rest of my life?

**Charles:** (Responds in a dramatically quieter voice.) It sounds as if you have not made up your mind completely yet about this surgery.

**Mr. Clancy:** I still think my legs can get better.

**Charles:** Let's talk about what the doctor said yesterday and review the information those tests are telling us. Then we can call Dr. Marin and ask if he can spend some time with you if you need to . . . However, this is your decision and you have the right to refuse to have the surgery done.

Later Charles and Marie are discussing Mr. Clancy's case.

**Marie:** I never know what to say when patients get angry and upset. You handled Mr. Clancy very well.

**Charles:** It's hard to know what to say when someone is so upset. But there are some very good principles that come from communication I always remember. First, don't get into the emotions. Second, just listen and look at the nonverbal information the client sends you. Third, be human and try to get at the root of the problem from the client's perspective. Then also, I review what has worked well and what hasn't.

**Marie:** Yes, I remember some of those skills from school. I guess review and practice will make me more competent in dealing with those emotional situations.

**Charles:** Even now, I try to go to seminars and read about how to handle difficult situations. It helps!

# Effective Communication ▪▬▬▬▬▬▬▬▬▬▬

Scenarios such as the one involving Charles, Marie, and their patient Mr. Clancy are repeated many times and in many ways in a nurse's professional life. To be effective in delivering nursing care, nurses need not only to be good communicators but also to be able to skillfully defuse situations such as Mr. Clancy's. Communication is the tie that binds in human relationships and the glue of human interaction. Communication is an essential need of humans, a universal characteristic of life and living. Students of human communication have attempted to determine what is helpful or not helpful, what is detrimental, what promotes growth and satisfaction, and what blocks understanding.

The skill of communication was introduced to you in your previous nursing studies. It is one you continue to use in your clinical practice and everyday life. Many seasoned nurses say that they, like Marie, feel helpless in many circumstances. Like Charles, nurses are aware that communication is a skill that needs review and practice for a nurse to become caringly competent. This chapter contains a review of the concepts of communication (verbal and nonverbal), a review of caring and how it affects communication, and tips for effective communication with clients.

## Basic Communication Revisited

The process of communication is not a simple one. It is helpful to review the simple two-person communication model developed by Berlo (1960) **(Figure 10-1)**. This model involves many variables that affect the sender, the message, and the receiver. It all begins with a message and the sender's desire to be understood. The sender communicates the message by **encoding** verbal and nonverbal signals to the receiver. The receiver **decodes** the message, that is, tries to understand the meaning of the message. **Feedback** is given to the sender, from the receiver, and the process continues. There are many pre-existing factors that influence communication, including the physiologic and biologic characteristics of the participants. Psychological, sociocultural, and environmental variables can also alter the clarity of communication. Anywhere in this model, a breakdown in the message can happen, causing miscommunication or an inaccurate message to be conveyed between the two participants.

## Therapeutic Communication

Therapeutic communication is an essential skill for nurses in all areas of healthcare. "Therapeutic communication facilitates interactions focused on the client and the client's concerns" (Craven & Hirnle, 2003, p. 344). Communication is the medium through which all nursing services are provided.

Effective communication also is recognized as the basis of working productively with team members or work groups in the planning and provision of patient care. Nurses need more than a theory basis for pathology, patient behaviors and symptoms, and the requisite nursing care. They also must be able to communicate patient observations, make referrals, and participate in nursing care-planning conferences and interdisciplinary care conferences. Nurses must be able to provide effective and accurate reports about patient status, interpret

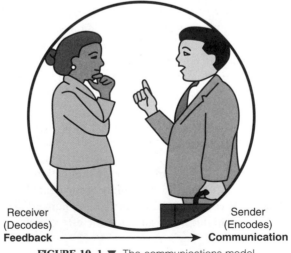

Receiver
(Decodes)
**Feedback** ⟶

Sender
(Encodes)
**Communication**

**FIGURE 10–1 ▼** The communications model.

**TABLE 10-1**
CHARACTERISTICS OF SOCIAL AND THERAPEUTIC RELATIONSHIPS

| Social | Therapeutic |
|---|---|
| Self-serving | Client goal oriented |
| Polite | Respectful, sincere, patient |
| Superficial content | Feelings and emotional content |
| Sympathy | Empathy |
| Lacks clarity/validation | Clarity/validation essential |
| Minimal problem solving | Effective problem solving/coping |

policies and procedures relating to nursing care, give directives to other caregivers, and coordinate the care provided by a number of members of the healthcare team. Nurses must also use newer technology in promoting communication. The use of videotapes, faxes, computers, and cellular phones has had an impact on how nurses go about the care of clients.

## Characteristics of Therapeutic Communication

The characteristics of therapeutic communication can be identified as nonsocial (therapeutic), client goal oriented, occurring at a feeling level, promoting problem solving by the client, empathic, and respectful. There is a difference between the social interaction reinforced by cultural beliefs, such as politeness, and therapeutic communication (**Table 10-1**). In a social interaction, communicating individuals generally attempt to fulfill self needs. Often individuals in a social conversation are not aware of or concerned about the other's feelings and needs. Most social communication dwells on factual information, which is usually of a superficial nature, rather than feelings or emotions. When emotions are discussed in a social conversation, the needs of both participants are addressed.

In contrast, therapeutic interaction involves a helping person, such as a nurse, assisting someone in physical or emotional need to gain better understanding and satisfaction of that need through verbal and nonverbal techniques. The nurse plans interaction that focuses on the client's needs, rather than the nurse's needs. This interaction is designed to empower the client to see his or her needs better and thereby change behaviors for more effective and satisfying living. To promote this process, nurses must learn and update effective caring techniques.

## NCLEX–RN Might Ask 10-1

The use of therapeutic communication by the nurse in client interaction is *primarily* done to

    A. foster dependence on the nurse.
    B. discuss the client's inner secrets.
    C. allow the client to trust the nurse.
    D. obtain information required for goal-oriented nursing care.

• *See Appendix A for correct answer and rationale.*

# Characteristics of Effective Therapeutic ▬▬▬ Caring Nurses

Therapeutic relationships are more effective if the nurse demonstrates caring behaviors. These are displayed by the nonverbal and verbal cues the nurse uses to establish, promote, and terminate the relationship. **Display 10-1** lists caring characteristics used by successful nurses to help patients problem solve.

## Trust

The nurse must establish trust with the client to be an effective communicator and change agent. Keeping promises, being there, and using therapeutic communications that accept the client's feelings as valid can establish trust. The client needs to trust that what happens to him/her is kept in judicious confidence. The nurse needs to respect the client and show genuineness in his/her treatment. Patience and understanding shown by the nurse can be helpful when the client's verbalization of feelings is often painful and time consuming.

## Empathy

A distinction between sympathy and empathy is helpful. Sympathy is common in social relationships. It is described as being sorry for the individual with the need, reacting to the situation as a friend would under the same circumstance. In contrast, empathy is attempting to understand the situation without being judgmental or experiencing the emotional involvement of being immersed in the situation. The nurse tries to understand the client by mentally placing himself/herself in the client's situation.

## Therapeutic Humor

Humor can be a powerful tool physiologically and psychologically when used in both patient and staff communication. Done with common sense and in good taste considering the individual, laughter and humor have been known to stimulate the immune system, increase pulmonary volumes, and promote coughing as well as increase cardiac exercise by increasing the heart rate (McGhee, 1998; Cousins, 1983). Psychologically, well-timed humor can diminish anger and frustration and lead to the release of tension.

---

> ### Display 10-1 | Caring Characteristics

| | |
|---|---|
| Trustworthy | Warm |
| Knowledgeable | Patient |
| Nonjudgmental | Authentic |
| Empathetic | Respectful |
| Genuine | Understanding |
| Accepting | Use of humor |

A smile and a relaxed attitude are the easiest to present initially but can be hard to do on a very busy day. However, they help to set a positive tone to the conversation and show caring early in the relationship. There are many other ways to enhance humor appropriately. Cartoons, toys and props, joke books, and videotapes can be provided to promote therapeutic humor. Many hospitals now encourage the use of clowns and volunteers to cheer clients and provide diversion from pain. Many websites promote the use of professional, therapeutic humor in the workplace.

Negative humor can be harmful or offensive to the client. **Display 10-2** lists times when humor and laughter are inappropriate and may be perceived as unprofessional. There are no hard, fast rules with laughter and humor, but considering individual variations in taste, humor is best approached in a test-the-waters manner. Go slowly and try a few light comments, noting the nonverbal and verbal reactions in the client. If the client is open to the approach, more techniques may be added but always with observation of the client's reaction.

# Two Forms of Communication: Nonverbal and Verbal

In the model of communication (see Figure 10-1), the sender and receiver impart both nonverbal and verbal messages (or cues), which are exquisitely interrelated. Nonverbal behaviors support, emphasize, or contradict what the verbal part of the message implies. Although the predominant cultures of the United States emphasize and consciously recognize verbal communication as most important, most communication is nonverbal. There needs to be congruency and consistency between the verbal message the nurse is trying to express, or trust in the nurse may not be established. Techniques that can be successful in promoting effective communication include active listening, judicious use of silence, speaking clearly and distinctly, maintaining eye contact and open body gestures, simplicity of word use, and caring touch **(Display 10-3)**. Nurses are usually aware of their verbal statements but may be unaware of what they "telegraph" or tell the client with nonverbal cues.

---

**Display 10-2**  |  **Inappropriate Situations for the Use of Humor**

Timing is important for the effect of humor to be a positive experience. The nurse should use caution when engaging in humorous, playful behavior when the client is

- Trying to communicate something important
- Receiving unexpected and unwelcome test/diagnostic results
- In the same room with a patient who is very ill
- New and the nurse hasn't established a trusting relationship yet
- Offended by content (i.e., age, religion, sex, race)
- "Put down" by the nurse's use of sarcasm
- Showing nonverbal signs of wanting a more serious relationship
- Experiencing pain from the act of laughter (abdominal or chest sutures)

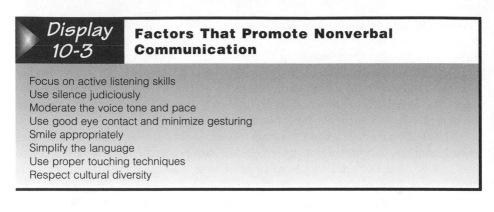

Display
10-3

**Factors That Promote Nonverbal Communication**

Focus on active listening skills
Use silence judiciously
Moderate the voice tone and pace
Use good eye contact and minimize gesturing
Smile appropriately
Simplify the language
Use proper touching techniques
Respect cultural diversity

# Nonverbal Communication

## ACTIVE LISTENING

"Successful communication occurs when you hear what people mean, not just what they say" (Fontaine & Fletcher, 1999, p. 91.) Active listening helps establish and maintain the trust and genuineness necessary in the helping relationship. It is the most therapeutic aspect a nurse can use. The nurse's attitude is paramount for active listening. The nurse needs to convey readiness to hear and understand what the client wants to say without argument, judgment, or interruption. Although silence is passive, active listening is not. As the name implies, it requires intense action and concentration on the part of the nurse. Nonverbal and verbal information are processed and understood. Active listening behaviors can be observed and learned from a seasoned nurse mentor but must be actively practiced to work effectively within the nurse's practice.

Behaviors a nurse can perform to enhance attentive listening are called the "posture of involvement." The nurse should turn toward the client and lean slightly forward. To convey an open and less threatening position, the nurse should make an attempt to be at the client's eye level when possible. This will make the client feel less like he is being talked "down to" or being "talked at" and more like an equal partner in the communication. Moving closer to the client without violating his body space will help lessen the distance from formal to therapeutic.

Timing is critical with active listening. Every effort should be made to decrease interruptions at this time. In the home setting, it may mean to turn off televisions or radios. In the hospital it may mean drawing the curtain and pulling up a chair momentarily. Decreasing interruptions allows both nurse and client to focus on emotions, facts, and problem solving.

## SILENCE

Silence can be both a nonverbal and a verbal technique of enhancing quality discussion. Silence on the nurse's part allows full concentration on the client and promotes a caring, attentive attitude. The proper use of silence decreases the pace and allows the nurse to observe and interpret the client's meaning. The nurse may miss valuable information and cues if the sometimes uncomfortable void of silence is full of meaningless conversation.

## PARALANGUAGE

Clarity, quality, pitch, tone, and tempo of the spoken word are called paralanguages. Paralanguage deals with "how" a word or words are said, independent of "what" is said. Speak to the client in a clear, moderate voice at a medium rate of speed. Mumbled, indistinct, fast communication can be misinterpreted, even in clients without special needs. It may also contradict caring behaviors the nurse wants to foster. Speaking clearly presents a clear message. Try to stick to one subject at a time. Use verbal checks periodically throughout the conversation to determine if your intentions have been clear to the client.

## EYE CONTACT, BODY POSTURES, AND GESTURES

Eye contact and moderate body gestures can enhance the quality of effective nurse–patient interaction. Friendly, open eye contact by the nurse promotes interest and caring. Comfortable eye contact is not glancing, darting, shifting, or fixed. An inability by the nurse or patient to maintain eye contact may convey anger, mistrust, or even suspicion.

The nurse must be culturally sensitive when using eye contact. In Asian and Hispanic cultures, direct eye contact can indicate disrespect. Patients from these cultures may not look at the nurse directly and may give the impression that they are not sincere. The nurse needs to be culturally sensitive when deal with nonverbal messages from other cultures. Chapter 12 contains more information on cultural sensitivity.

Although eye contact is dictated by cultural norms, facial expressions are not. Charles Darwin (1872) noted facial expressions as having universal meanings. Laughing, smiling, frowning, and crying convey similar emotions transculturally. The nurse needs to adopt a friendly, open facial expression initially. The nurse who frowns or nervously paces the room indicates nonverbally she/he has terminated the interaction. Warmth and caring can be displayed by a relaxed stance and posture, with shoulders level and flexible and hands unclenched.

Gestures are motions made with the body and hands that have culturally defined meanings. Uplifted hands with the head cocked may mean the communicator isn't sure in one culture but may mean something vastly differently in another. As a rule of thumb, the nurse should use a minimum of gestures if she or he is not sure of the audience's cultural heritage.

## SIMPLICITY

Nurse–client relationships require that a client interpret and understand words that have taken the nurse many years of study to understand. Clients are not unlike strangers in a land where a foreign language is being spoken. It is the nurse's role as the advocate and the healthcare worker with the most patient contact to find a way to explain words and medical problems in a way the client, family, or community can understand. Use of complex words to describe treatment, medications, or complications can confuse the client and lead to feelings of anger and frustration. The nurse should use simple terms or concrete layman's examples when describing the more complex medical protocols.

## APPEARANCE

Clients and nurses can communicate much about grooming, hygiene, and emotional and mental status by their appearance. The nurse needs to unravel the complexities of the client's nonverbal cues and correct that with verbal questioning. The nurse also needs to be acutely aware of her or his own nonverbal cues. A nurse who has clean, neatly tailored and pressed clothes, neatly manicured nails, and a prominently worn name badge conveys a strong professional self-concept as she or he enters the room. This nurse is using nonverbal cues to express a definite professional image.

There is an adage: "Looks can be deceiving." A nurse needs to question further and not make snap judgments about a client's status based on appearance alone. A client who enters a community clinic dressed in worn clothes and with untrimmed hair but who is essentially clean and has no body odor may, at first glance, convey the impression of being homeless. However, the nurse may find this client is employed but barely making ends meet. The person may also convey a high self-esteem in that he can't afford new clothes on a regular basis but is making every effort to keep up social appearances.

## TOUCH

Although touch is listed last, it is a very important nonverbal communication because it involves sensory input from the body's largest organ—the skin. Touch can be a powerful communicator of caring and acceptance. Clients are touched as a part of every nursing procedure. How the nurse performs vital signs assessment, a bed bath, or administers a medication conveys the nurse's basic philosophy about those in her or his care. Touch, like humor, should be used in small amounts with close observation paid to the client's reaction. If the nurse invades the client's "safety zone," the nurse needs to step back, increasing physical distance to restore respect and comfort (Fortinash & Holoday-Worret, 2000, p. 152).

### ► Thinking Critically

Referring to the example of the patient vignette in the introduction, visualize Mr. Clancy and the nurses. Write down the nonverbal communication Mr. Clancy is conveying to the nurses.

# Verbal Communication

Verbal communication deals with the content of "what" is said during a therapeutic interaction. Although there are many different techniques, and you have been introduced to some in your previous training, the nurse needs to refine them periodically to enhance professional effectiveness. Verbal communication is a lifelong learning skill. The nurse may use general leads, open-ended questions, sharing observations, restating, clarifying, use of silence, and summarizing in promoting effective interaction. A summary of these techniques is included in **Table 10-2**.

**TABLE 10-2**
SUMMARY OF VERBAL THERAPEUTIC COMMUNICATION TECHNIQUES

| Technique | Examples |
|-----------|----------|
| 1. General leads | "I see..." |
| | "Go on..." |
| | "I hear what you are saying." |
| 2. Open-ended relevant questions | "Where would you like to begin?" |
| | "Tell me more about what happened to you." |
| | "Can you describe what you were feeling?" |
| 3. Sharing observations | "Are you uncomfortable when you.....?" |
| | "I noticed that you have a hard time when you..." |
| | "You seem to be in more pain today...." |
| 4. Restating | *Client:* "I'm sorry about doing that." |
| | *Nurse:* "You're sorry." |
| | *Client:* "I'm angry about taking all of these pills!" |
| | *Nurse:* "You're angry about taking pills." |
| 5. Clarification | "I'm not sure I understood...." |
| | "I didn't follow that part about...." |
| | "Did I understand you to say...." |
| | "Could you give me an example of how this affects you?" |
| 6. Silence | *Client:* "I'm afraid of losing both of my legs." |
| | *Nurse:* Stops, sits down in a chair by the bed, leans close to the client, and takes an offered hand. |
| 7. Summarization | "So far we have talked about...." |
| | "I think the main ideas you have told me are...." |
| | "Have I got this straight about your problem with...." |

## GENERAL LEADS

General leads are brief words or phrases to tell the listener that reception is occurring; these leads encourage the client to communicate further. Phrases such as "I see," "Oh, then what happened," "Tell me more," and "I follow what you are saying" are useful in concentrating on promoting more informational exchange.

## OPEN-ENDED RELEVANT QUESTIONS

Open-ended questions encourage the client to elaborate on a subject. They do not require a "yes" or "no" answer. They may be useful in situations in which the client is guarded or resistant to talk. Questions may begin with "who," "what," "when," or "where." "Why" questions are usually avoided because they tend to place the client on the defensive. Open-ended questions add depth and relevance to the communication.

## SHARING AN OBSERVATION

To perform this technique, the nurse needs to observe behaviors in the client. Some examples of this include: "I haven't seen you drink anything today.... Am I wrong?" or "You seem sleepier today." Such questions are neutral and allow the client to confirm or deny the nurse's observation. They can often be used to initiate a conversation.

## RESTATING

When restating what a client has said, the nurse uses a segment of what the client has said exactly. An example is: *Patient*: "I'm afraid to do this dressing here at home." *Nurse*: "You are afraid to do this at home?" As with general leads, this technique lets the client know the nurse is following the intent of the interaction. This technique should not be relied on frequently, or the client may feel the nurse is mocking or making fun.

## CLARIFICATION

Clarification is essential to ensure effective communication. An individual may make a statement that is unclear to the interviewer. In such a situation, the interviewer must clarify the meaning of the statement. Leads such as "I don't quite understand," "Could you explain that again," and "I hear you saying" are examples of clarification. It is tempting for the novice interviewer to believe it is best to pretend to understand and hope the meaning will become clear later in the interaction. However, such an approach is usually not effective.

## SILENCE

Silence can be an effective tool in communication. Silences provide time for both participants in an interaction to analyze what has been said and plan for the next step. Silence helps the client express his or her thoughts more completely, particularly a client who tends to be quiet. A frequent deterrent to effective communication is the lack of pauses for planning. If the interviewer is unable to tolerate silence, a common habit is to talk to fill the anxiety-provoking silence. Once the interviewer recognizes the value of silence and finds the silence easier to tolerate, the client is usually able to express his or her thoughts more completely.

## SUMMARIZATION

A helpful way to conclude an interview or a therapeutic interaction is to summarize the ideas developed, clarify goals, and list the actions to be taken by the individual (summarization). Mutually acceptable goals are important in some situations. In other circumstances, the helping person must be able to accept client actions and decisions with which she or he does not agree.

---

# NCLEX–RN Might Ask 10-2

The nurse is interviewing a client. The most effective therapeutic technique a nurse can use in the communication process is

    A. general leads.
    B. active listening.
    C. using open-ended questions.
    D. a professional appearance.

• See Appendix A for correct answer and rationale.

# Verbal Communication Blocks

Verbal blocks in communication are words spoken by the nurse that decrease the ability of the nurse to get at the heart of the client's needs. They are words or phrases that are frequently used in the social setting and may be used out of sympathy. Blocks in communication include providing false assurance, giving advice, being moralistic, and changing the subject.

## False Assurances

One of the most frequently used blocks in therapeutic communication is providing false assurance to the client. "It's OK, everyone feels that way" and "You'll see, everything will be just fine" are phrases the nurse might say after a client reveals a major problem or concern. Unintentionally, the nurse has belittled the client's fears and concerns. The client may perceive that the nurse does not take him or her seriously because these statements trivialize what the client is experiencing. Each client is unique and wants the nurse to recognize his or her experience as such.

Instead of false assurances, the nurse should respond with neutral statements, such as "Tell me more about. . ." or "You sound worried or fearful about. . . ."

## Giving Advice

Although clients frequently ask the nurse what she/he would do, giving advice may prematurely end the interaction with the client. Clients are really not asking for advice; they are using the nurse as a sounding board to process through decision making. The client may feel that the nurse is controlling the client by telling her or him what to do. Giving advice also fosters a feeling of dependency and leads the client to believe the nurse knows what is best for the client. Statements that indicate advice giving include "The best thing for you do is. . .," "Why don't you. . .," and "If I were you I'd. . . ."

The best way to eliminate this behavior by the nurse is to be aware of it as a pitfall to the client. Alternatives to giving advice include "I wonder if you've considered. . . ." and "Maybe we should look at. . . ." In this way the nurse, instead of imposing her or his will, is asking the client to explore options.

## Being Moralistic

When a nurse responds with a moralistic statement, she or he is adopting a judgmental attitude. Like giving advice, it negates the client's right to choose and belittles feelings the client may express. The nurse needs to be aware of personal values and how they can affect client interaction. Transcending these values will allow the client the respect and right to choose what he or she wants. Moralistic statements, such as "I'm glad you've come to your senses" and "You should never feel that way," should be revised to be more neutral in tone—for example, "You sound upset" or "Tell me more about how you feel."

## Changing the Subject

Changing the subject is introducing an unrelated topic into the discussion. This diverts the client from revealing intended feelings and thoughts. The nurse may react by changing the subject when the content is sudden and a surprise or when the subject is too painful for the nurse to discuss. This block in communication tells the client the nurse is no longer listening, and it is a very quick way to end the interaction. A sample of this block would be:

> *Client:* "I want to kill myself right now."
> *Nurse:* "Did you have any visitors today?"

One of the easiest ways to deal with surprise revelations is the use of silence. The adage, "If you don't know what to say, don't say anything" may be helpful for the nurse to keep in mind. However, silence cannot be the nurse's only communication tool, or the client will question the nurse's competence.

A summary of types of blocks in communication is included in **Table 10-3**.

# Process Recordings

Newer technologies provide ways for nurses to practice and improve their therapeutic communications. Interactive videotape, role playing, and computerized learning scenarios can safely simulate the proper use of therapeutic techniques until the student gains comfort. In your class work, you may be asked to videotape or audiotape your interaction with another student and analyze that conversation. It may be helpful to use a checklist **(Display 10-4)** to fine-tune your use of therapeutic techniques.

A common teaching tool used to refine therapeutic communication used in nursing programs is a process recording. According to Varcarolis (2002), "process recordings are written records of a segment from the nurse–client session that reflect as closely as possible the verbal and nonverbal behaviors of both the nurse

---

**T A B L E   1 0 - 3**
**SUMMARY OF BLOCKS IN COMMUNICATION**

| Technique | Examples |
| --- | --- |
| 1. False assurances | "Don't worry."<br>"Things will all work out for the best." |
| 2. Giving advice | "I think you should..."<br>"Everyone I know does this when this happens." |
| 3. Being moralistic | "You should be ashamed of your behavior."<br>"Someone your age should..." |
| 4. Changing the subject | *Client:* "I have been very depressed for about a week."<br>*Nurse:* "Come, let's play a nice game of checkers."<br>*Client:* "When my baby died, I thought I couldn't go on."<br>*Nurse:* "How many other children do you have?" |

> ### Display 10-4
> ### Therapeutic Communications Performance Checklist
>
> The following checklist can be used by a student to evaluate the use of therapeutic interventions during a client interaction or videotape of a client interaction.
>
> | | Yes | No |
> | --- | --- | --- |
> | 1. Introduces self and states the purpose of the visit | | |
> | 2. Identifies goals for the day and termination time | | |
> | 3. Maintains eye contact and minimizes gestures | | |
> | 4. Maintains consistency between nonverbal and verbal communication | | |
> | 5. Avoids dominating the conversation with personal details | | |
> | 6. Asks open-ended questions | | |
> | 7. Promotes expression of client feelings | | |
> | 8. Clarifies and restates main ideas | | |
> | 9. Offers alternatives to the plan of care | | |
> | 10. Avoids the use of blocks in communication | | |
> | 11. Summarizes the content of the exchange | | |
> | 12. Terminates the relationship by identifying | | |
>
> **Goals accomplished** _____
>
> _Comments_
>
> _____
> _____
> _____

and client" (p. 245). A sample of a process recording is included at the end of this chapter (**Display 10-5**).

Once the student has reviewed nonverbal and verbal communication techniques and blocks, the phases of the nurse–patient relationship need to be examined.

# Phases of the Nurse–Patient Relationship

The four phases of the nurse–patient relationship have been described by Sundeen, Stuart, Rankin, and Cohen (1998) as preinteraction, introductory or orientation, working, and termination.

## Preinteraction Phase

In the preinteraction phase, the nurse explores his or her feelings about the patient situation, analyzes his or her abilities, gathers patient data, and plans for the first patient meeting.

## Display 10-5   Sample Process Recording

Client initials: _____     Student name: _____

Client diagnosis: _____     Date: _____

Setting: _____     Instructor: _____

Clinical site: _____

| Nonverbal and Verbal Data | Thoughts / Feelings | Analysis of Client / Student Communication Techniques |
| --- | --- | --- |
| | | |

## Orientation Phase

The orientation phase includes determining patient needs and establishing trust and acceptance with the patient. This is essential to help the patient explore feelings and thoughts and identify problems and goals. The nurse and patient mutually determine actions, responsibilities, and expectations for each other. Open communication (being able to share feelings without perceiving censure) must be established at this phase. To establish an environment in which open communication can flourish, the caregiver must convey to the patient that she or he will accept the patient's feelings and beliefs as important and will not judge them.

## Working Phase

During the working phase, stressors are analyzed and resistance behaviors are explored and overcome. The nurse promotes development of insight and use of more constructive coping behaviors by the patient.

## Termination Phase

The termination phase consists of reviewing progress and exploring the client's feelings associated with separation, such as rejection, loss, sadness, or anger. This phase also includes self-evaluation by the nurse of the relationship and its effectiveness. Peer evaluation is included in this phase. Self-evaluation is needed for a person to review his or her behavior and seek improvement in communication. Peer evaluation provides the nurse with an objective view of the communication techniques by another caregiver about how the interaction proceeded and whether or not it was effective.

The nurse who is working with other staff also may use the idea of the phases of communication. For example, consider a situation in which a nurse wishes to discuss a concern about caregiving with another nurse. The concepts of preparation, setting goals for the interaction, working on or discussing the issue, and summarizing the action to be taken can all promote the development of higher quality decision making by the nurses.

Although the primary focus of therapeutic communication skills is in the basic nurse–client interaction, such communication techniques are appropriate for peer interactions commonly encountered throughout the workday. For instance, a co-worker who is worried about completing a task may seek assistance from you. Your ability to help that co-worker be successful in that task may help create the trusting and cooperative atmosphere that is conducive to good work relations.

## Competence in Communication ▬▬ Across the Life Span

The communication skills that have been covered are general and can be useful in communicating with any clients, families, co-workers, or groups. However, there are times when specific techniques are useful, such as when the nursing care of children, adolescents, or older adults is involved.

Infants and children are very sensitive to nonverbal communication. The tone of voice and gestures used can startle or frighten a small child. Comforting techniques such as cuddling, patting, or rocking in the presence of the primary caregiver are important to adopt. When caring for older children, it is important to talk to the primary caregiver and to the child. When children are very young, the caregiver may be the only accurate source of needed information. Using simple words and short sentences and talking to the child at eye level are important tips to remember.

The adolescent stage of development can be a trying time for the nurse as well as the caregiver. One of the most important techniques for this age group is to listen first and remain nonjudgmental. A sense of give and take should be maintained, and thoughtful, creative, firm limit setting may be needed. This will encourage the adolescent to express himself and show tolerance and respect for his/her budding individuality. Every effort should be made to give the adolescent a sense of modesty and privacy.

Communication with the older adult presents other challenges for the nurse. Assessment of the client is very important. Hearing and seeing difficulties accentuate the need for the nurse to face the client, talk directly to him or her, and use simple nonverbal gestures to help facilitate clear interaction. Establishing priorities for what is necessary for the client to know can assist the client in retaining needed information. The nurse should stick with one topic at a time and allow time for the client to respond with an answer. Selecting a time in which the client is less fatigued or stressed will help facilitate communication. Knowing the client's previous experiences with health-related issues can help the nurse relate what the client is experiencing in the present. Consistent thought and consideration for the dignity of the older client is paramount, so the nurse should address such clients in the manner they request.

# Conclusion

This chapter introduces several concepts essential to the nurse's role as communicator. The importance of recognizing nonverbal and verbal adjuncts to communication and barriers to communication is discussed. Factors that promote effective communication, including therapeutic communication techniques, are explained. Phases of the therapeutic relationship are discussed, and mechanisms of communication are explained. Suggestions for use of communication concepts throughout the life span are made.

## Student Exercises

SITUATION ONE

Nurse Frederick is caring for Mr. N., a patient who has recently received a diagnosis of multiple sclerosis. As Nurse Frederick enters the room, Mr. N. is sitting on the side of his bed, staring vacantly into space. His bath water is set up on his bedside table, and his washcloth is unused. When she says "Hello," he does not respond. She stands by his bedside and looks at the flow sheet on her clipboard. She asks, "How's the appetite?" without looking at him. A low "OK," in a monotone voice is the reply. "Have you had a BM?" The nurse is still not looking at him. "Yes." The low monotone voice and vacant stare continue. Next Nurse Frederick takes Mr. N.'s vital signs. Quickly glancing at him, she records them on the flow sheet. "Looks good," she says and leaves the room.

1. Identify the nonverbal communication of nurse and patient.
2. Identify the barriers to communication demonstrated by the nurse.
3. Suggest some verbal and nonverbal techniques the nurse could have used to encourage Mr. N. to verbalize his concerns.

SITUATION TWO

Student Nurse Reese reports off duty to her charge nurse. She says, "Mrs. Jones slept a little, complained of chest pain twice, and ate very little lunch. She received a PRN medication and weighed 110 lb."

1. Discuss some areas the nursing student omitted in her report. Why do you think these areas were omitted?
2. Suggest some therapeutic techniques the nursing student might have used to elicit the needed data from Mrs. Jones.
3. Write the response you would use if you were the charge nurse to help the nursing student elicit the needed information.

SITUATION THREE

A nursing team is discussing the care of Mrs. Jones, described in the previous situation. Student Nurse Susan is the group leader. She says, "Mrs. Jones' highest priority problem is her anxiety." Student Nurse Daniel replies, "Explain how she demonstrates her anxiety."

1. Write a response demonstrating how you would answer Daniel.

2. Suggest some nursing interventions that would be included in the nursing care plan for Mrs. Jones related to the anxiety.

SITUATION FOUR

Steven Shortledge, 68 years old, is walking into your community clinic for treatment of new onset of depression. The nurse's goal is to get Steven to participate in a support group for grieving spouses. Using the techniques for older adults, explain the assessments and interventions you will be using with Mr. Shortledge to accomplish the goal of his visit.

## References

Berlo, D. (1960). *The process of communication: An introduction to theory and practice.* New York: Holt, Reinhart & Winston.

Cousins, N. (1983). *Anatomy of an illness: As perceived by the patient.* New York: Norton.

Craven, R., & Hirnle, C. (2003). *Fundamentals of nursing: Human health and function* (4th ed.). Philadelphia: Lippincott Williams & Wilkins.

Darwin, C. (1872). *The expression of emotions in man and animals.* London: John Murray.

Fontaine, K., & Fletcher, J. (1999). *Mental health nursing* (4th ed.). Menlo Park, CA: Addison-Wesley.

Fortinash, K. M., & Holoday-Worret, P. A. (2000). *Psychiatric mental health nursing* (2nd ed.). St. Louis: Mosby.

McGhee, P. (1998). Rx: Laughter. *RN, 61*(7), 50–53.

Sundeen, S. J., Stuart, G. W., Rankin, E., & Cohen, S. (1998). *Nurse–client interaction: Implementing the nursing process* (6th ed.). St. Louis: Mosby.

Varcarolis, E. M. (2002). *Foundations of psychiatric mental health nursing* (4th ed.). Philadelphia: WB Saunders.

## Suggested Reading

Cherry, B., & Jacob, S. (2002). *Contemporary nursing: Issues, trends & management* (2nd ed.). St. Louis: Mosby.

Keltner, N. L., Schweck, L. H., & Bostrom, C. E. (2003). *Psychiatric nursing* (4th ed.). St. Louis: Mosby.

Riley, J. B. (2000). *Communication in nursing* (4th ed.). St. Louis: Mosby.

Tate, D. M. (2001). 10 tips for effective communication. *Nursing Spectrum, 10,* 12PA, 11. *http://community.nursingspectrum.com/MagazineArticles/article.cfm?AID=4263*

*On the Web*  · · · · · · · · · · · · · · · · · · · · · · · · · · · · · · · · · · · · ·

*ideanurse.com/aath*: The American Association of Therapeutic Humor

*www.jocularity.com*: Journal of Nursing Jocularity

*www.laughterremedy.com*: The Laughter Remedy

*www.nfb.org*: National Federation for the Blind

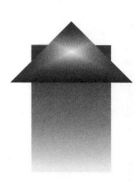

# C H A P T E R *11*

# The Nurse as Teacher

## LEARNING OBJECTIVES

*By the end of this chapter, the student will be able to:*

1 Explain why client education is an important nursing responsibility in an ever-changing healthcare setting.
2 Describe the differences between teaching and learning.
3 List principles of teaching–learning and relate them to client education planning.
4 Describe internal and external influences that affect client learning.
5 Differentiate teaching methods appropriate for cognitive, affective, and psychomotor learning.
6 Relate the steps in the teaching–learning process to the nursing process.
7 Specify assessment data necessary to determine client learning needs.
8 Formulate nursing diagnoses for identified client learning needs.
9 Outline the essential components of a teaching plan.
10 Describe how to implement client education.
11 Explain how to evaluate client education.
12 Discuss the essential elements of documenting client education.

## KEY TERMS

andragogy
affective learning
cognitive learning
compliance
deficient knowledge
feedback
learning
learning need

learning style
motivation
noncompliance
pedagogy
psychomotor learning
reinforcement
teaching

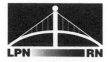

## VIGNETTE

Mary has been an LVN for 2 years and has just graduated from an associate degree program. She is working on a busy medical–surgical unit with another LPN and two unlicensed assistive personnel (UAPs). Mary entered the nursing station at 10 AM and sat down, exasperated.

**Mary:** How am I going to teach my patients anything when there isn't enough time?

**Alice (Head Nurse):** What's the problem Mary?

**Mary:** Mr. Martinez in 203 isn't doing very well with his insulin injections because he doesn't speak or understand English very well. And he's going home today. Mrs. Duncan is going to surgery in 1 hour, and I haven't taught her how to deep breath and cough yet. Mr. James is upset about the medication changes Dr. Lotte made and won't take his new heart medications until he knows more about them. Mr. Willis is afraid to take his wife home tomorrow because he can't put her back brace on by himself. I need to change Mrs. Lewis' dressing, but Dr. Craig has ordered a new IV antibiotic and her IV is infiltrated. Some time this morning, I have to irrigate Mr. Martin's colostomy! Writing a teaching plan was one of my strong points in school. Now, I barely have time to explain things to patients as I dash from room to room. My LPN and my UAPs can't help because this is what I have been trained to do, not them.

**Alice:** Yes, it does seem like teaching is taking a back seat these days, but I think the importance of teaching is getting greater. Teaching on the run and early discharge planning are the ways to go these days and will continue to be the most practical approach in the future.

**Mary:** When will we get those standardized teaching plans everyone has been talking about, Alice? Maybe they would give me some new ideas and reduce the paperwork that's burying me.

**Alice:** They should be available in a week or so, but I hope they get used and don't turn into chart stuffing.

**Mary:** Well, I need something. I won't have time to write a teaching plan for all my patients today. I'll just have to hope the nurses on the next shift can figure out what needs to be done next from my charting.

**Alice:** You need to chart, Mary. Legally, you have to chart what was taught and how well the patient understood. Come on, I'll give you a hand.

**Mary:** Thanks, Alice. I sure appreciate the help.

# The Challenge of Client Education

Mary is right to become concerned about her client teaching. Teaching is such an important legal and professional responsibility that teaching responsibilities are included in most state nurse practice acts and the American Nurses Association's *Stan-*

*dards of Nursing Practice* (American Nurses Association, 1998). Nurses who fail to provide proper client education not only increase their risk of civil liability, but also, and more importantly, are negligent in their nursing practice. Another challenge to completing competent client education is the downsizing of professional nursing staff positions and the substitution of such positions with UAP staff. Although there is help with the simple physical care, clients are sicker, there is less client contact for assessment, and clients are confused about the roles of their healthcare providers. Nurses are challenged daily by the increasing demands of the work setting to meet their teaching responsibilities. With the advent of managed care, patients and families are presented with the challenge of managing more complex health problems at home. Learning now must occur in a shorter time and in situations and environments that are not always ideal for learning.

Nurses like Mary are busier managing larger caseloads with clients who require more complex treatments and nursing care. New professionals must have clear communication and documentation skills to make the transition from the healthcare setting to home more safe and efficient for such clients. In cases like that of Mr. Martinez, the nurse must be a worldwide citizen who is flexible and open to clients' learning needs, especially needs not previously encountered by the nurse. In addition, nurses are legally bound to protect client confidentiality, so family members of clients who do not speak English should not be used as interpreters. With the advent of economic downsizing, the nurse is accountable for work that is done by others less skilled in client communication. As an LPN/LVN, you could help with basic assessment skills but now you are legally, morally, and ethically responsible for the entire process of client education. Teaching is an integral part of all ongoing nurse–client interactions, such as answering a client question or explaining the purpose of a nursing action.

Research has shown how valuable health teaching is for the healthcare recipient. Health teaching shortens hospital stays, minimizes complications, and reduces symptoms of illness and surgery (Rankin & Stallings, 2001). Given a willing client, the extent of client education that can be accomplished is limited only by the depth and breadth of the nurse's knowledge, the constraints of the setting, and the circumstances in which the nurse–client interaction occurs.

# Teaching and Learning Defined ▬▬▬▬

Client teaching is an ongoing process whereby the nurse organizes experiences in varied ways to facilitate client learning. The basic purpose of teaching is to help clients become confident and independent in managing their health. According to Redman (2001), "instruction is the deliberate arrangement of conditions to promote attainment of some intentional goal" (p. 3). When appropriately used, client teaching is a powerful means for achieving nursing's goals to prevent illness, promote or restore health, and facilitate coping with chronic and terminal illness.

Learning is "a process by which a person acquires or increases knowledge or changes behavior in a measurable way as a result of an experience" (Taylor, Lillis, & LeMone, 2001, p. 375.) To promote learning, the nurse must have understanding and be able to apply teaching–learning principles.

# Teaching–Learning Process: Principles of Teaching

Principles of teaching and learning provide basic guidelines for the nurse assuming the role of teacher. The teaching process and principles closely follow the communication process presented in Chapter 10. They are necessary for planning individualized client teaching and selecting teaching materials and methods that best meet client education needs **(Display 11-1)**.

## Trust

Establish client trust and acceptance. People learn best when they are accepted. Clients must trust their nurse, and nurses must respect the client's ability to learn for the teaching–learning process to succeed. Nurses must identify all signs of client frustration and hostility to their instructions. Client attitudes vary from pleasant and accepting to hostile, bitter, or rejecting. Nurses must be sensitive to these attitudes and adapt their teaching approach so that learning can occur.

## Partnering With the Learner

Include the client in the development of learning objectives. The teaching–learning process will be more effective if the client is included in the planning of the learning experience. Including the client in the teaching–learning process tells the nurse what the client is willing and unwilling to do. Compliance is the adherence of the client to his/her healthcare teaching. Compliance is best attained when the nurse and client agree upon goals and an action plan. Unless the learning goals center around what the client values and is willing to achieve, little learning will take place. Noncompliance occurs when the client or family does not follow the plan of care. Careful reassessment must be done to determine the reasons this has occurred.

---

**Display 11-1** | **Principles of Teaching and Learning**

1. Establish trust
2. Partner with the learner
3. Client motivation signifies readiness to learn
4. Vary teaching style to the client's needs
5. Individualize strategies and materials
6. Capitalize on client strengths and resources
7. Simplify language
8. Consider developmental stage
9. Modify the environment
10. Judiciously use content sequencing
11. Provide repetition and practice
12. Relate new learning experiences to client's past
13. Reinforce newly learned behaviors

# Motivation

Motivation can be defined as the internal reasons/forces that cause a person to initiate and maintain a behavior. What motivates one individual may annoy another, resulting in no change in behavior. A key concept the nurse must remember is that the "best laid plan" may be ineffective if the targeted learner lacks the motivation to learn (Doak, Doak, & Root, 1996).

The nurse needs to identify emotional, physical, and experiential factors that signal a client is able, motivated, and willing to learn. The emotional state of the client can motivate a client to learn or inhibit such learning. Emotions such as anxiety, depression, denial, and fear can require a great deal of the client's energy and distract from learning. However, anxious parents of a sick child may be receptive to learning special techniques that allow them to participate in their child's care.

Assess for physical barriers to learning, such as pain, acuity of illness, or prognosis of illness. A client in pain, very weak, or preoccupied with thoughts about illness may be unable to concentrate on instructions and attend to learning.

A client's background, skills, knowledge, and attitudes regarding a health situation provide the necessary foundation for developing the teaching plan. A client who has cared for a frail elderly relative after a stroke will be better able to cope with a spouse convalescing from a heart attack than a client who has always depended on others to care for ill family members.

Client attitudes and values can facilitate or inhibit the learning that can be achieved. A client recovering from knee replacement surgery will be more successful in learning to use a walker if she values independence and accepts direction and help from others than will a client who wants to be helped and feels safe in a wheelchair.

# Learning Style

The nurse should remember that different people learn differently, and material should be presented in varied ways. Learning is a complex process affected by people's responses to varied sensory input and their orientation to learning. Some individuals learn in a singular mode, by doing, feeling, thinking, or seeing, and others learn via a combination of modes, such as seeing and doing. Nurses are more effective teachers if they get to know their client learners and how they learn best before teaching begins.

---

## NCLEX–RN Might Ask 11-1   **?** **?** **?**

The nurse is assessing a client's motivation to learn. Which of the following factors could block that client's motivation to learn?

    A. Severe pain
    B. Successful past experiences
    C. Strong family support system
    D. A positive attitude

• See Appendix A for correct answer and rationale.

Regardless of the client's learning style, nurses will be more successful if they vary and combine the different types of sensory input when teaching. Information presented in a variety of ways is understood and remembered better than that which is only seen or heard.

Another aspect of learning style to consider is the client's way of understanding the situation. Some prefer to look at the big picture and then learn about its segments, whereas others like to take one piece at a time learn about the whole situation. A client who prefers to see the whole may respond to segmental teaching with the plea, "Would you get to the point; what does all this mean?" A client who likes to take things segmentally might respond to an explanation of the big picture by saying, "This is very confusing. Can you explain it one step at a time?"

# Teaching Materials

Use charts, models, pictures, diagrams, videotapes, television programs, and the Internet to enhance learning. Hospitals and ambulatory care settings may use their own commercially packaged educational channels on television for general and specific client education. However, be careful not to use literature and audiovisuals as a substitute for the nurse–client interaction. With less time and fewer resources available, it is common to see instructional pamphlets or video programs used to teach about medical conditions, such as diabetes, and health education topics, such as breastfeeding. Clients, such as Mr. Martinez in our opening vignette, may not understand written instructions because of language differences, age, or functional illiteracy. Thus, it is important to assess the reading ability and fluency of English language at the onset of a client teaching relationship.

Illiteracy is common and affects individuals of all races and socioeconomic levels. According to Taylor et al. (2001), about 20% of adults are functionally illiterate, meaning they cannot read beyond a fifth grade reading level. According to Canobbio (2000), to be effective, teaching materials need to be geared at the sixth to eighth grade reading levels. The nurse should always assess client literacy level when client teaching.

Direct testing would be the best method for assessing client literacy, but is not very practical in clinical settings. A less accurate but expedient method might be to observe and ask clients about their favorite materials for pleasure reading. Assess the client for an inability to focus on reading materials, a tendency to focus on detail, consistent tendency to interpret literature literally, and lack of ability to concentrate on dominant themes. These are common assessments found in clients who have difficulty reading. In addition, a functionally illiterate client may be slow to interpret information. Again, careful assessment is the key.

Provide several options (reading, watching, and listening) and then ask simple questions about the content and descriptions of any materials provided. Reduce the amount of reading involved by using gestures, pictures, videotapes or audiotapes, and diagrams to get across important learning concepts. Make learning sessions involve small, usable chunks of information. Monitor the client's understanding frequently by return demonstration or questioning him or her.

## NCLEX–RN Might Ask 11-2

In the home care setting, the nurse is assessing the reading skills of a client with newly diagnosed diabetes. The *best* way the nurse could assess this skill is by

    A. asking the client to take a literacy test.
    B. checking the client's type of pleasure reading
    C. making the client read a complex instruction sheet.
    D. asking the client's husband the last year of school the client completed.

• *See Appendix A for correct answer and rationale.*

## Client Learning Strengths and Resources

Determine the client's learning strengths and resources to facilitate learning. Client strengths are the internal physical, psychological, social, and spiritual resources a person mobilizes to cope with problems. See **Display 11-2** for examples of strengths that nurses can use to develop a teaching plan.

Resources are external forces such as support systems, housing, income, transportation, and education that influence a person's ability to meet his or her needs. These resources must be considered for teaching to be effective. For example, if Mr. Martinez, our non-English speaking, Hispanic, client with diabetes has a language barrier and vision loss, he will never achieve any degree of independence in self-injection unless Mary works to resolve these issues. A hypertensive client such as Mr. James, who has a limited income and lack of housing, may not be able to comply with the medication regimens and diet modifications that would more effectively control the disease.

### ► Thinking Critically

Select three clients mentioned in the Vignette. What resources should you identify that would be useful for these clients?

## Language and Cultural Background

Take into consideration the client's language, education, socioeconomic background, and cultural factors when deciding what vocabulary to use in teaching. Be sensitive to the client's unfamiliarity with medical terms and jargon. This is such a pervasive healthcare need that one of the four objectives listed by Healthy People 2010 is the need for simple language that is understandable by the general public.

Define terms you will use, such as "ambulation," and try to use terminology with which the client is familiar because of work or daily experiences, such as walk or stroll. If a client does not speak English well, the nurse should obtain a knowledgeable translator to assist with the instruction.

Use analogies, comparisons, examples, and illustrations to promote understanding. Common analogies include comparison of the heart to a pump, the bladder to a reser-

## Display 11-2  Examples of Client Strengths

▶ **PHYSICAL STRENGTHS**

Maintains good health through daily exercise
Moves about with ease
Maintains skin integrity
Sleeps well
Eats nutritional diet
Breathes effectively
Blood pressure stable
Independent in activities of daily living

▶ **PSYCHOLOGICAL STRENGTHS**

Resolves developmental tasks favorably
Demonstrates good problem-solving skills
Verbalizes confidence in philosophy of life
Expresses knowledge about health condition
Has a sense of humor
Shows insight into personal situations
Communicates willingness to learn
Reports ability to cope with health concerns
Verbalizes positive feelings of self-esteem

▶ **SPIRITUAL STRENGTHS**

Actively participates in church
Expresses spiritual peace
Verbalizes confidence in religious faith

▶ **SOCIAL STRENGTHS**

Relates well with spouse, children, and others
Has a strong support system of family and friends
Uses personal/family resources appropriately
Seeks out appropriate healthcare resources (e.g., insurance, Weight Watchers, health club)
Accepts help from family and friends
Is a dedicated employee
Contributes to financial security of family

voir tank, the eyes to a camera lens, a heart valve defect to a leaking washer, and the joints to a hinge.

## Developmental Considerations

To individualize teaching and ensure optimum learning, consider the client's developmental level when planning client teaching. Pedagogy is the science of teaching children and adolescents. Children have varying limitations in attention, concentration, and cognitive and psychomotor skills related to developmental level.

Andragogy is the study of how adults learn. Adults generally are motivated learners but sometimes lead busy lives and might lack self-confidence in trying something new. Adults also learn best when they see clear and immediate need for information to be integrated into their lifestyle.

The process of aging changes many neurosensory body systems. The elderly may have hearing and visual impairments and reduced motor abilities. If the client has difficulty understanding you, shorten the length of the teaching session, establish priorities for teaching the information, and repeat the material as necessary. **Table 11-1** gives commonly used techniques for effective learning techniques across the developmental continuum.

## Environment

Determine environmental factors that influence client learning. Careful attention should be paid to time constraints, the physical environment, client activity schedules, and client privacy. For example, it may be unrealistic for a nurse to give instructions for self-injection to a patient with diabetes during the morning medication period, when the nurse is rushed and responsible for administering multiple drugs to several clients. It would be better to schedule such teaching in the afternoon. For clients who do not speak English, the nurse must arrange to have an interpreter present and additional family support. If a client's learning needs can be anticipated, such as relaxation techniques for childbirth or preoperative instructions, arrange for the client to come for instruction in advance of the situation. Perhaps home care visitation can be scheduled at a time the client can be with the care provider, who then can be an additional resource for the client. The nurse needs to be a skillful manipulator of the environment to enhance teaching.

## Sequence

Plan for a series of instructions that builds on previous knowledge and lays the groundwork for future learning. Teach from easy to difficult, known to unknown, well to ill, normal to abnormal, and step by step for complicated topics.

**TABLE  11-1**
**DEVELOPMENTAL LEARNING STRATEGIES**

| Child | Adult | Older Adult |
|---|---|---|
| Visits to healthcare agency | Contracting | Connect past to present |
| Dress-up | Emphasize immediate | Give more time to learn |
| Use toys, dolls | Draw upon previous | Assess for sensory changes |
| Use coloring, storybooks | Emphasize independence | Promote independence |
| Health fairs | Allow time to practice | Make fonts bigger |
| Include caregiver | Emphasize use for social roles | Consider resources/support systems |

Instruction in self-injection of insulin and then routine glucose monitoring at home is an example of sequential instruction. Clients are first taught about the insulin, then the steps in preparing the injection; finally, they are taught the injection technique. When teaching a client to perform blood glucose testing, set up a sequence that begins with the purpose of testing, progresses through equipment operation and maintenance, the testing procedure, and finally quality assurance and troubleshooting problems. Such sequencing of complex procedural steps leads to optimal learning.

## Repetition and Practice

Repeat, summarize, and ask questions after each segment of instruction. Reviewing material covered in previous teaching sessions or an earlier segment of the teaching period reinforces the learning, rewards the client, and helps the nurse to evaluate learning. To provide motivation and enhance incentive, reinforce small successes, especially with the challenging learner.

Provide frequent and repeated opportunities to practice new skills, especially with adults; adult learners learn by doing. Generally, several practice sessions spaced over a period of time are more effective than one long practice session, during which client fatigue may impede performance.

## Past Experiences

Keep in mind that in all developmental levels, new learning is contingent upon a client's previous life experiences. Use the knowledge of the client or family as a base on which to build. For example, you may use a garden hose as an analogy for blood pressure if the client is a gardener, or the analogy of flushing a radiator to describe how to prime an IV line if the client works on cars.

## Reinforcement

Many learning theorists consider rewarding the learner for making the desired response to be the primary basis for learning. The nurse should praise, compliment, or provide a tangible reward when the client achieves the desired learning objective. The type of reward should be appropriate to the client and immediately follow the desired behavioral response. For example, providing a favorite video game might be effective for a diabetic child, whereas verbal praise and a smile would be more appropriate for an elderly diabetic client who correctly self-administers an insulin injection.

### ▶ Thinking Critically

Apply the previous principles of teaching if you were the nurse caring for the clients in the Vignette. Compare and contrast your application of these principles with those of your classmates and formulate an ideal approach for these clients.

# Teaching Interventions

The nurse can use many approaches to client teaching to meet the client's learning needs **(Display 11-3)**. Choosing the right strategy, based on a thorough assessment and mutually acceptable goals, will make the experience enjoyable and effective. The method or strategy chosen depends not only on the setting in which teaching will occur, but also the type of learning that needs to take place (affective, cognitive, or psychomotor). If one approach is unsuccessful, changing or combining modalities, such as seeing, doing, and hearing, may achieve the desired learning outcome.

## Lecture

Lectures, with which we are all familiar, are an effective and efficient way to teach several people at once. The lecture approach works well with groups who are seeking information on common healthcare issues, such as diabetes management, prenatal care, and parenting classes. One of the problems with the lecture is that it does not promote active listening. The nurse should not confuse telling with learning. When using lecture, the nurse cannot be sure learning is taking place unless he or she evaluates the learner. Lectures are less effective for affective and psychomotor learning or in most acute care hospital settings, where the ill client needs shorter and more individualized instruction.

## Discussion

Discussion works well for the cognitive and affective domains of learning. This approach is useful for individual or group instruction in classroom, home, community,

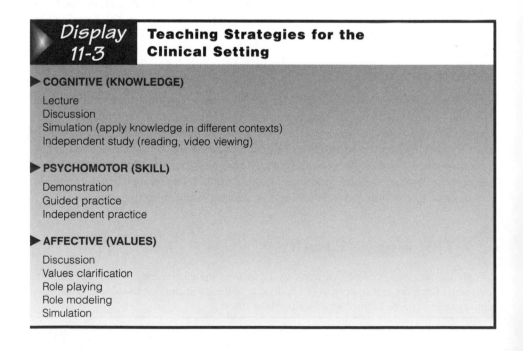

**Display 11-3   Teaching Strategies for the Clinical Setting**

▶ **COGNITIVE (KNOWLEDGE)**

Lecture
Discussion
Simulation (apply knowledge in different contexts)
Independent study (reading, video viewing)

▶ **PSYCHOMOTOR (SKILL)**

Demonstration
Guided practice
Independent practice

▶ **AFFECTIVE (VALUES)**

Discussion
Values clarification
Role playing
Role modeling
Simulation

or bedside situations. Teacher and learner discussions more commonly involve the exchange of information, ideas, and feelings during brief encounters, such as preparing a patient for a diagnostic procedure or when the nurse administers medications. Nurses involved with family support groups and organizations such as stroke and ostomy clubs also frequently use this approach.

## Thinking Critically

Explain how the clients in the Vignette might benefit most from a discussion approach versus a lecture approach in meeting their learning needs.

## Simulation

The simulation strategy teaches and evaluates client learning. Because of its interactive nature, simulation promotes partnership in the learning process. Application of information in different scenarios gives the client experience with the subject and lets the nurse evaluate what was learned. For example, a nurse could teach and evaluate how well a hypertensive client learned dietary modifications by giving a sample menu and asking the client to order a meal that best meets sodium and fat restrictions. Reinforcement would be provided if the client chooses correctly, or instruction could continue if an incorrect choice was made.

## Independent Study

Many clients prefer self-paced learning through independent study of printed, audiovisual, or online resource materials. A newer trend in healthcare education is the use of the Internet as a resource for health information. Independent study should not be used in isolation but as a stimulus or precursor to a nurse–client learning interaction. Allowing a client to view a program on breastfeeding before a discussion or the nurse-directed experience of feeding of a newborn can spark client questions and make the nurse–client interaction more successful. Careful assessment of client literacy and language should always be considered when using independent study materials.

As with preprinted materials, screening of the Internet resources is critical. There is no standard or assurance that materials obtained by the client/family are from a reliable source. The nurse can be helpful in showing the client where reputable sources may be obtained.

## Demonstration

Demonstration is the ideal way of teaching procedures, techniques, exercises, and use of special equipment. Models of body parts, medical practice models, and teaching simulators, such as resuscitation dolls, breast models, and injection manikins, are available to help clients learn independent healthcare practices. Providing step-by-step instructions in short, sequential teaching sessions usually works best for complex procedures, such as ostomy care or self-injection of insulin. Return demonstration by the client provides opportunities to evaluate and praise the client's learning.

# Practice

Client practice, independent and guided, should always be considered in conjunction with the demonstration strategy for psychomotor learning. After explaining and demonstrating a skill, sufficient time should be planned for the nurse to direct or guide the client through each step of procedures, such as changing sterile dressings or operating a glucose monitor. Additional independent practice with or without the nurse present will help the client move to more independent functioning. Written materials or videotapes should be given to provide the client with resources for review.

> ### ► Thinking Critically
>
> In the Vignette, Mr. Martinez was having difficulty learning self-injection. Assuming that the nurse was using demonstration and practice as teaching strategies, what principle of learning needs emphasis in revising Mr. Martinez's teaching plan so he can be more successful?

## Self-disclosure

Seeing a nurse who has overcome health challenges can help the client change attitudes and values associated with health issues. A nurse who has struggled with a weight issue or giving up an addiction to tobacco or caffeine may be able to share personal insights that are helpful to a client. Nurses who were former smokers have been excellent role models for clients who are trying to quit smoking to improve their health.

## Role Playing

Acting out feelings or behaviors gives the learner a chance to experience, relive, or anticipate a situation. Role playing emphasizes the cognitive and affective domains of learning. The client can experiment with different responses to a situation, while the nurse offers guidance and feedback.

Play with puppets and dolls has proven effective in preparing young children for procedures and helping them express negative feelings about hospitalization. Role playing in prenatal class is effective and necessary to help couples get through transition in childbirth. One disadvantage of using role play is adults may feel uncomfortable when using this process. Every effort should be made to help them feel safe to explore feelings and assure them that the exercise will be helpful in meeting their learning needs.

## Values Clarification

Encouraging clients to explore and identify their values about health, sickness, and healthcare issues helps remove barriers to learning new or different approaches to managing health and illness. Identification of values in different aspects of a client's life might serve as a stimulus for changing behaviors in healthcare practices. A nurse might help a client see the value of routine follow-up visits for hypertension through values clarification for a client who values regular maintenance of a classic car or regular health maintenance of a pet. Such transference of a common value is an important achievement regarding personal health.

# Steps in the Teaching–Learning Process ▬▬

Client teaching is most effective when approached through the nursing process, as outlined in **Table 11-2**. Rather than think of client education as a separate and unique nursing function, nurses must integrate client education into their general approach to client care and address learning needs in every aspect of the nursing process. The nurse should be aware and take advantage of all client interactions to determine learning needs and guide teaching. In some situations, the nurse can anticipate a whole series of learning needs, such as the standardized preoperative teaching topics needed by Mrs. Duncan in the Vignette, whereas other situations are incidental to ongoing nursing care, such as teaching the purpose and side effects of a newly prescribed drug, as was needed by Mr. James in the Vignette before administration of the medication.

## Assessment

An organized and thorough assessment is the first and most essential step for effective learning (London, 2001). When a client's condition and situation are assessed, be sure to determine what the client or family needs to know or learn. A basic educational assessment should include motivation level, comprehension ability, current knowledge level, attitudes about health, and factors that will affect teaching, such as sensory, physical, and mental abilities and language. Ideally, this information should be obtained on admission or during early periods of client contact, when the nurse interviews the client for the nursing database. In addition, the nurse should remain vigilant about obtaining information about the client's learning needs as revealed through the client's questions and behaviors when the nurse is giving care.

**TABLE  11-2**
NURSING PROCESS VERSUS TEACHING–LEARNING PROCESS

| Nursing Process | Teaching–Learning Process |
|---|---|
| Assessing | Determine learning needs |
| Diagnosing | Identify learning needs<br>Nursing diagnoses of learning needs |
| Planning | Specify learning objectives<br>Select teaching method<br>    Informal teaching<br>    Formal teaching<br>    Standardized teaching plans<br>Select teaching strategies |
| Implementing | Implement teaching plan<br>    Prepare materials<br>    Structure teaching sessions<br>Control environment |
| Evaluating | Evaluate teaching<br>Evaluate learning |

A basic educational assessment can be accomplished by answering the following questions during client interactions:

- What does the client know?
- What does the client need to know?
- What does the client want to know?
- How does the client feel about the situation and about managing the situation independently?

Answers to these questions help the nurses in **Display 11-4** discover why Mr. Martinez was having difficulty mastering his insulin injections and exactly what Mr. Wallis needed to be less afraid to take his wife home.

## Diagnosis

After collecting the necessary data, the nurse analyzes the information and identifies the nursing diagnosis that most clearly describes the client's learning needs. According to

---

### *Display 11-4*   Case Studies

▶ **MR. MARTINEZ—HISPANIC, INSULIN-DEPENDENT DIABETIC CLIENT**

In preparation for Mr. Martinez's discharge, Mary visits him and arranges for a hospital interpreter to be present during the sessions. During their conversation, Mary concentrates on speaking to Mr. Martinez, not the interpreter. She learns that Mr. Martinez's mother is very knowledgeable about diabetic diet management because she also has diabetes. His mother is also a respected curandira or local healer. Mary arranges for Mr. Martinez's mother to be included in the teaching and arranges for the afternoon nurse to carry on training in the evening. Mary learns that Mr. Martinez is very knowledgeable about the signs and symptoms of hypoglycemia and hyperglycemia but has difficulty mixing and preparing his insulins. Part of the problem is he can't see well. Because of this, Mary contacts the local Visiting Nurses Association for follow-up teaching at home and refers him to the walk-in clinic for vision testing for presbyopia.

▶ **MRS. WALLIS—CLIENT UNDERGOING POSTOPERATIVE LAMINECTOMY**

Mary's visit to Mrs. Wallis is equally revealing. Mr. Wallis has never had to be responsible for an ill family member before. Mrs. Wallis has always cared for their children when they were ill, "nursed" his invalid mother for 5 years after a stroke until her death 2 years ago, and has cared for him after five major surgeries during the past year, including his colostomy care. Mr. Wallis can explain the principles, purpose, and instructions for applying his wife's brace but has avoided handling the brace or practicing its application before Mrs. Wallis' surgery. When Mary asks for his assistance in applying the brace so Mrs. Wallis can get up to the bathroom, his manipulative skill in arranging the brace for application is very good, but he becomes extremely shaky and clumsy when attempting to apply the brace on his wife. During further conversation, Mr. Wallis expresses fear of hurting his wife or not being "a good nurse" like she was during his recovery from surgery. Mary arranges several more supervised practice sessions before discharge; these sessions include a lot of praise from both the nurses and Mrs. Wallis. Eventually, Mr. Wallis becomes the preferred "nurse" in managing the brace because of his consistent and tender approach.

the guidelines of the North American Nursing Diagnosis Association (NANDA, 2001), there are two approaches to diagnosing learning needs. If the learning need is keeping the client from functioning optimally, the problem statement "deficient knowledge" can be used with additional clarification and etiology, as in the following examples:

**Mr. Wallis:** Deficient knowledge (application of orthopedic brace) related to inexperience and concern about home care management

**Mrs. Duncan:** Deficient knowledge (postoperative exercises) related to lack of information about postoperative care

**Mr. Martin:** Deficient knowledge (ostomy care) related to unfamiliarity with home management of colostomy

Deficient knowledge also may be the etiology of the healthcare problem in other NANDA taxonomy categories of human response patterns, such as ineffective health maintenance, anxiety, risk for infection, ineffective coping, and noncompliance. Thus, lack of knowledge, knowledge deficit, lack of understanding, or insufficient information may be used as the etiology of the nursing diagnosis, as in the following examples:

**Mr. James:** Ineffective health maintenance related to lack of understanding about disease process, treatment regimen, and home care management

**Mr. Martin:** Delayed surgical recovery related to insufficient knowledge of colostomy irrigation, peristomal skin care, and incorporation of ostomy care into activities of daily living

When *deficient knowledge* is used as the problem in the nursing diagnostic statement, the nurse supports the belief that giving information can change behavior. This approach directs nursing care to resolve cognitive learning needs but does not necessarily focus on a client's affective learning needs. However, when the learning need "deficient knowledge" or lack of understanding is used as the etiology, nursing care can be directed toward the affective factors that block the client's ability to maintain health and manage self-care (Carpenito, 2002). For example, Mr. Martinez's care plan needed to develop his confidence in mixing insulin correctly, rather than merely providing additional information about insulin injections.

The nurse must choose which style of diagnosis to use. Regardless of which style the nurse uses, both approaches give direction to nursing care and education interven-

---

## NCLEX–RN Might Ask 11-3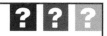

Which of the following nursing diagnostic statements would be most accurate in writing a "deficient knowledge" etiology?

   A. Anxiety related to upcoming surgery
   B. Impaired Verbal Communication related to insufficient information and inexperience in mixing insulins
   C. Risk for Infection related to lowered immune system
   D. Ineffective Individual Coping related to stress of job change

• See Appendix A for correct answer and rationale.

tions. To comply with legal and professional nursing standards, every nursing care plan must include at least one nursing diagnosis addressing client education.

Although the term "noncompliance" is a widely accepted nursing diagnosis, it has a very negative connotation in the eyes of the client. It can imply that the healthcare worker has made a judgment about the client, negating the client's choice. The nurse may want to consider substituting the terms "difference of opinion" or "different values" when talking about the client's learning needs, especially in public.

# Planning

Writing a teaching plan or emphasizing the teaching component of the client's general nursing care plan is a major nursing responsibility. When the client's learning needs are identified and presented in a diagnostic statement, the nurse (in collaboration with the client) develops a client-centered teaching plan that establishes goals and appropriate interventions. The nurse may develop an individualized teaching plan or individualize a standardized (or model) teaching plan with stated goals (behavioral objectives) and nursing interventions (teaching strategies) that reflect the individuality of the client.

## INDIVIDUALIZED PLANS

Individualized teaching plans are generally a component of the client's overall nursing care plan. Educational outcome criteria and teaching interventions are included as one of three approaches (diagnostic, therapeutic, and educational) to resolve an identified human response pattern problem. This type of plan requires more composing and writing time for nurses, but this is the preferred method for ensuring the unique needs of clients will be addressed.

## STANDARDIZED TEACHING PLAN

Standardized teaching plans or model teaching plans have evolved in clinical settings in which teaching situations frequently recur. The standardized preoperative teaching plan is one of the most common. Specialty areas such as prenatal clinics, maternity centers, emergency rooms, outpatient ambulatory care centers, and client education clinics are developing others to lessen the nurse's work and make client education documentation easier.

Standardized plans are available in books or preprinted guides. They usually include checklists, blank lines, or empty spaces for the nurse to individualize goals and nursing interventions and document the teaching provided. This type of plan should be used as a guide because it does not address the client's individual needs and can cause the nurse to focus only on predictable problems and miss cues to unique client problems.

Nurses must always assess the client's knowledge level first to determine if all the information included in the model plan is needed and then individualize the plan to meet the client's specific needs. Most nursing care planning guides include teaching outcomes and interventions in a general abbreviated form, and nurses need to personalize the teaching plan in more detail for specific clients (**Display 11-5**).

# Display 11-5 | Nursing Care Plan for Post-operative Laminectomy

## ▶ ASSESSMENT FOR MRS. WALLIS:

Before using the standardized model teaching plan, Mary carefully assessed what Mr. and Mrs. Wallis knew and were able to do regarding positioning, activity precautions, and back brace management. In her assessment, she found Mrs. Wallis could independently log roll when changing position in bed and maintained proper body alignment while lying in bed, sitting, and standing with her walker. She was cooperative and showed personal responsibility in adhering to the 15-minute limitation on sitting and did not need any reminders from the nursing staff. Mrs. Wallis needed assistance in applying the back brace when getting out of bed, and Mr. Wallis became extremely shaky and appeared awkward when trying to align and comfortably position the brace for Mrs. Wallis. Mr. Wallis always called for the nurses to assist Mrs. Wallis with the brace, and he left the room during his wife's dressing period.

| Standardized Plan | Individualized Plan |
| --- | --- |
| **Nursing Diagnosis:**<br>Risk for injury related to lack of knowledge of postoperative position restrictions and log-rolling technique | **Nursing Diagnosis:**<br>Risk for injury related to lack of knowledge and skill in use of back brace |
| **Outcome Criteria:**<br>1. The client will demonstrate correct positioning and log-rolling techniques.<br>2. The client will verbalize feeling necessary activity precautions. | **Learner Objective:**<br>1. Client will demonstrate correct application of back brace.<br>2. Mr. Wallis will express a feeling of confidence in assisting Mrs. Wallis in donning the back brace.<br>3. The client will demonstrate proper application and use of back brace. |
| **Intervention:**<br>1. Teach client to use arms and legs to transfer weight properly when getting out of bed.<br>2. Encourage walking, standing, and sitting for short periods as soon as permitted after surgery.<br>3. Teach the client precautions to maintain proper body alignment:<br>  a. Log-rolling techniques.<br>  b. Side-lying position in bed<br>  c. Positions to avoid<br>  d. Standing and weight bearing<br>4. Teach the proper use of a back brace, if indicated.<br>5. Teach client to avoid:<br>  a. Prolonged sitting<br>  b. Twisting the spine<br>  c. Bending at the waist<br>  d. Climbing stairs<br>  e. Automobile trips | **Intervention:**<br>1. Demonstrate the proper use of a back brace:<br>  a. Explain the mechanism and purpose of the back brace.<br>  b. Show Mr. Wallis proper positioning of brace while it is being worn by Mrs. Wallis.<br>  c. Demonstrate how to secure the back brace.<br>  d. Demonstrate and explain how to minimize skin irritation from wearing the brace.<br>  e. Show pictures and describe skin breakdown to be assessed each time the brace is applied and removed.<br>  f. Demonstrate skin care and massage after brace removal.<br>2. Encourage Mr. Wallis to discuss his concerns about responsibilities in helping his wife put on back brace.<br>3. Give verbal praise each time Mr. Wallis participates or takes charge in assisting his wife to put on her back brace. |

## GOALS/LEARNING OBJECTIVES

Learning goals are similar to the goal statements used for nursing care plans in general. Learning goals should be client centered, measurable statements of what the client will say or do to give evidence of learning. Learning goal verbs should be consistent with the three domains of learning:

- **Cognitive learning objectives** use verbs describing results of the thinking process: "The client *will state* how diet intake affects his blood sugar levels."
- **Affective learning objectives** use verbs that disclose the client's feelings, attitudes, and values: "The client *will express* feelings about his colostomy stoma."
- **Psychomotor learning objectives** use verbs that clarify client actions and skills: "The client *will demonstrate* aseptic technique when self-administering an insulin injection."

The more specific the goals or desired outcomes, the easier it will be for the client to pursue learning and for the nurse to evaluate progress. A single general goal, such as Mr. Martin will become independent in colostomy care, may be accurate but is too global and provides too little direction for meeting the client's individual needs. Having several objectives (refer to **Display 11-6**) can make the teaching plan easier to implement segmentally, gives the nursing team clearer direction, and enables the nurse to evaluate client learning better.

## Interventions

When learning objectives have been identified, the nurse chooses teaching strategies appropriate for the type of content, the client's learning style, and the outcomes to be achieved. As discussed, any number of teaching methods and materials may be available, but they will not be effective if misapplied. A demonstration will not facilitate a change in attitude or values if there is no opportunity to express feelings; the best-planned and delivered lecture will not achieve psychomotor skills if there is no opportunity to practice. In most client situations, integration of several teaching methods may be required. Nurses must use their own creativity to develop and use teaching interventions to implement their teacher role.

## Implementation

When the teaching plan is implemented, the nurse should stay alert and sensitive to the client's needs and responses. If the nurse or client becomes frustrated with the process,

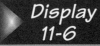

| Display 11-6 | Objective Goals for Mr. Martin's Individualized Teaching Plan |
|---|---|

1. Mr. Martin will empty and change colostomy bag using proper technique.
2. Mr. Martin will perform colostomy irrigation independently.
3. Mr. Martin will accurately assess skin area and describe management of skin irritation if it occurs.
4. Mr. Martin will describe plans for resuming his preoperative lifestyle.
5. Mr. Martin will discuss feelings about the stoma with significant others.

the nurse should take a step back and review the goals and interventions. Were they made with the client? Be prepared to adjust the teaching approach and modify the pace or setting according to the client's progress. The client may have more discomfort or fatigue than expected, so the teaching session may need to be delayed or shortened. Learning a new skill, such as dressing changes, ostomy care, or self-injection, may be more complex for the client than anticipated, so additional practice sessions will need to be provided.

When possible, include family members and support people in the teaching plan and instructional sessions. Their involvement will help them assist in the client's home care and can reinforce the client's learning.

## Evaluation

Do not assume that learning has occurred without some type of validation. Evaluation of an individual teaching plan should include achievement of desired outcomes or goals, adequacy and appropriateness of teaching materials and methods, and effectiveness of the nurse as a teacher. Such evaluation of learning flows logically from the goals and objectives of the teaching plan if the teaching–learning process is developed systematically from the nursing process.

Learning can be evaluated in a variety of ways, including written tests, questionnaires, oral questioning, observation, and return demonstration. The method of evaluation should be consistent with the type of learning: Cognitive learning can be evaluated by questioning (written or oral), affective learning through client responses, and psychomotor by client return demonstrations. Although questionnaires are sometimes used to evaluate group learning, written tests are not commonly used in clinical settings.

To be effective, evaluation should occur throughout the teaching–learning process and at completion. The nurse should always be alert for staff frustration, client confusion, inaccurate information, and improper actions. Early correction will ensure that the client does not learn misinformation or practice skills incorrectly.

Evaluation of learning also should include assessment of the adequacy and appropriateness of the materials and methods used. If the assessment shows that the resource library contains adult education materials only in English, it might be necessary to get more materials (printed and audiovisual) that include pictures or languages appropriate to other client populations.

Just as with other nursing roles, teaching requires practice and experience. The nurse should always complete a self-evaluation to improve his or her approach. Some questions the nurse might ask include:

1. Did the client achieve the learning objective?
2. How was I the most (or least) helpful to the client's learning?
3. What factors facilitated (or blocked) the client's success?
4. How could I improve this teaching session next time?

Nurses also should seek client feedback about the teaching–learning experience. Much can be learned from the client's perception. An anonymous questionnaire using a standardized form in an objective format (requiring circled or checked responses) should be provided to the client on discharge. Communication of the results should be shared with staff.

# Documentation of Client Teaching

Documenting client teaching is an important nursing responsibility required by the following:

- State nurse practice acts
- State home health agency licensure laws
- Medicare and Medicaid program regulations
- The American Nurses Association, which established a standard of care that includes teaching as a measure of accountability for quality of nursing care rendered, which must be demonstrated through documentation
- The Joint Commission on Accreditation of Healthcare Organizations (JCAHO), which requires that teaching must be shown by documentation for a facility to receive accreditation

Documentation of teaching and learning is set by agency policy and procedures. Each agency must determine the method of documentation and the types of clinical records that meet the agency's requirements for client teaching. Teaching may be written on a care plan, in nursing notes, or on a separate teaching record, but it must be part of the client's official record. Generally, documentation of client teaching should include:

- Learning needs
- Teaching interventions planned
- Teaching interventions implemented
- Client outcomes achieved or not achieved
- Revisions or changes in teaching methods used

Whatever charting format or record is used, the nurse's charting must be clear, concise, accurate, and complete. The charting entries must show what was taught and how well the client or significant other demonstrated learning. An example of documentation of client learning is shown in **Display 11-7**.

---

**Display 11-7** | **Focus on Charting: Client Teaching**

Problem: Requested nurse change newborn son's wet and soiled diaper after circumcision procedure. Asking many questions about how to care for circumcised son, including diaper change and bathing instructions.

Intervention: Taught postcircumcision care with diaper change; explained and demonstrated cleansing circumcised penis. Answered questions. Will supervise mother in next diaper change and reinforce teaching.

Evaluation: Mother returned demonstration of diaper and circumcision care as taught.

# Clinical Applications of the Teaching–Learning Process

Now that we have reviewed important principles of teaching and learning and applicable teaching strategies for varied clinical settings, we will use the teaching–learning process to help Mary in the Vignette complete Mrs. Duncan's preoperative teaching. (See **Display 11-8**.)

**Assessment for Mrs. Duncan** ▼ Before using the hospital's guidelines for preoperative teaching (standardized plan), Mary assessed Mrs. Duncan's previous experiences with surgical experiences and hospitalizations, knowledge about the procedure to be performed, and her emotional state regarding surgery. In her assessment, Mary found Mrs. Duncan had two previous hospital experiences (childbirth at the age of

**Display 11-8   Individualized Preoperative Teaching Plan for Mrs. Duncan**

▶**NURSING DIAGNOSIS:**

Anxiety related to insufficient knowledge about current anesthesia side effects and pain control management practices

***Goals:***

1. Before surgery, Mrs. Duncan will effectively verbalize specific fears and concerns regarding surgery and anticipated recovery.
2. Before surgery, Mrs. Duncan will verbalize postoperative pain management routine with use of patient-controlled analgesia.

***Interventions:***

1. Provide an environment with privacy and minimal disruptions to encourage expression of feelings and concerns.
2. Listen actively, and clarify and reflect feelings as expressed by client.
3. Explain preoperative and postoperative activities with emphasis on use of patient-controlled analgesia.

▶**NURSING DIAGNOSIS:**

Deficient Knowledge (deep breathing and coughing) related to unfamiliarity with postoperative care activities

***Goals:***

1. Mrs. Duncan will verbalize knowledge of perioperative care before surgery.
2. Mrs. Duncan will demonstrate correct deep breathing and coughing techniques before surgery.

***Interventions:***

1. Explain usual preoperative and postoperative activities and expectations for Mrs. Duncan's procedure. Include family members and how the hospital staff will keep them informed of Mrs. Duncan's situation.
2. Demonstrate deep breathing and coughing using abdominal splinting technique. Have Mrs. Duncan return practice and demonstrate techniques.

26 years and appendectomy at age 14 years), which she found to be satisfying and uneventful, except for postanesthesia nausea and vomiting after her appendectomy. Mrs. Duncan cannot recall what the nurses and physicians expected of her after surgery, but she is apprehensive about pain management and nausea after surgery and the postoperative length of stay because she has no sick leave accrued from her new job as a legal secretary and needs to return to work as soon as possible. Mrs. Duncan gives a good description of her surgeon's instructions regarding her procedure and potential complications that may arise with her surgery. She expresses confidence in her physician and trust that the nurses will give her good care. On physical examination, Mary finds Mrs. Duncan's lungs are clear to auscultation and learns that she was a moderate smoker for 10 years but has not smoked in the last 2 years. Based on her assessment and the efforts of Mary and Mrs. Duncan's family, the nurse and client developed and implemented the individualized teaching plan outlined in Display 11-8.

# Conclusion

This chapter focuses on the nurse as teacher. To institute sound teaching effectiveness, the nurse must be a good communicator first. Through proper application of the principles of communication, teaching, and learning, the nurse gains the trust and respect of her or his clients in meeting their many self-care needs for the maintenance and promotion of health and recovery from illness or injury. Respect for the client's unique needs is necessary for a successful teaching–learning experience. When possible, the client and the nurse must work as a team toward meeting mutually agreed upon objectives, goals, and interventions. The nursing process provides an effective framework for assessing, planning, implementing, and evaluating client learning. Use of varied strategies with direct personal interactions between the nurse and client is essential to the client's learning. Nurses as health professionals must play a major role in meeting the public's health education needs. The nurse–client interactions provide an excellent opportunity for ongoing client health education.

## References

American Nurses Association. (1998). *Standards of clinical practice* (2nd ed). Washington, D.C.: Author.

Canobbio, M. M. (2000). *Mosby's handbook of patient teaching* (2nd ed.). St. Louis: Mosby.

Carpenito, L. J. (2002). *Nursing diagnosis: Application to clinical practice* (9th ed.). Philadelphia: Lippincott Williams & Wilkins.

Doak, C. C., Doak, L. G., & Root, J. H. (1996). *Teaching patients with low literacy skills* (2nd ed.). Philadelphia: Lippincott Williams & Wilkins.

London, F. (2001). Take the frustration out of patient education. *Home Health Nurse, 19*(3), 1–15.

North American Nursing Diagnosis Association (NANDA). (2001). *Nursing diagnoses: Definitions and classifications.* Philadelphia: Author.

Rankin, S. H., & Stallings, K. D. (2001). *Patient-education* (4th ed.). Philadelphia: Lippincott Williams & Wilkins.

Redman, B. (2001). *The process of patient education* (9th ed.). St. Louis: CV Mosby.

Taylor, C., Lillis, C., & LeMone, P. (2001). *Fundamentals of nursing* (4th ed.). Philadelphia: Lippincott Williams & Wilkins.

## Suggested Reading

Craven, R. F., & Hirnle, C. J. (2003). *Fundamentals of nursing: Human health and function* (4th ed.). Philadelphia: Lippincott Williams & Wilkins.

Deering, C. G. (1999). To speak or not to speak: Self-disclosure with patients. *American Journal of Nursing, 99*(1), 34–38.

Donovan, H., & Ward, S. (2001). A representational approach to patient education. *Journal of Nursing Scholarship, 33*(3), 211–216.

Griggs, S. A., & Dunn, R. S. (Eds.). (1998). *Learning styles and the nursing profession.* New York: NLN Press.

Kozier, B., Erb, G., Berman, A., & Burk e, K. (2000). *Fundamentals of nursing: Concepts, process and practice* (6th ed.). Upper Saddle River, NJ: Prentice Hall Health.

Mennies, J. H. (2001). Teaching adult patients with learning disabilities. *Nursing Spectrum, 10*(21), 15–18.

Potter, P., & Perry, A. (2001). *Fundamentals of nursing* (5th ed.). St. Louis: Mosby.

*Patient teaching made incredibly easy.* (1998). Springhouse, PA: Springhouse.

Wagner, J. (2001). Patient education: Teaching older adults. *Advance for Nurses, 3*(20), 15–17.

Ward-Collins, D. (1998). 'Noncompliant': Isn't there a better way to say it? *American Journal of Nursing, 98*(5), 27–32.

## On the Web

*www.literacyvolunteers.org*: Information on functional illiteracy

*www.healthAtoZ.com*: Consumer health information; maintained by health care professionals

*www.betterhealth.com*: Australian site for clients; maintained by health care professionals

*www.osu.edu/units/osuhosp/patedu*: Ohio State University site; has teaching guides

*www.cbsnews.com*: Up-to-date client health information

*www.americanheart.org*: Mostly cardiovascular education sites

*www.pharmweb.net*: Medication information

# Manager of Care

# CHAPTER *12*

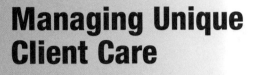

# Managing Unique Client Care

## LEARNING OBJECTIVES

*By the end of this chapter, the student will be able to:*

1  Provide examples of the following: culture, subculture, customs, beliefs, attitudes, values, and ethnocentrism.
2  Define the concepts of culture relevant to health and health-seeking behaviors.
3  Discuss how values, beliefs, and attitudes affect the nurse–client relationship.
4  Use communication skills that allow open discussion of similarities and differences with each client.
5  Use a variety of techniques to perform an accurate assessment of the unique variables for each client.
6  Apply concepts of uniqueness in the nursing care planning process.
7  Recognize the influence of beliefs, attitudes, and values on the nursing care planning process.
8  Develop a knowledge base to increase the appreciation of unique differences among clients.

## KEY TERMS

attitudes
beliefs
cultural competence
cultural relativism
cultural sensitivity
culture

customs
enculturation
ethnocentrism
subculture
uniqueness
values

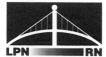

**VIGNETTE**

With the nursing shortage at its peak, Sacred Heart Hospital administrators have recruited Jose Cruz, LPN, from his native Puerto Rico to help staff their community hospital. Jose has been enjoying his orientation to the telemetry unit and has made a valuable contribution, especially with the large Hispanic population. The nurses within the hospital have welcomed Jose and other actively recruited Puerto Rican nurses. Jose has made plans to enter the RN program at a local community college and is talking to one of his professors about his situation.

**Professor:** How are things going at the hospital, Jose?

**Jose:** I'm very happy to be in America. The conveniences and the living are much easier than in Puerto Rico. We have been having some problems communicating with the Anglo nurses and physicians. They talk so fast and they use a lot of slang words. All of the medications are different; we don't have as many in Puerto Rico. There have been multiple transcription and medications errors. Even though we speak the same language, it is a difficult time adjusting.

**Professor:** What would be most helpful for you considering this?

**Jose:** I think if people would just slow down and be more patient. Maybe if they would go to another country and work. Then they would be able to be more aware of our needs.

**Professor:** I think that would be a good plan. Could you help us understand your culture in class? Would you be willing to share what is happening to you and what you have found helpful to communicate?

**Jose:** Sure. I want people to learn how different but also how much the same everyone is.

Nurses strive to assess, plan, and intervene based on an individual's response to illness. You have spent most of your time learning about the various anatomic and physiologic responses to illness. You have, no doubt, worried about the intricacies of hormonal regulation, adverse reactions to medications, and the variations in laboratory values and testing procedures. You know what to assess and how to plan and intervene while working with a client. You are aware of the resources available to blend variables such as age and chronic conditions into a plan of care. However, nurses interact with clients and other nurses, like Jose, from different cultural, social, and religious backgrounds and need to be **culturally competent** to care for diverse client populations.

# Uniqueness

Now you are given another piece of the nursing care plan puzzle: uniqueness. We define **uniqueness** as a combination of customs, beliefs, and values that each individual brings into the healthcare setting. Each of these customs, beliefs, and values is the result of an individual's life experience. Each person belongs to various social groups (i.e., **cul-**

**tures**) that form her or his life experience). The life experience of the nurse also is a significant variable that affects the nurse–client interaction.

## Definitions ▄▄▄▄▄▄▄▄▄▄▄▄▄▄▄▄▄▄▄▄▄▄▄▄▄▄▄▄▄▄

Anthropologists and other social scientists define human culture as learned behavior acquired by individuals as members of a social group. Each human society has a body of norms governing behavior and other knowledge to which an individual is socialized or enculturated, beginning at birth or at the time the individual becomes a member of the social group.

The United States is composed of many cultures. Many social groups (**subcultures**) come together to form a larger social group (dominant culture). The nurse needs to assess the unique elements of culture the client possesses. These elements are customs, beliefs, attitudes, and values.

**Customs** are learned behaviors. These behaviors are shared and practiced by individuals who belong to a particular group. Examples of the cultures to which an individual may belong are family units, nationality, religions, social classes, and professions. Customs are based on beliefs, attitudes, or values. The importance of a custom is related to the importance of the belief, attitude, or value on which it is based.

The customs that are important to a particular client are easily assessed because they can be observed or elicited by direct questioning. For example, a custom in the nursing profession is to wear the pin signifying the school from which the nurse graduated.

**Beliefs** include opinions, knowledge, and faith. A belief is the acceptance of truth or reliability of something with or without proof. Another term for a belief is *supposition*. A dominant American belief is the right of the individual is most important.

An **attitude** is a feeling tone directed toward a person, object, or idea. Attitudes are made up of many beliefs. If the nursing staff working with Jose believe he has made multiple errors in transcription, then they may conclude he is a bad nurse and shouldn't be allowed to practice. Judgments of good and bad derive from attitudes.

**Values** are a set of personal beliefs and attitudes about the truth, beauty, and worth of any thought, object, or behavior. They are action oriented and give direction and meaning to life. Values develop from associations with people, the environment, and self. They are derived from life experiences. Values that are important to Americans include individualism, accumulating items for self, nuclear family, and competition. These values are vastly different than the Native American culture, in which dependence and bonding to the family or group, sharing with others, extended family relationships, and cooperation are more highly valued (Luckmann, 1999).

## Self-Assessment ▄▄▄▄▄▄▄▄▄▄▄▄▄▄▄▄▄▄▄▄▄▄▄▄▄▄

People naturally think that their way of viewing the world is the only right way. This narrow view is called **ethnocentrism**. Stepping out of one's own comfort zone to learn about another culture is the opposite of ethnocentrism and is called **cultural relativism**. Learning more about your own cultural background is the first step in the understand-

| Display 12-1 | Suggestions to Enhance Cultural Sensitivity |
|---|---|

- Engage in student foreign exchange programs
- Take a foreign language course
- Visit other countries on guided tours
- Talk to nurses from other countries about their experiences
- Read books and journals
- View videotapes and movies with cultural themes

ing of culturally diverse client populations. **Display 12-1** gives suggestions on how a nurse can become more culturally sensitive.

### Thinking Critically

Make a list of the culture/subculture to which you belong. Write down what you value most about communication, space, social organization, and time. Try to find another friend, student, or nurse and ask him/her to do the same. What is the same? What is different?

One challenge for the registered nurse is the assessment of each client's uniqueness. As discussed in Chapter 11, nursing care planning must be individualized for each client. The following provides some suggestions for data collection strategies to assess each client's unique characteristics.

**Customs:** The most easily identifiable unique behaviors are those that can be observed or elicited by questioning.

**Beliefs:** An individual's beliefs can be ascertained in discussion.

**Values:** Distinct values, those that form the basis for beliefs and customs, are most difficult to uncover during conversation or observation. The nurse must be sensitive to a client's values, even if they differ from her or his own.

Read the scenarios that follow to see how sensitive assessments are performed.

## E X A M P L E   1

■ A 3-year-old Hmong child is hospitalized for dehydration. As the nurse prepares to start an intravenous (IV) line, she notices an embroidered cloth bracelet on the child's wrist.

The nurse sees the bracelet and wants to remove it so that he can start the IV on the forearm without interference. His attitude is the sterile insertion of an IV is extremely important so that the child can receive fluids and get better. Before snipping the bracelet, the nurse performs an assessment: "Tell me about your bracelet." He learns by direct questioning that placing a bracelet on a child is a Hmong custom. The nurse pursues the discussion and learns that the custom is based on the belief that the child will be protected from harm. The nurse is sensitive to this belief and allows the bracelet to remain and starts the IV in the opposite arm. ■

# E X A M P L E   2

■ A 6-month-old Mexican infant is brought by her mother to the clinic for immunization.

　　The admitting nurse says, "Your baby is so beautiful!" To which the mother responds, "Oh, this is the ugliest, naughtiest child." The nurse questions, "What makes you say such things about your baby?"

　　By direct questioning the nurse learns that it is the custom to say negative things about an infant. The mother believes that this will ward off the mal-ojo or evil eye. She explains that admiration of infants by strangers attracts this curse. The nurse uses this information and acts in a way that is sensitive to the beliefs of the mother. ■

To incorporate uniqueness into the plan of care, the assessment skills used by the nurses in these examples were finely tuned. In both cases, the nurses used wide-angled observational skills (the bracelet, the comments). Their communication was open, accepting, and free from judgment. The nurses did not ask "why" questions or judge the worth of the stated customs.

　　Remember, your best source of information about the particulars of social, cultural, sexual, and spiritual uniqueness is the client. To assess the impact of unique characteristics on the plan of care, you must communicate effectively and develop a self-awareness and sensitivity to similarities and differences among individuals.

## ▶ Thinking Critically

*This exercise is designed to stimulate discussion about how the attitudes, beliefs, and values of the nurse may affect the caring, collaborative relationship when the client holds different beliefs and attitudes.*

　　Role play three situations: One person will play client, another nurse, and a third the observer/recorder. Change roles for each situation.

### Situation 1

*Client:* You are a 30-year-old lesbian hospitalized for a total abdominal hysterectomy. You are crying when the nurse walks into the room.

*Nurse:* Use therapeutic communication to allow your client to express her feelings.

*Observer:* Note the nonverbal techniques that are used; note any statements that are judgmental or effectively neutral.

### Situation 2

*Client:* You are a 43-year-old confirmed speed (amphetamine) abuser. You are not interested in giving up your lifestyle. You are hospitalized for a skin staphylococcal infection from IV drug use.

*Nurse:* Teach the client the causes and preventive measures for infections.

*Observer:* Note the nonverbal techniques that are used; note any statements that are judgmental or effectively neutral.

### Situation 3

*Client:* You are 56 years old. You are 5 ft 2 in tall, weigh 220 lb, and have been hospitalized with low back pain.

*Nurse:* Discuss the impact of increased weight and the complications associated with low back pain.

*Observer:* Note the nonverbal techniques that are used; note any statements that are judgmental or effectively neutral.

After completion of this exercise, have each member of the group answer the following questions:

1. How did it feel to play the client character? What was difficult for you?

2. How did the interaction affect you and your responses? Did you feel your character was supported in her or his unique problems?

3. What approach did you take during the interaction as the nurse?

4. What statements or questions were easiest for you to answer? What other information did you gather?

5. What communication techniques were used during the interaction? Which techniques were facilitative and which blocked the interaction?

---

The nursing process begins with accurate assessments and continues as the nursing care plan is evaluated and reassessments are made. The rest of this chapter presents a framework for assessing unique client systems, thereby enriching the level of nursing care provided.

The client is viewed from four different sets of assessment variables. These variables look at the client as a member of smaller social groups or subcultures. The four groups considered are cultural, personal (interpersonal and intrapersonal), sexual, and spiritual. Accurate assessment of these variables in each client provides the basis of information necessary for holistic nursing care planning.

As you become more adept at recognizing the uniqueness of each client, you will develop your own sensitivities. Your personal experiences will give you a list of assessment variables much longer than any chapter or book could contain.

# The Client as a Member of a Cultural Group

A client may be of a particular cultural group, such as a Japanese man or a Muslim woman. He or she may identify solely with that culture or group or may have adopted or blended values and customs from another group into his or her lifestyle. This blending or adaptation is called **enculturation**. An example of enculturation would be a Muslim woman coming to the United States and adopting a Western style of dress but continuing to practice Islam. The nurse needs to demonstrate **cultural sensitivity** in this situation, that is, to assess this woman based on the client's individual beliefs and values, not on preconceived ideas about Muslim women.

## Impact of Physical Characteristics

Physical characteristics are an apparent set of variables. "You can't judge a book by its cover" is a saying to keep in mind when looking at each physical feature. Each client will display physical characteristics (e.g., skin, eye, and hair color; facial shape) attributable all or in part to a definite racial or ethnic group or gender. A sensitive assessment of the accuracy of your assumptions will allow you to uncover the unique aspects of the individual.

A client may resemble a particular group but possess cultural characteristics that resemble a different group. The nurse's initial assumption based on these attributes can be incorrect and incomplete. An example is assuming a dark-skinned client with the last name of Rodriguez speaks Spanish when she really is Portuguese and has married an Hispanic man. A careful interaction with this client would have made apparent her primary language.

Another example is that of an African American woman who, when registering at the emergency room, is asked for her welfare card. The woman, who holds a doctorate in economics and is a faculty member at the local university, must now wonder what other false assumptions will be made during her treatment.

## Impact of Language

There are many variations of idiomatic expression. The classic example is "bad" meaning something is exceptionally good. English-speaking populations have great variation. For example, the term "bloody," has quite a few meanings, depending on where one resides. Consequently, when caring for a client, it is important to clarify meanings. If the client requires a language translator, it is important to get a translator who can interpret idiomatic phrases. If your client is from Puerto Rico, he or she may have a hard time understanding a Spanish-speaking translator from Spain.

Language also includes nonverbal communication. Head nodding while smiling can be interpreted as signifying an understanding. However, among some groups, these nonverbal messages are a sign of respect only.

## Impact of Customs, Beliefs, and Values

This chapter has already discussed how customs, beliefs, and values are assessed. This is an area in which mistakes in assessment data can be made. In the Arab/Muslim culture, it is taboo for a woman to be uncovered for a physical examination or to be examined without the presence of her husband. It is impolite among certain Native American people to look into someone's eyes. Time, personal space, customary healing foods, and rituals for the dead are some of the issues around which poor assessment techniques can have deleterious effects. If the nurse is sensitive to the customs, beliefs, and values of the client, she or he will be able to provide optimum care.

## NCLEX–RN Might Ask 12-1

The nurse is caring for a Hindu client. The nurse would be culturally sensitive to this client if the nurse

- A. bases interactions on preconceived knowledge about Hindus.
- B. assesses this client for individual preferences.
- C. assigns this client to another nurse.
- D. teaches him to change his diet based on Western ideas.

• *See Appendix A for correct answer and rationale.*

## The Client as a Social Being

The social aspects of each person include interpersonal relationships, educational status, and intrapersonal sense.

### Impact of Family, Friends, and Community

When we use the word "client" we refer to an individual, a family, or a community. Each person plays a particular role, and each role affects the other client systems.

A man may be the main homemaker and caregiver of the children, which is considered nontraditional in North American society. A nursing care plan developed to allow him to express his concerns about the daily management of household chores in his absence may be appropriate. The client who is ill may not only be taking care of her children, but may also be the caregiver of elderly parents. When planning discharge teaching, the nurse needs to know what family, friend, or community support is available. It also is important to assess the beliefs and values the individual holds about independence versus dependence.

### Impact of Economic Status

Each client has a unique means of financial support. When planning nursing care, we must understand how the client's financial support will be affected by her or his illness. Loss of the ability to earn money is a major concern. Many households are managed by single parents, whose incomes pay the rent and buy food. Elderly clients may not be able to pay for the medications or nutritional supplements that are prescribed or suggested.

When assessing economic status, the nurse can learn through direct questioning and by careful listening to the client's concerns. The nurse should not be lulled into false assumptions by material trappings. The client may be well dressed but may have lost her or his job recently. It is appropriate to ask: How will you purchase medications?

### Impact of Self-esteem

The client who feels lack of control over the situation may not be able to participate in care. A client who feels he or she deserves to be ill will be an unwilling participant on the road to recovery.

At particular risk are people in violent relationships, people with addictions, and people with chronic diseases that require lifestyle changes to remain healthy. When assessing in this area, the nurse needs to listen for clues. A client may say, "I can't," "I shouldn't," or have excuses for the inability to agree with a plan of care. Often this is a sign that the person does not have the ability to make independent healthy decisions. Psychosocial interventions in the form of counseling or therapy groups may be necessary before the client is willing to take control of her or his own life.

# The Client as a Sexual Being

Sexuality is a personal and unique experience. It is value laden for most people. In other words, we all have attitudes and opinions about sexuality based on our own experiences. Sexual needs are basic in Maslow's hierarchy. Gone are the days when nurses interacted solely with parents of the traditional family. Single-parent households, homosexual couples, multigenerational families, and biracial families present challenging situations for the nurse to manage. The nurse needs to be accepting and open when assisting the client with sexual issues. Sexuality can be such an emotional issue that occasionally nurses may use another health team member to obtain accurate, factual assessments.

## Variations in Expression

A person's sexuality is expressed in the context of her or his own culture. Openly discussing sexual matters may be comfortable to one person and intimidating to another. The nurse needs to be knowledgeable about her or his own attitudes toward sex before she or he can be comfortable with a client's ability to express sexual concerns. Often the first step is to give permission to the person to discuss sexual concerns in an open way.

## Variations in Orientation

Individuals may be heterosexual, homosexual, or bisexual. Sexual variations are often not apparent. When interviewing, it is important for the nurse to use questions

---

## NCLEX–RN Might Ask 12-2

The nurse is caring for the child of a biracial couple. Recognizing that this couple's choice is based on a value system different from the nurse's is known as

    A. prejudice.
    B. enculturation.
    C. ethnocentrism.
    D. cultural relativism.

• See Appendix A for correct answer and rationale.

that are neutral. For example, one common question asked of people in their repro-ductive years is: "What type of birth control do you use?" This question assumes a partner of the opposite sex. This assumption does not allow the homosexual client to discuss health related to sexual practices. A neutral question that would elicit more information would be: "What precautions do you take when practicing safe sex?"

# The Client as a Spiritual Being

We are all spiritual beings. Spirituality is an individual's journey to find the purpose behind his/her life. Religion and spirituality are often thought of as the same. However, religion is an organized system of beliefs, a part of spirituality. The nurse needs to be open and accepting. The best way to become open to others' ideas is to know and be comfortable with your own spirituality. As you become open, the client is allowed to be open. It is this intersection of communication in which each person (the nurse and the client) is touched in some way by the other.

## Impact of Religious Beliefs

Each organized religious group has its own values and beliefs. Occasionally these affect either the client's ability to participate in her or his own care or the nurse's ability to give care. The nurse must clarify her or his values and be able to help the client clarify values.

## Impact of Personal Beliefs

The use of a crystal or an herbal remedy is therapeutic when supporting a client's per-sonal belief system. Spiritual healers, acupuncture, meditation, or Reike therapists are examples of personal belief choices a client might consider therapeutic. Incorporating these into the plan of care will promote the health of the client by respecting her or his belief system.

# Nursing Care Planning

Uniqueness affects the nursing process in the following ways.

## Assessment

The ability to obtain a full assessment depends on communication skills. Asking ques-tions in an open way will allow the nurse to gain valuable information about the way each individual will achieve a state of health that is personally satisfying.

> *Display 12-2*   **Assessment of Cultural Uniqueness**

1. What are your views of health and healthcare?
2. Tell me about your family and community relationships.
3. What is the language spoken at home?
4. Do you have ties to another country or another part of this country?
5. Describe some of the types of foods you usually eat.
6. What religion are you? How much of a part of your life is it?
7. Tell me about how you view childbirth and child rearing? Who is the decision maker at home?
8. What are your views about death/death rituals?

The way in which the questions are worded and which questions are asked are important. **Display 12-2** provides some questions to start with in a cultural assessment.

## Diagnosis

The North American Nursing Diagnosis Association (NANDA) uses nursing diagnoses to include cultural, spiritual, and social variations (**Display 12-3**).

## Planning and Goal Setting

True planning and goal setting require collaboration between the client and the nurse. This collaboration must include a sensitivity to the nurse's and the client's values and beliefs. Behavior that one nurse might interpret as noncompliant might actually be behavior that signifies respect.

## Interventions

The impact of uniqueness during this phase of the nursing process should be clear. Why include warm foods in your plan of care when your client has the belief that cold foods have healing properties when one has a fever? How can an intervention be written to

---

# NCLEX–RN Might Ask 12-3    ❓❓❓

The nurse is formulating a nursing diagnosis for a client who speaks only Chinese. Which of the following nursing diagnoses would be most appropriate?

    A. Knowledge Deficit related to surgical procedure
    B. Impaired Communication related to inability to speak and read English
    C. Social Impairment caused by inability to hear
    D. Spiritual Distress caused by hopelessness

• *See Appendix A for correct answer and rationale.*

| Display 12-3 | Cultural/Social/Spiritual Nursing Diagnoses |
| --- | --- |

Powerless related to inability to make verbal needs known
Spiritual Distress related to limited access to spiritual advisor
Impaired Communication related to inability to speak and read English
Role Strain related to recent divorce

monitor vaginal bleeding if the female client holds spiritual beliefs that allow her to show her body only to a relative? **Display 12-4** gives interventional strategies that can be used by the nurse to be more culturally sensitive.

## Evaluations

When uniqueness is considered throughout the nursing care planning process, the evaluation phase will reflect satisfactorily. If the evaluation of the plan is unsatisfactory, one should consider that there are unique factors at play. If the client is not able to express the reasons for using insulin, you must assess the impact of educational level on understanding health teaching or the cultural beliefs about using medications. Evaluation always leads back to the assessment phase of the nursing process. Review the areas of uniqueness that might need to reassessed when goals are not met.

## Conclusion

This chapter provides an overview of the management of unique client systems. The nurse can better assess and individualize care planning by viewing the client as a member of a cultural group, a social being, a sexual being, and a spiritual being. Several clinical examples and exercises are provided. The nurse's ongoing clarification of her or his own values fosters a greater sensitivity to those of the client.

| Display 12-4 | Interventions for the Culturally Sensitive Nurse |
| --- | --- |

- Be aware of how your ethnocentric tendencies color your world.
- Listen with a sensitive ear.
- Use a "wide-angle lens" with observational skills.
- Speak slowly and try not to raise the voice tone.
- Avoid medical terminology and slang.
- Use gestures, pantomime, or pictures.
- Incorporate practices/ideas from the client's healthcare beliefs.
- Use the dominant family member for support.
- Respect food preferences when possible.
- Use a nonfamily, culturally similar interpreter, if needed.

## Reference

Luckmann, J. (1999). *Transcultural communication in nursing.* Albany, NY: Delmar Publishers.

## Suggested Reading

Andrews, M., & Boyle, J. (1999). *Transcultural concepts in nursing care* (3rd ed.). Philadelphia: Lippincott.

Bowers, P. (2001). Cultural perspectives in childbearing. *Nursing Spectrum, 10*(14PA), 17–20.

Catanzaro, A., & McMullen, K. (2001). Increasing nursing students' spiritual sensitivity. *Nurse Educator, 26*(5), 221–226.

Choudhry, U. (1998). Health promotion among immigrant women from India living in Canada. *Image: Journal of Nursing Scholarship, 30*(3), 269–274.

Giger, J. N., & Davidhizar, R. E. (1999). *Transcultural nursing: Assessment and intervention* (3rd ed.). St. Louis: Mosby.

Kersey-Matosiak, F. (2001). An action plan for cultural competence. *Nursing Spectrum, 10*(7), 21–24.

Lowe, J., & Struthers, R. (2001). A conceptual framework of nursing in Native American culture. *Journal of Nursing Scholarship, 33*(3), 279–283.

McGee, C. (2001). When the golden rule does not apply. Starting nurses on the journey to cultural competence. *Journal for Nurses in Staff Development, 17*(3), 1–25.

O'Neill, D., & Kenny, E. (1998). Spirituality and chronic illness. *Image: Journal of Nursing Scholarship, 30*(3), 275–280.

Rivera-Andino, J., & Lopez, L. (2000). When culture complicates care. *RN, 63*(7), 47–49.

### *On the Web*  · · · · · · · · · · · · · · · · · · · · · · · · · · · · · · · · · · ·

*www.tcns.org/journal:* Journal of Transcultural Nursing

*www.diversityrx.org:* Diversity Rx is an organization promoting language and cultural competence to improve the quality of healthcare for minority, immigrant, and ethnically diverse communities.

*www.opening-doors.org:* Opening Doors: Reducing Sociocultural Barriers to Health Care is a national program that supports service and research projects to identify and break down nonfinancial, culturally based barriers to healthcare.

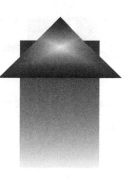

CHAPTER *13*

# Managing Care: Managing Time, Conflict, and the Nursing Environment

## LEARNING OBJECTIVES

By the end of this chapter, the student will be able to:

1   Summarize factors that influence time management.
2   Describe strategies to manage time more effectively.
3   Discuss various contexts in which conflict occurs.
4   Identify the process for conflict resolution.
5   Apply the guidelines for conflict resolution to a hypothetical situation.
6   List the steps in the decision-making process.
7   Compare the role of the registered nurse (RN) to that of the licensed practical/vocational nurse (LPN/LVN) in decision making.
8   Recognize the role of the nurse in cost-containment activities.
9   Analyze the role of the nurse in managing a safe environment.
10  Give examples of the LPN/LVN-to-RN role transition in managing client care.

## KEY TERMS

conflict
conflict resolution
cost containment
decision making
delegation

effectiveness
efficiency
time management
unlicensed assistive personnel
worksheet

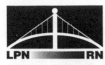

## VIGNETTE

**Mary:** (Enters the nursing station at 10 AM and sits down exasperated into the chair.) How am I going to care for my patients when there isn't enough time?

**Alice (head nurse):** What's the problem, Mary? You look frustrated and upset.

**Mary:** I just can't seem to get ahead. Mr. King in 203 isn't doing very well with his insulin injections, and he's going home today. Mrs. Duncan is going to surgery in 1 hour, and I haven't taught her how to deep breath and cough, and I haven't completed the pre-op checklist. Mr. James is upset about the medication changes Dr. Lotte made and won't take his new heart medications no matter how I explain it to him. So I'll have to call Dr. Lotte and let him know of Mr. James' refusal. I need to change Mrs. Lewis' dressing and irrigate Mr. Martin's colostomy before lunch. Dr. Craig wants Mrs. Lewis to have a different IV antibiotic as soon as it arrives from the pharmacy and her IV infiltrated. Miss John needs to get OOB, and my 0900 vital signs are still not done.

When I was an LPN, I was very organized and could complete everything by the end of my workday. Now, I barely have time to finish things as I dash from room to room.

**Alice:** Yes, there is so much more to do and so little time to do it in. You are working with another LPN and an aide. Let's look at your daily plan and see if anyone can help out. If not, I'll ask Grace, the other RN to help, and I'll pitch in and get you caught up.

**Mary:** Thanks Alice, I could use the help... Now about that plan, I don't use one.

**Alice:** Let me show you how to do one. I have several types of plans you could use. Planning is one of the most important things to do to complete your work.

Today's healthcare system requires that registered nurses (RNs) be prepared to assume the management of care for groups of clients. This includes the maintenance of a safe environment for all clients, supervision of unlicensed personnel, adherence to cost-containment issues, and the coordination of client care with other healthcare disciplines. The frustration Mary is feeling is not uncommon in a new nurse's transitioning from licensed practical/vocational nurse (LPN/LVN) to RN.

Managing client care requires that the nurse be able to assess the needs of the clients; plan, organize, and direct the implementation of care; and evaluate its effectiveness. The definition of manager of care is centered around a combination of care roles: care provider, coordinator, and overseer. It also involves the ability to organize time effectively, establish priorities, delegate appropriately, and ensure effective and efficient client care. The concepts of conflict management and decision making are important components of the manager of care role.

In this chapter, you are introduced to strategies to manage your time more effectively while providing and managing client care. You also learn about methods to deal with issues of conflict and conflict resolution in the work setting. Other aspects of managing client care involve decision making and managing resources. This chapter is designed to provide you with a better understanding of organizational and management skills as you change roles and expand your responsibilities.

# Managing Time

**Time management** is "the accomplishment of specified activities during the time available" (Huber, 2000, p. 125). One of the most difficult aspects of managing client care is the effective use of time. In managing client care, the task of time management becomes more complex and extremely variable. The process of time management is similar to the nursing process. It involves assessing current activities to do; determining an estimated time to do them; planning and setting goals and priorities; and evaluating the results (**Table 13-1**). In the next few pages, methods for examining time usage are described.

# Time Assessment

In your role as a student nurse, you recognize that managing your time with respect to client care is dictated by the number of clients to whom you are assigned and the role that you have for that particular clinical day. For example, if you are assigned to two clients, you are able to plan the care based on the needs of those two people. Although your time is somewhat controlled by what else happens with your clients or by having to wait for an instructor to supervise you in a procedure, you are able to complete the requirements of the assignment with appropriate planning. As an LPN/LVN, you also are familiar with caring for a larger number of clients and not having as much flexibility in planning your time. The shift is dictated by predetermined schedules for care and procedures and by multiple interruptions.

As you move into the RN role, you will have very little free time, time that is not dedicated to assessment, implementation, accomplishing tasks, and evaluating the results of those tasks. When assessing your time as a manager of care, it is helpful to formulate a chart with times listed every 15 minutes for the shift you work (Ellis & Hartley, 2000). **Display 13-1** shows an example of this type of log. After you have listed the hours appropriate to your shift, indicate the activity in which you were

---

**T A B L E   1 3 - 1**
**COMPARISON OF TIME MANAGEMENT AND THE NURSING PROCESS**

| Time Management | Nursing Process |
|---|---|
| 1. Assess daily jobs to be done and who will do them | 1. Assessment of the client |
| 2. Develop a daily plan | 2. Diagnosis |
| 3. Set priorities | 3. Planning |
| 4. Complete assignment tasks | 4. Interventions |
| 5. Set new priorities as needed | 5. Evaluation |
| 6. Evaluate the results of the plan | |

## Display 13-1 | Time Assessment

| | Day 1 | | Day 2 | | Day 1 | | Day 2 |
|---|---|---|---|---|---|---|---|
| Time | Activity | Time | Activity | Time | Activity | Time | Activity |
| 7:00 | _____ | 7:00 | _____ | 11:45 | _____ | 11:45 | _____ |
| 7:15 | _____ | 7:15 | _____ | 12:00 | _____ | 12:00 | _____ |
| 7:30 | _____ | 7:30 | _____ | 12:15 | _____ | 12:15 | _____ |
| 7:45 | _____ | 7:45 | _____ | 12:30 | _____ | 12:30 | _____ |
| 8:00 | _____ | 8:00 | _____ | 12:45 | _____ | 12:45 | _____ |
| 8:15 | _____ | 8:15 | _____ | 13:00 | _____ | 13:00 | _____ |
| 8:30 | _____ | 8:30 | _____ | 13:15 | _____ | 13:15 | _____ |
| 8:45 | _____ | 8:45 | _____ | 13:30 | _____ | 13:30 | _____ |
| 9:00 | _____ | 9:00 | _____ | 13:45 | _____ | 13:45 | _____ |
| 9:15 | _____ | 9:15 | _____ | 14:00 | _____ | 14:00 | _____ |
| 9:30 | _____ | 9:30 | _____ | 14:15 | _____ | 14:15 | _____ |
| 9:45 | _____ | 9:45 | _____ | 14:30 | _____ | 14:30 | _____ |
| 10:00 | _____ | 10:00 | _____ | 14:45 | _____ | 14:45 | _____ |
| 10:15 | _____ | 10:15 | _____ | 15:00 | _____ | 15:00 | _____ |
| 10:30 | _____ | 10:30 | _____ | 15:15 | _____ | 15:15 | _____ |
| 10:45 | _____ | 10:45 | _____ | 15:30 | _____ | 15:30 | _____ |
| 11:00 | _____ | 11:00 | _____ | 15:45 | _____ | 15:45 | _____ |
| 11:15 | _____ | 11:15 | _____ | 16:00 | _____ | 16:00 | _____ |
| 11:30 | _____ | 11:30 | _____ | | | | |

(Adapted with permission from Ellis, J., R., & Hartley, C. L. (2000). *Managing and coordinating nursing care*. Philadelphia: Lippincott Williams & Wilkins.)

engaged for that quarter hour; be as specific as possible. It is helpful to do this for several days to determine what interruptions you experience and what happens when the unexpected occurs. Keeping a log for several days also helps you to analyze how you cope with interruptions, what strengths you have in keeping things organized, and when you are the most productive. You will be able to identify how you save time and how you waste it. In the next section, strategies for managing time more effectively and common ways time is wasted are described.

## Planning

The notion of planning when working as a manager of care is sometimes viewed as unnecessary or useless because the work is already dictated by time constraints and unit policies. One of Mary's problems in the Vignette was that she failed to plan. However, in nursing care, one shift never mirrors another, and careful planning is one of the best ways to maximize efficiency. It can actually assist you in dealing with the unexpected and changing gears as needed. At the beginning of a shift, you should take a few minutes to examine what needs to be done (goal setting) and then develop a plan to accomplish those goals. It is important to estimate the time required to complete assigned tasks. As you gain experience in the RN role, being realistic with time requirements for the work to be done will become easier. Obviously this daily plan cannot account for crises, but it should allow for flexibility and reorganization if needed.

## Identifying Necessary Activities and Setting Priorities

When developing a daily plan, the activities that need to be accomplished will obviously emerge. Many nurses find it useful to make a **worksheet** from the daily plan (**Display 13-2**). This worksheet simply lists what must be done. It also assists you to establish priorities by determining what is essential and what is important but not critical. It often is beneficial to indicate what absolutely must be done by highlighting or designating such items with different color ink or highlighter. Although this seems rather simplistic, if you are in hurry, this can save some time by being able to glance at the list quickly. Items to perform can also be separated into the "do now," "do later," "do whenever," and "don't do" priorities.

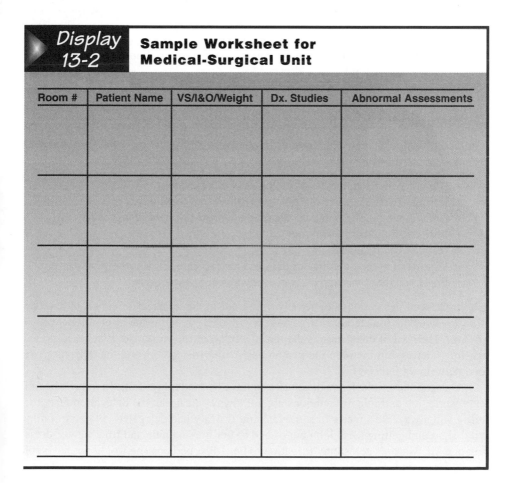

| Display 13-2 | Sample Worksheet for Medical-Surgical Unit | | | |
|---|---|---|---|---|
| Room # | Patient Name | VS/I&O/Weight | Dx. Studies | Abnormal Assessments |
|  |  |  |  |  |
|  |  |  |  |  |
|  |  |  |  |  |
|  |  |  |  |  |
|  |  |  |  |  |

Another aspect of developing and maintaining a worksheet is to get in the habit of writing things down. Although some nurses have an ability to remember everything, most nurses find it useful to write things down. The worksheet is an excellent place to do this, either beside the listed items or on the back of the paper. This information can include abnormal assessment findings, laboratory results, and PRN medications given. It is not meant to replace appropriate documentation, but it is a method to assist you in being accurate and continually updating the establishment of priorities for critical tasks.

A final aspect of the worksheet is to determine who needs to be doing what. This is an essential component of managing client care and an important aspect in your role transition.

### Thinking Critically

Divide into groups of three or four. Share with the group examples of daily plans and worksheets that you have seen in your work as an LPN/LVN. Discuss the various formats, paying attention to each suggestion so that all formats are viewed as having merit. When you have completed this discussion, formulate as a group the ideal daily plan and worksheet for a clinical unit where you have been assigned as students. Determine what is needed, what you would find useful if employed there as a new associate degree nurse graduate, and how this method might assist you in your role as a student nurse.

## Delegation

The process of delegation often proves troublesome for new nurses and for those who are making the transition from LPN/LVN to RN. The reasons for this are:

- Lack of understanding about the process of delegating
- Inability to assess what should be delegated and to whom
- Guilt about not doing as many tasks as the rest of the team members
- Desire to be liked by everyone
- Inability to organize
- Distrust of others' abilities or the need to take care of everything personally
- Being caught in the trap of "we've always done it that way"

The process of delegation is extremely important in the manager of care role. **Delegation** involves the transference of "a task or procedure to someone else" (Huber, 2000, p. 231). The goal of delegation is the redistribution of the workload. It is based upon a trusting relationship between the person delegating (delegator) and the delegatee (the one performing the task).

Delegation must be learned, just as you have learned other skills. In today's healthcare world, job and role expectations are not always clear, but the delegation responsibility will always be a factor in some fashion. If Mary had delegated obtaining routine vital signs and getting Miss John out of bed to her nursing aide and Mrs. Lewis' dressing and Mr. Martin's colostomy irrigation to her LPN, perhaps she would not have gotten so far behind.

---

**Display 13-3** | **When to Red Flag Delegation to Unlicensed Assistive Personnel**

1. When the client's needs are other than the standard or routine
2. When the outcomes of the procedure/task are unpredictable
3. When the skill is not within the realm of the job description
4. When the client's response is threatening his or her mental health

---

As a first step in delegating, the nurse assesses the skill and responsibilities of those assigned to provide client care. The use of unlicensed assistive personnel (UAPs) has increased greatly in the 1990s and 2000s. As an LPN/LVN, you are familiar with the scope of practice for LPN/LVNs in your state, but you will need to increase your knowledge of the changing responsibilities of UAPs and what you are able to delegate to them. It is your job as manager of care to determine your resources and to match those resources appropriately with the work that needs to be done. Each person also will have strengths and weaknesses that need to be identified. As a new RN, you may not have that knowledge, so it is important that you know the scope of practice for each person and what you are able to delegate. In Chapter 15, you learn more about the issue of legal accountability. Remember that you are accountable for delegating the appropriate tasks and responsibilities to the appropriate person. In addition, tasks may be delegated but nursing practice may not **(Display 13-3)** (Cherry & Jacob, 2002).

A second part of delegation is communicating the assignment effectively to co-workers and other healthcare team members. This involves supervising the activities of the team members so that tasks are completed, directions are followed, and standards of care are maintained. It also is important to recognize that this supervision does not imply control. Once you have delegated to a person, you must trust that person has the ability to carry out the assignment. If you do not have this trust, you need to examine why. As you make the transition to the RN role, you must learn the skills of delegation to provide optimal client care.

A last component of delegation is accountability. The RN must monitor the performance and provide feedback to the delegate. If the performance does not meet the standard, intervention to bring the performance to the standard must be sought (Cherry & Jacob, 2002). **Display 13-4** summarizes the four "A"s of delegation. In the Vignette,

---

**Display 13-4** | **The Four "A"s of Delegation**

**Assessment:** Patient needs, skills of the delegate
**Assignment:** Clearly communicate needed tasks
**Authority:** Give the delegate the power to do the task
**Accountability:** Correct performance within the standard of care

From Eason, F. (2001). The four 'A's' of delegation: A primer delegation is a recognized and essential nursing skill. Available at *www.advancefornurses.com/CE_Tests/delegation.html.*

Mary would need to check on the vital signs and both procedures to see they had been done and what the results were. Once a nurse has assessed, assigned, and evaluated the performance of the delegates, she needs to master another component of time management: the ability to use time efficiently and effectively.

## Efficient and Effective Use of Time

Some of the components of managing time assessment, planning, setting priorities, and delegation are essential to being efficient and effective. However, some other factors can assist you to manage your time. Zerwekh and Claborn (1997) distinguish between "efficiency" and "effectiveness" in the following way: **Efficiency** is the process of doing something right; **effectiveness** is doing the right thing right. As simplistic as this may seem, as a nurse, you have to make choices about what needs to be accomplished and then do it right **(Display 13-5)**.

One of the best methods for increasing effectiveness is to know yourself. Assess your own energy levels as they relate to the time of day. Are you a night owl or a morning lark? You probably can determine at what time of day you are the most productive, allowing for some variation regarding the time of year and the multiple demands on your time. Although you may not always be able to work according to your time clock, it is useful to pay attention to the high-energy periods and plan to do the things that require more energy at those times. It also is helpful to recognize that your efficiency may not be as great at the low-energy times, even though you need to accomplish some

## Display 13-5   Tips for Personal Effectiveness

• Pay attention to your basic human needs (sleep, nutrition, exercise)
• Plan frequently (daily, weekly, yearly)
• Declutter and organize any work areas
• Work as a team when possible
• Delegate appropriately
• Handle paper only once

important tasks. During these times, you may work with less speed and focus. Methods to augment your energy needs include providing for basic human needs, such as eating appropriately, sleeping adequately, and planning regular exercise.

A second method for increasing effectiveness is to be careful about assisting others or asking for help. Although this may seem to be in direct conflict with the notion of teamwork, effective time management means that you have to learn to ask for help, just as you need to learn when it is not appropriate to provide assistance. As you may recall from Chapter 1, having the ability to say "no" or the recognition that you need help will assist you in coping more efficiently and effectively with time management.

One of the issues that you face as you make the transition from LPN/LVN to RN is related to the need to demonstrate that you can do everything without help. You may have felt overburdened with work as an LPN/LVN and are determined not to impose on other members of the team. What was difficult to appreciate at the time was the need for the RN to manage client care, make judgments, make decisions, and delegate. The RN needs time to reorganize, set priorities, delegate the appropriate tasks to the best people, and generally manage time. You will accomplish this by "asking for help appropriately and responding appropriately to requests from others" (Ellis & Hartley, 2000, p. 136).

A final method for increasing efficiency and effectiveness is to assess the paperwork dilemma. One way to do this is to reduce the amount of paperwork to which you attend. You cannot avoid the requirements of the agency for which you work, but you can decrease the amount of paper. For instance, if you use a worksheet, limit yourself to one piece of paper so that you are not dealing with multiple pieces and having to shuffle through them. Keep the worksheet easily accessible so that you know where it is and are not spending valuable time looking for it. Create a worksheet that meets your needs and improves the efficiency in managing the care for a group of clients. If you think that paperwork issues could be more streamlined, develop and suggest methods to do that. Often changes are made because someone is able to demonstrate a more streamlined approach. Marquis and Huston (2000) have the following suggestions: Gather all of the supplies that you will need before engaging in an activity or group them in the same area, if possible. In addition, use time estimates to complete tasks and document them as soon as possible. Remember nursing care is frequently "around the clock." You may not always be able to complete everything in your allotted time. It is important to communicate to the following nurse what remains to be done and its priority.

Handling paperwork more efficiently will make you more effective in managing client care **(Display 13-6)**.

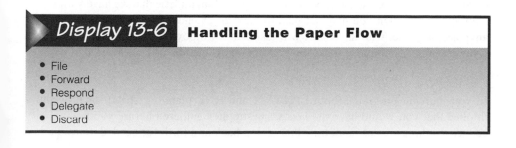

**Display 13-6**  **Handling the Paper Flow**

- File
- Forward
- Respond
- Delegate
- Discard

| Display 13-7 | Common Time Wasters |
|---|---|

- Interruptions
- Socialization
- Poor communication (lack of information or feedback)
- Meetings
- Paperwork

## Identifying Time Wasters

The last aspect of managing time is the identification of things that waste time or decrease your ability to be efficient and effective. You undoubtedly are able to identify factors that waste time or generally impede your ability to get a job done. Some of these things are personal time wasters, and others are outside factors. In the following paragraphs, some of these issues are highlighted with suggestions on how to control or minimize the things that interfere with your efficiency and effectiveness **(Display 13-7)**.

### INTERRUPTIONS

An interruption can be defined as any time you are stopped in the middle of one activity to give attention to another. Some of these interruptions are necessary and essential to the well-being of a client or to the general management of a group of clients. Other interruptions are less urgent and should be limited for greater efficiency. The task for the nurse is to determine which interruptions are positive. Many cannot be avoided but are part of your job. For example, if a call bell is on, it is more prudent to answer the call, just as it is necessary to answer the telephone to speak with family members or the physician. The use of mobile handheld telephones is common and can allow the nurse to manage telephone calls while performing other tasks and decreasing travel time to a stationary phone. However, personal phone calls (nonemergent) are negative interruptions and should not interfere with your job performance. You must determine how to deal with interruptions. You need to stay focused as much as possible on completing what you start and moving on from there. With multiple interruptions, you may start many things but never complete any.

### SOCIALIZING

Socializing is possibly the major factor in wasting time. All of us participate in a variety of social conversations while at work and enjoy the camaraderie that we have with fellow employees. Although you may not plan to have an extended conversation, it can occur anyplace, anytime, with anyone. It will take some willpower on your part and perhaps some planning to minimize socializing except on planned breaks and outside of work.

### PERSONAL DISORGANIZATION

In your nursing programs (both LPN/LVN and RN), planning ahead for procedures implied that you would have the necessary supplies gathered before you begin a procedure. Nothing wastes more time than going back and forth for needed items. Patient units in many hospitals have tried to minimize this issue by having some commonly used supplies in the client's room. However, careful planning will still help to alleviate wasted steps. Saving time also can be accomplished by combining several requests from clients into one trip. Personal organization is further reflected in how you organize your work. The use of a worksheet or other plan will assist you in being more organized.

## PROCRASTINATION

Marquis and Huston (2000, p. 90) define procrastination as putting "off something until a future time, to delay needlessly" (p. 90). Although there are times when delaying a particular task is advantageous, waiting to complete something generally will have only negative results. For example, if there is a particular procedure to be done sometime during the shift, it is more beneficial to do it as soon as you have time because the unexpected may occur, preventing you from getting it done. In addition, tasks that are delayed often become bigger than they were when they first needed to be done. There are several things to do to avoid procrastination. First, start early; break a task into small steps that seem more manageable (sometimes called "chunking"); remember that perfection is not always necessary as long as standards are maintained; and finally, reward yourself for accomplishing the dreaded chore.

## SUMMARY

The management of time is crucial as you make the transition from LPN/LVN to RN. Although you may be naturally good at keeping everything organized, you may have to acquire or improve your time management skills. Managing care for a group of clients requires that you are knowledgeable, flexible, thorough, responsible, and accountable. Take the time to assess your time management abilities and identify methods that will help you to be more skilled in this area. This activity will prove invaluable in your role transition.

In the following sections, you are introduced to other components of managing client care. The RN role requires that you have the ability to manage conflict, make decisions, and manage resources. The critical thinking activities give you an opportunity to consider issues you may encounter as you move into the RN role.

---

# NCLEX–RN Might Ask 13-2

The RN should be efficient and effective in delivering client care. A common time waster a nurse should avoid is

    A. socialization.
    B. handling a paper once.
    C. organizing supplies ahead of time.
    D. calling physicians to report changes in clients' assessed condition.

• *See Appendix A for correct answer and rationale.*

# Managing Conflict ▬▬▬▬▬▬▬▬▬▬

**Conflict** can be defined as tension or disharmony between individuals or groups when there is a difference about ideas, values, or beliefs. In general, conflict is an inevitable part of life. When two or more people work together, the potential for conflict is strong. Conflict is not necessarily a negative phenomenon, although it may be viewed as damaging to the relationships in a work environment. Examples of positive outcomes of conflict include innovative change, exchange of ideas, and a greater understanding of another person's feelings. However, conflict is uncomfortable; it produces tension and may cause people to engage in uncharacteristic behaviors.

When managing client care, you will be faced with a variety of conflicts related to care of the client and to other healthcare workers. This conflict may lead to antagonism and incompatibility between individuals or groups and can be disruptive. Unfortunately, conflict is common within healthcare agencies. It may be that the business of taking care of clients produces a certain amount of tension at all times. Whatever the reason, nurses are often in the midst of conflict-producing situations. The types of conflict that a nurse may experience are role, goal, personality, and ethical conflict.

## Types and Causes of Conflict

Types and causes of conflict within nursing are numerous. Zerwekh and Claborn (1997) have identified some common factors that contribute to conflict in nursing.

### ROLE CONFLICT

Conflict can occur when people share similar responsibilities, but the boundaries are not well delineated. For example, shift-to-shift conflict about who is responsible for particular procedures during certain hours is common. Role conflict may also occur when a community nurse enters a home for a visit. Decisions need to be made with the patient and family on who will do what in the care of the client. This conflict may be ongoing or related to a specific treatment.

### COMMUNICATION CONFLICT

This type of conflict has several levels. One is that communication is not understood or is misinterpreted. Another is that differences are recognized but not discussed between the individuals or groups. The final one is that information is not communicated because it was forgotten or overlooked. Whatever the reason, because communication involves two or more parties, a break in the process may lead to conflict. The conflict becomes greater when it is not discussed with the appropriate person but with everyone else instead.

### GOAL CONFLICT

In some situations, an individual may place a higher priority on achieving personal goals than on working for the goals and objectives of the group or organization. A patient's goals need to be taken into consideration in formulating nursing goals, or goals will not be achieved.

## PERSONALITY CONFLICT

This factor is unfortunately common. No one has a perfect personality, and there are instances when we may not deal with a situation appropriately. In addition, some individuals seem to lack a sense of humor, rarely display common courtesy, or have other social interaction shortcomings. There will always be difficult people in the work setting.

## ETHICAL OR VALUE CONFLICT

This type of conflict can pose a real dilemma. For example, disagreement about the code status of a client or the type of treatment to be used for a terminally ill client can be a source of conflict. In Chapter 16, you examine ethics as they relate to nursing practice. You will have more opportunity to discuss the potential for conflict in relation to ethics and values.

The factors described in the preceding paragraphs contribute to conflict within nursing. In the next paragraphs, guidelines for resolving and dealing with conflict are examined.

# Conflict Resolution

Resolving conflict within a healthcare setting is not easy and is a situation in which you may not want to participate. However, as you move into the RN role, it will become more imperative that you deal with conflict. Some individuals are selective about the conflict in which they engage, and others seemingly enjoy conflict for conflict's sake. Some methods for dealing with conflict include accommodation, avoidance, competition, compromise, and collaboration. Choosing or participating in any of these methods will be determined by the situation, your comfort level, and your reaction to the conflict. An examination of these various methods follows.

## ACCOMMODATION

In this approach, the nurse suppresses anger about the conflict but does not address the issue directly. The nurse may be doing this to lessen the disruption that the conflict has caused. The nurse may also do this if there is a large power differential between her/him

---

### NCLEX–RN Might Ask 13-3   ❓❓❓

An RN has delegated the obtaining of vital signs on a six-client assignment to a UAP. When the RN checks the vital sign sheet, only four have been recorded. When the RN draws the UAP's attention to this, the UAP states, "I thought I only had these four to do." This type of potential conflict is known as a(n) _____ conflict.

    A. role
    B. communication
    C. goal
    D. personality

• *See Appendix A for correct answer and rationale.*

and another individual (such as a cardiothoracic surgeon). The underlying concept is "a little sugar goes a long way." This method also may be chosen because the individual wants time to plan a solution to the conflict.

## AVOIDANCE

This method also is referred to as "denying" conflict. Generally, nurses who are uncomfortable with conflict avoid addressing conflict situations. There are times when avoiding conflict is preferable, such as when insufficient information is available or when the particular problem represents a minute portion of the overall difficulty. The main idea here is to "leave it alone, and it will go away." However, in most instances, avoiding conflict is not a positive way to deal with issues.

## COMPETITION

Resolving conflict in a competitive manner usually means that a person wants to force the issue or achieve personal goals. In this situation, the person or group has a strong need to win the conflict and asserts this desire by out-talking, outshouting, and possibly threatening the opponents. Someone always loses in this approach. A competitive approach may be beneficial if the conflict warrants moving beyond a deadlock, but it rarely does much to resolve a problem.

## COMPROMISE

The method of compromise or negotiation implies that a conflict will be resolved by considering all aspects of the conflict and creating solutions that are agreeable to all participants. It also ensures that the issues are handled in a more direct way because all parties are aware of what is transpiring.

## COLLABORATION

This method builds on the method of compromise yet is more committed to creating a solution to the conflict that all participants feel good about and can support. This method requires a lot of effort but has long-reaching benefits.

You may recall from Chapter 1 that a method of win/win was used to reach agreements with significant others. When considering the conflict resolution methods discussed, collaboration has the most potential to produce a win/win agreement (**Display 13-8**).

In the following thinking critically activity, you build on the conflict that you presented or created with your classmates and determine the benefits of the various methods used to resolve the conflict.

### ▶ **Thinking Critically**

Recall a conflict that you or your classmates have had recently. Develop possible methods of resolving this conflict using accommodation, avoidance, competition, compromise, and collaboration. Contrast the advantages and disadvantages of each method for resolving the conflict.

> ### Display 13-8 | Conflict Resolution Strategies
>
> **Accommodating:** "A little bit of sugar goes a long way"; schmoozing.
> **Avoidance:** "Leave it alone... it will go away."
> **Competition:** "I win.... You lose."
> **Compromise:** "One for you...one for me... Two for you.... Two for me."
> **Collaboration:** "The more heads, the better!"

## Guidelines for Dealing With Conflict

Resolving daily conflict when managing client care may seem to be unrealistic. However, you will encounter many situations that require using conflict resolution methods. It is wise to use the following behaviors when dealing with conflict.

- Deal with issues, not personalities.
- Take responsibility for yourself and your participation.
- Communicate openly.
- Listen actively.
- Sort out the issues.
- Identify key themes in the discussion.
- Weigh the consequences (Zerwekh & Claborn, 1997, p. 178–179).

Managing client care involves a greater responsibility for the RN to deal effectively with conflict. The method that you select will depend on what meaning the conflict has for you and how it affects the nature of the care being provided to the client or group of clients. Successful resolution of conflict requires that the nurse be committed to resolution and that communication and trust are maintained. In the rest of this chapter, other issues related to managing client care are presented. These issues build on the use of conflict resolution methods.

## Making Decisions

As you make the transition from LPN/LVN to RN, an important element in your role is the ability to make decisions for client care based on information that has been reported to you or that you have observed. Decisions involve judgments, and these judgments can affect client care negatively or positively. **Decision making** usually involves values, life experiences, personal perceptions of the issue, possible risks involved, and personal approaches to making decisions. Decision making incorporates personal ability with learned skills. As the healthcare system becomes more concerned with cost containment and client outcomes, the need to be an effective decision maker will become more important.

The process of making a decision consists of six steps (Ellis & Hartley, 2000). The first step is to identify the problem or concern. This identification will be based on the nurse's perception of the issue. Another nurse may view the same situation differently.

Once the problem has been identified, the nurse will obtain more information to be more knowledgeable. This process is similar to the assessment step in the nursing process, in that assessment and communication skills are important. Part of gathering more data includes analyzing the information. The third step is to establish goals. In developing goals, the nurse determines what is realistic and if the measure would produce an improvement or positive change. Seeking alternative solutions or strategies ensures that the issue is being considered from all sides. Analysis of each strategy will help you determine whether it is beneficial and cost effective, and whether the resources needed are available. The selection of a strategy will be based on the methods of implementation available, time involved, and resources. The next step is to implement. This step may be done by the nurse or be delegated. That is part of the decision-making process. However, the nurse generally will be accountable for overseeing the implementation. The final step of the process is evaluation. As with any evaluation, the nurse compares the results of the implementation with the goals.

For many of the decisions they must make, nurses do not have the luxury of time to conduct such a formal process. Many decisions must be made within seconds. However, when learning to make more effective decisions, it is useful to use the decision-making process as much as possible. This process will enable you to be more efficient and effective, particularly as you gain more experience with it.

### Thinking Critically

As a new nurse in a long-term care facility, the oncoming charge nurse tells you that you spend too much time giving report. Although your feelings are hurt, you also face the dilemma of needing to shorten report and passing along what you feel to be essential information. Using the six steps of the decision-making process, make a decision that will solve this dilemma.

Managing client care involves being effective in making decisions. The quality of client care is affected by the quality of decisions made. Other aspects of decision making and managing client care include managing resources.

## Managing Resources

Resources by definition are things that are necessary to do a job. Resources include work space, supplies, equipment, available budgeted funds, and services available. In today's healthcare world, the attention to resource management has greatly increased. The expectation is that high quality care will be delivered to a large number of clients by fewer people (particularly professional people) with a cost-conscious use of resources. In addition, the environment will be conducive to maintaining high standards and a safe environment. This is an enormous responsibility for nurses and other healthcare workers and one with which you will be more acquainted as you gain experience in the RN role. This section gives you a brief overview of managing resources.

One of the first steps in managing resources is to develop cost awareness. This involves having an understanding of budgetary constraints related to salaries and resources. Many healthcare agencies have developed strategies to deliver client care services in a different way so that fewer professional services are needed. There also is more emphasis on conserving supplies and equipment. Knowledge of the standards for client care is important as you learn to balance client safety, environmental safety, and cost awareness. It will be helpful for you to gain a greater understanding of what is involved in cost savings measures in the agency where you will be employed.

A second step in managing resources is related to **cost containment**. This term applies to any efforts that are made to reduce rising healthcare costs. It may include decreasing ineffective use of resources and time, finding more efficient and cost-effective methods to deliver care, and developing more businesslike approaches to managing the care of clients. Ellis and Hartley (2000) state:

> Cost containment, in terms of time and materials, begins at the bedside. The nurse carefully balances the quality of care with conservative management of available resources. It is the legal responsibility of the nurse to maintain the standard of care and not jeopardize patient safety (p. 66).

The future of healthcare will continue to be linked to financial concerns. Your role as an RN will combine the need to continue to provide high quality, safe, and responsible care to clients with the necessity of being cost conscious and efficient. Standards of care and safety will need to be followed and not compromised. This is the continuing challenge, which also may prove to be ethically challenging. Theoretically, if safety and standards are maintained, client care will be cost effective.

# Conclusion

The role of the RN as manager of client care is crucial in healthcare today. The changes occurring in healthcare are geared to cost containment and to the use of less skilled and less trained personnel. Registered nurses will be required to manage the care of larger groups of clients and will be less supported by professional staff. As LPN/LVNs moving into the RN role, you will discover that this transition will mean that your skills as managers and your ability to provide expert clinical care will be highly valued.

Your role as an RN is that of a decision maker, deciding who is qualified to provide a particular aspect of care, what will best preserve a client's dignity in the face of increased technology, and how to restore hope when fear and suffering threaten to overcome clients. Your role will be one of problem solving, managing time in a cost-effective and efficient manner, resolving conflict so that clients receive optimal care, and ensuring that the client environment is safe in all respects.

The role of the RN will continue to expand. It will be your job to maintain the caring components of nursing practice so that the client is not forgotten in the quest to contain costs and to provide support in a cost-effective way. Your role as manager of client care will be complex and challenging. Acquisition of management skills is as important as the skills that you have acquired to provide client care.

## Student Exercises

Consider the following scenario:

A new associate degree nursing graduate named Diane is working on a 30-bed adult surgical unit, where she had previously been employed as an LPN. After completion of her orientation, she has been working 3 evenings a week. When Diane arrives at work one evening, she is assigned to team lead for half of the unit, which currently has 12 clients. On her team is one LPN and two patient care technicians. During report, she learns that there are five new postoperative clients, all of whom are having problems with nausea. Two clients are scheduled for surgery in 1 hour. The postoperative client from yesterday who had a colon tumor removed just tore off his colostomy bag and is screaming that the nurses are trying to kill him. Four of the clients are elderly and require much assistance for activities of daily living. The client in Room 4 has just fallen out of bed. The unit secretary for the floor has called out sick, and the float unit secretary cannot be in for 1 hour. Diane tells the charge nurse that she is concerned she will not be able to attend to everything. The charge nurse is orienting a new team leader and tells Diane that she will be there but cannot be too available. The charge nurse thinks that Diane's experience on the unit as an LPN will help her to get through and that she will not need any more help.

1. What does Diane need to do to get organized?

2. What should the work plan or worksheet include?

3. What should a client care assignment look like in this situation?

4. What does Diane need to know about the people assigned to her team?

5. Does Diane need additional personnel? If yes, what skill level does she require?

6. What is Diane's role in this situation? What should her assignment include?

7. What advice would you give to Diane?

8. What might you discuss with the charge nurse if you were in this situation?

## References

Cherry, B., & Jacob, S. (2002). *Contemporary nursing: Issues, trends and management* (2nd ed.). St. Louis: Mosby.

Eason, F. R. (2001). The four 'A's' of delegation: A primer delegation is a recognized and essential nursing skill. Available at *www.advancefornurses.com/CE_Tests/delegation.html*.

Ellis, J. R., & Hartley, C. L. (2000). *Managing and coordinating nursing care*. Philadelphia: Lippincott Williams & Wilkins.

Huber, D. (2000). *Leadership and nursing care management* (2nd ed.). Philadelphia: WB Saunders.

Marquis, B. L., & Huston, C. J. (2000). *Management decision making for nurses* (3rd ed.). Philadelphia: Lippincott Williams & Wilkins.

Zerwekh, J., & Claborn, J. C. (1997). *Nursing today: Transitions and trends* (2nd ed.). Philadelphia: WB Saunders.

## Suggested Reading

Fisher, M. (2000). Do you have delegation savvy? *Nursing 2000, 9,* 58–59.

Forman, H. (2001). Difficult people? What's the problem? *Nursing Spectrum, 10*(12), 10.

Goleman, D. (1998). *Working with emotional intelligence.* New York: Bantam Books.

Lyon, B. (2001). Positive situation focusing: Pollyanna or a powerful stress prevention strategy? *Reflections on Nursing Leadership, 27*(2), 38–39.

Minar-Baugh, V. (1998). Survival strategies: Improving time management skills. *Ostomy/Wound Management, 44*(5), 79.

National Council State Boards of Nursing. (1995). *Delegation: Concepts and decision-making process.* Chicago: Author.

Pagana, K. (1994). Teaching students time management strategies. *Journal of Nursing Education, 33,* 381.

Parsons, L. (1997). Delegation decision-making: Evaluation of a teaching strategy. *Journal of Nursing Administration, 27*(2), 47–52.

## On the Web

*www.nurseadvocate.org*

*www.crazyladyco.com*

*www.dayrunner.com*

*http://daytimer.com*

*http://compasnet.org*

*http://ncsbn.org*

*http://nursingworld.org*

*http://familytime.com*

*http://supercalendar.com*

# *C*

# Member of the Discipline of Nursing

# CHAPTER 14

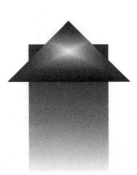

# Professional Responsibilities

## LEARNING OBJECTIVES

*By the end of the chapter, the student will be able to:*

1   Recall the four qualities of the professional discussed in Chapter 1.
2   Discuss the commonalities of, and differences between, the licensed practical/vocational nurse (LPN/LVN) and the registered nurse (RN) in the role of member of the discipline of nursing as outlined by the National League for Nursing.
3   Describe areas of responsibility of the RN in the role of member of the discipline of nursing.
4   Critique your verbal statements and behaviors and those of others for their portrayal of how nursing is valued and their subsequent impact on nursing's image.
5   Describe areas of professional growth to which the RN is committed as a member of the profession.
6   Delineate your professional growth needs to respond to societal changes.
7   Describe ways in which the RN promotes and maintains standards of nursing practice.
8   Describe the role of the RN in clinical practice regarding generating questions for research and applying research findings to practice.
9   Describe the RN's role in professional stewardship and the advancement of nursing.
10  Compare and contrast the roles of the LPN/LVN and the RN as a client advocate.

## KEY TERMS

| | | |
|---|---|---|
| accountability | image | professionalism |
| advocacy | integrity | referrals |
| bilingual | mentor | responsibility |
| client advocacy | modeling | role modeling |
| clinical research | multiculturalism | self-regulation |
| evidence-based | peer review | stewardship |
|   practice | proactive | valuing |
| global community | profession | |

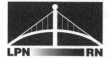

## VIGNETTE

Jennifer and Courtney have been friends since LPN school 5 years ago. They have maintained their friendship via e-mail despite the distance and time factors. Jennifer is in her second semester of RN school as an advanced placement student, and Courtney is considering returning to school. This is an e-mail transmission of their conversation.

**Courtney:** Sometimes I get so discouraged. It seems like we are going nowhere in nursing. The work is hard, the hours are difficult, and you hit a ceiling where you can't make any more money no matter what you do. Is it fruitless for me to go back to school?

**Jennifer:** You sound very down right now. The professional responsibilities of an RN are really awesome. I never imagined the responsibility to the public we have. Right now, RNs are very respected in the public eye, and we want to keep it that way. We are also moving more toward peer review, shared governance, and evidence-based practice. These are all hallmarks of a professional. What the two of us have been doing for years is networking. Now, thanks to school, I have other RNs and teachers who are networking with me as well as mentoring me. School is also teaching me more about power and how to intervene effectively in speaking for the client. I feel a renewed sense of spirit in all of my nursing endeavors. School has truly been an eye-opening experience.

**Courtney:** You sound so excited and positive. I hope this will "rub off" on me. I need a shot of something to help me from getting so down. I don't really see the need to get more education when I see very little difference in what an RN does and what I do now!

**Jennifer:** Well, one thing we need to do is keep in touch. I can also help you by sending you some other online sources to help you get excited and maintain that energy level. These documents talk a lot about the differences in roles from an LPN to RN. I am attaching them now to this.

**Courtney:** Thanks, Jen. You've really made my day and restored my confidence in nursing and its future role. I'm going to also work on that application to nursing school now and send it in.

The conversation Jennifer and Courtney are having is not a new one. In fact it is probably one you had several times with many LPNs before you applied to nursing school. What is the difference in practice between the LPN and RN? Is it worth my while to pursue further education? This chapter provides you with the opportunity to reflect on what you have learned in previous chapters and to answer such questions as: What are my professional responsibilities as an RN? In what ways and how will I assume a more expanded role with greater accountability within the profession? What role will I play in research and stewardship of the profession as an RN?

It may be helpful to look at the National League for Nurses' (NLN, 2000) *Educational Competencies for Graduates of Associate Degree Nursing Programs* **(Display 14-1)**. Both graduates practice within their respective scopes of practice and adhere to legal and ethical standards. Both practitioners are client advocates and engage in continuous learning and professional growth. However, the associate degree nurse (ADN) has more formalized education in communication skills, assessment, and teaching–learning. Much more time is spent in knowing not just how but also why a nurse performs certain skills. The RN also organizes, collaborates, and manages care using the nursing process as a model. She or he is a role model to other members of the nursing team and assumes a proactive role in governance, self-regulation, and advancement of the profession. Some of the documents Jennifer sent Courtney involved role differentiation. Until the LPN/LVN "steps into the RN's shoes," he or she may not be aware of the RN's level of functioning.

This chapter presents RN responsibilities in the role of member of the discipline of nursing **(Display 14-2)**. Responsibilities are presented in seven major areas:

1. modeling and valuing nursing,
2. professional growth,
3. standards of nursing practice,
4. nursing research,
5. professional stewardship and the advancement of nursing,
6. client advocacy, and
7. legal and ethical practice.

Legal and ethical issues are presented in more depth in Chapters 15 and 16.

---

### Display 14-1   RN Core Competencies

| | |
|---|---|
| Professional behaviors | Collaboration |
| Communication | Managing care |
| Assessment | Teaching–Learning |
| Clinical decision making | |

Adapted from National League for Nursing (NLN). (2000). *Educational competencies for graduates of associate degree nursing programs.* Boston: Jones and Bartlett Publishers.

**Display 14-2** | **Registered Nurse Responsibilities in the Role of Member of the Discipline of Nursing**

Responsibilities of the registered nurse in the role of member of the discipline of nursing include the following:

1. Modeling and valuing nursing
2. Making a commitment to ongoing professional growth
3. Ensuring that high standards of nursing are practiced
4. Contributing to and using nursing research in practice
5. Practicing professional stewardship to support the advancement of nursing
6. Serving as a client advocate
7. Practicing within the legal boundaries and ethical framework of nursing

# Modeling and Valuing Nursing

Perhaps the most important responsibility you will have in the role of member of the discipline of nursing as you transition to the RN level is that of modeling and valuing nursing. The image of nursing within the healthcare industry and in the eyes of the public affects policy development, decision making, funding, recruitment of new nurses, autonomy and development of the profession, and nursing's role in the structure and governance of healthcare systems. In its *Code of Ethics for Nurses with Interpretive Statements*, the American Nurses Association (ANA, 2001) states that nurses are client advocates who work to protect the health, rights, and safety of the clients they serve.

## Nursing's Image

The nursing profession has struggled over time to portray accurately who a nurse is and what a nurse does. Kalisch and Kalisch (1982, 1995) and Kalisch, Kalisch, and Scobey (1981) have done extensive work on the image of nursing. As they report, the public forms its view of nursing from the media, particularly through television and films, but also from books.

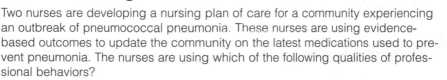

## NCLEX–RN Might Ask 14-1

Two nurses are developing a nursing plan of care for a community experiencing an outbreak of pneumococcal pneumonia. These nurses are using evidence-based outcomes to update the community on the latest medications used to prevent pneumonia. The nurses are using which of the following qualities of professional behaviors?

    A. Tradition, shared personal values, and autonomy
    B. Intellectual activities, service to society, and autonomy
    C. Licensure, tradition, and accountability
    D. Coalition building, professional dependency, and tradition

• *See Appendix A for correct answer and rationale.*

In the 1950s and 1960s, the nurse, nearly always a woman, was portrayed as a hand-maiden to the physician. The nurse as an independent care provider, decision maker, patient teacher, manager, and member of a profession was noticeably absent from the media. In addition, the nurse was not represented in such advanced roles as clinical specialist, educator, researcher, and administrator. Nursing's image was further compromised in the 1970s, when in addition to being under-represented in the media, the profession was grossly misrepresented, with nurses portrayed as overbearing and sadistic. Muff (1982), in examining the portrayal of nurses in the media and novels, identified several categories into which the nurse fell: ministering angels, handmaidens, battle-axes, fools, and whores. These portrayals also have been seen in children's books, comic strips, greeting cards, and other media, all-contributing to the denigration of nursing.

This low point in nursing's image during the 1970s heightened the need for nurses, acting as members of the discipline of nursing, to take a proactive role in strengthening nursing's image. Nurses learned from influences in the women's movement that they could play a pivotal role in political decision making and health policy and had the power to do so.

In 1982, the NLN formed the Task Force on Nursing's Public Image to provide leadership for nurses to take a proactive role in changing nursing's image. During the rest of the 1980s and into the 1990s, several media campaigns were launched and recruitment videotapes produced, which had a positive impact on the profession.

Nursing's image had improved in the late 1990s and 2000s. In June 1999, Sigma Theta Tau International consulted the Louis Harris Association to conduct a United States public opinion poll on 1,006 individuals considered to represent average Americans. This poll indicated that 92% of those polled trusted nurses as much as their physician with regard to information presented to them; 85% said they would be honored if their offspring chose nursing as a profession (*www.nursingsociety.org/media/exec*). Nurses need be active in political policy making and recognize their influence and power with the general public.

## The Nurse as Role Model

Each RN has a role to play as a member of the discipline to strengthen the image of nursing through modeling. As an LPN/LVN transitioning to the RN level, you will be assuming a lead role in nursing. Role modeling will become even more important. Each comment you make about nursing and all your actions or lack of action in matters dealing with nursing's image will have a positive or negative impact on the profession.

### ▶ Thinking Critically

What is your response when someone asks you what a nurse does and how you like being a nurse? How do you reply to the person (male or female) who is considering nursing as a career choice and asks you for your advice? How do your answers and the answers of thousands of other nurses affect the image and progress of the profession?

Your words, actions, conduct, and fulfillment of your nursing responsibilities demonstrate the degree to which you value nursing.

# Professional Growth

As a member of the discipline of nursing, the RN makes a commitment to ongoing professional growth. The NLN's *Educational Competencies for Graduates of Associate Degree Programs* (2000) states that an ADN graduate must:

* Participate in lifelong learning
* Develop and implement a plan to meet self-learning needs

You may be saying, "I already attend in-services and subscribe to nursing journals as an LPN." However, as you transition to the RN role you will assume a leadership role in the profession, including a broader scope of responsibility and accountability (as discussed in Units I and II). By making a commitment to professional growth at the RN level **(Display 14-3)**, the nurse continually strives to maintain a current knowledge base, remain technologically current, apply current research to practice, and respond to societal trends, such as those described in Chapter 4.

## Maintaining a Current Knowledge Base

Maintaining a current knowledge base in nursing is an ongoing challenge for any RN yet is a critical responsibility as a member within the discipline of nursing. On what areas should the nurse focus when seeking to update her or his knowledge base? Chapter 7 discusses RN competencies as a member of a professional discipline. As new information becomes available in the biological, physical, behavioral, social, and nursing sciences, each nurse must seek ways of gaining this new knowledge and applying it in each of the three nursing roles.

Maintaining a current knowledge base can be accomplished in several ways. In-service programs are available in most healthcare agencies, but the nurse should never wait for that to occur. If healthcare agencies cannot provide needed updating, the RN should take the initiative to attend. Local, state, regional, national, and international conferences are held regularly in nursing and in disciplines that support and inform nursing. Schools of nursing often offer courses, clinical updates, refresher programs, and some independent study options with an advisor, mentor, or preceptor. In addition, numerous nursing periodicals (journals) feature articles and case studies to maximize dissemination of new knowledge in nursing, and most journals offer online continuing education that can be accessed within the work or home setting.

| *Display* 14-3 | Areas for Professional Growth at the Registered Nurse Level |
| --- | --- |

The RN continually strives:

* To maintain a current knowledge base
* To remain technologically current
* To apply current research to practice
* To respond to societal changes

# Remaining Technologically Current

Equally important for professional growth is the nurse's need to be technologically current to practice competently in the care provider and manager roles. New technology continues to emerge, including cardiorespiratory diagnostic and supportive devices, pharmacotherapeutics, and computer-based treatment devices and client documentation systems. In-services are often provided as new technology is introduced in healthcare agencies, and schools of nursing may provide workshops or courses for technology upgrade.

# Applying Current Research

A third area of professional growth for the RN as a member of the discipline of nursing is the application of research to clinical practice. The usefulness of nursing research is presented later in this chapter. To meet the needs of clients and promote health, nurses must continue to incorporate nursing research into their practice. Nursing research expands the nurse's ability to use nursing process for nursing assessment and diagnosis, thereby providing comprehensive care planning.

In the last decade, **evidence-based practice** has been emphasized to try to change what nurses have done by tradition. "Evidence-based care is an approach to health care that realizes that pathophysiologic reasoning and personal experience are necessary but not sufficient for making decisions. This technique emphasizes decision-making based on the best available evidence and the use of outcome studies to guide decisions" (Craven & Hirnle, 2003, p. 122). In addition, the North American Nursing Diagnosis Association (NANDA) continues to update its list of nursing diagnoses based on research findings from clinical practice. This assists in providing a common language for the discipline of nursing, communicating nursing's domain to other healthcare professionals and the public, and establishing a framework for designing care standards.

# Responding to Societal Changes

When making a commitment to professional growth, the registered nurse strives to respond to societal changes to meet the needs of clients. As we enter a new millennium, a number of societal trends, as discussed in Chapter 4, influence nursing and have professional growth implications for nurses in clinical practice. Three important societal trends to note are changing demographics, the emerging global community, and the increasing amount, cost, and complexity of technology, especially in the healthcare industry (Heller, Oros, & Durney-Crowley, 2002).

## CHANGING DEMOGRAPHICS

American society is aging, and the ethnic population is growing. Within the next few decades, the population older than 85 years will dramatically increase. In some areas of the country, two of three clients are of minority populations, calling for nurses to think and act from a multicultural perspective. Such societal changes require RNs to seek professional growth to meet the needs of their changing client population. Many in-service programs, courses, conferences, and publications are available to assist the nurse with professional development in these areas.

- When caring for the elderly, the nurse must gain additional knowledge on the differing care needs of well, frail, and ill elders.
- What new research is available in geriatric nursing and the field of gerontology?
- What nursing intervention is needed for a client who is nearing 100 years of age?
- What safety and preventive measures are required to maintain health in this frail individual?
- What new information is available in the behavioral sciences to support nursing of elders?

Many new skills are needed by the nurse to address our multicultural population. Multiculturalism must be considered in every aspect of the care provider role. As the length of stay in healthcare facilities continues to shorten, communication skills and client teaching strategies must consider ethnic differences to meet increased self-care demands. At the RN level, these skills also are essential in the manager of care role, as the RN finds greater ethnic representation among her or his nursing team. Many RNs are learning a second language, finding that the nurse who is bilingual enriches her or his own life and is better able to fulfill nursing care responsibilities.

## GLOBAL COMMUNITY

As technology advances in the information and communication fields, nursing has become a discipline within a global community.

> Globalization is a broad term used to refer to international economic expansion as well as to the interdependent economic political and social processes that accompany the flow of people, capital, goods, information, concepts, images, ideas and values across increasingly diffuse borders and boundaries (Messias, 2001, p. 9–10).

Advances in distance education are creating the opportunity for nurses to participate in professional development activities with colleagues across the country and internationally through the use of fiber optics, satellite conferencing, and the worldwide web. This creates an exciting professional growth opportunity for RNs around the world. In addition, this challenges the RN to commit to professional growth to be a participating partner in confronting global issues, such as hunger, acquired immunodeficiency syndrome, bovine spongiform encephalopathy (mad cow disease), overpopulation, bioterrorism, and preservation of the environment.

## ADVANCES IN TECHNOLOGY

Technologic advances can be seen in every field, but the rapidly increasing amount, cost, and complexity of technology in the healthcare industry can be overwhelming to any nurse. As discussed, it is imperative that the nurse remain technologically current. The nurse must also be an astute observer and conserver of costly client resources. At the RN level in the manager of care role, this means ensuring that nursing team members are afforded opportunities to become comfortable and competent with new technology. It also means that every effort is coordinated to reduce costs.

In addition, the RN plays a leadership role in balancing "high tech" with "high touch." Nursing team members must believe the RN cares about them, is available, and listens to their needs. This also is true of clients. Numerous surveys to determine the satisfaction of clients at discharge from healthcare settings continue to rank personal, caring activities and listening as essential characteristics of the nursing staff. As flowers and personal belongings are set aside to make room for machines, and as supportive others have difficulty getting close enough to their loved one to touch, hug, or otherwise provide emotional support, the nurse must learn new ways to create the balance between high tech and high touch.

# Standards of Nursing Practice

A third major area of responsibility for the RN as a member of the discipline of nursing is ensuring that high standards of nursing are practiced. The ANA's (2001) *Code of Ethics for Nurses with Interpretive Statements* describes the nurse's role in safeguarding the client and public, using judgment in her or his own practice, and managing care provided by others.

## Promoting High Standards

Contributing to the establishment of high nursing standards and ensuring adherence to them is every nurse's responsibility. Chapter 7 describes standards of practice, differentiating them from regulations and policies. Chapter 4 discusses the role professional nursing organizations play in generating nursing standards. Participation in such organizations by individual practicing RNs generates standards that are comprehensive and based on daily nurse–client interactions in the clinical area. The healthcare settings in which nurses work have become more diverse, with a greater portion of clinical practice taking place in ambulatory and home care settings. Client care has shifted from a focus of providing hands-on care to one of client teaching for self-care. Standards for nursing practice must reflect such changes in the profession.

Nurses also participate in promoting high standards by contributing to the ongoing development of nursing diagnoses through activities sponsored by NANDA. This includes the generation and identification of emerging diagnoses with advances in nursing research assessment. It also means critiquing existing and recommended new diagnoses to ensure their applicability to clients of both genders, all ages, and with a diversity of socioeconomic, religious, cultural, and ethnic backgrounds.

Promoting high standards also means that RNs use as part of their autonomous practice such standards in writing and revising nursing orders and designing care plans. Nursing diagnoses, long- and short-term goals, and delineated nursing intervention activities must be clear, concise, and individualized to the client's condition and state of health. In addition, maintaining high standards means that nurses are current in their knowledge base and technical skills and incorporate current clinical research on preventive, therapeutic, and rehabilitative intervention strategies into nursing care plans.

Finally, RNs are mentors and teachers to other nursing staff to foster their knowledge and application of those standards.

## Accountability

As a member of the discipline of nursing at the RN level, the nurse maintains accountability for the standards of practice used by herself or himself and those to whom client care is delegated. Accountability extends beyond the responsibility of incorporating high standards into nursing care plans and assignments of delegated work. Accountability also involves evaluating the actual care implemented to ensure it is consistent with written standards and seeking consultation with healthcare provider colleagues and others as needed. (Accountability is discussed in more depth in Chapter 15.)

## Peer Review and Self-regulation

In its publication *Nursing: A Social Policy Statement* the ANA (1995) notes that nursing as a profession gains its authority from the social contract it holds with society. There is a social contract between society and the nursing profession. Under its terms, society grants the professions authority over functions vital to themselves and permits them considerable autonomy in the conduct of their own affairs. In return, the professions are expected to act responsibly, always mindful of the public trust. Self-regulation to assure quality in performance is at the heart of this relationship.

The major vehicle for the profession's self-regulation is through its professional organizations. Through activities and forums of these organizations, nurses are able to establish and maintain standards for nursing practice. This is discussed later in this chapter.

On the local level, RNs have a number of opportunities and responsibilities to engage in peer review to support standards of nursing practice. Some examples of these include peer nurse employee evaluation processes, nursing peer review panels, record audits, quality councils, quality assurance procedures, staffing ratio committees, and ethics committees. In addition, it is every nurse's responsibility to take the initiative to report behaviors or actions taken by nurse colleagues that are inconsistent with standards of nursing practice.

## Nursing Research ▬▬▬▬▬▬▬▬▬▬▬▬▬▬▬▬

A fourth major responsibility for the RN is in the area of research. The practicing RN plays three key roles in the area of nursing research. First, the nurse in clinical practice is in the position to generate questions for research. Second, the nurse can participate in clinical research studies that strengthen client care and health promotion. The practicing nurse notes possible relations between nursing intervention activities and client progress toward health. Third, the nurse in clinical practice fulfills the role of applying research findings to assist clients in regaining, maintaining, and promoting health. The new name for this is evidence-based research. Earlier in this chapter, information is provided on RN responsibilities related to professional growth, including a discussion on applying current research. Take a moment to review that section now.

> ### ▶ Thinking Critically
>
> Review some recent nursing journals. Synthesize one or two significant research findings presented. How can you apply these findings in your clinical practice to improve client care or strengthen client health?

## Professional Stewardship and the ▬▬▬▬ Advancement of Nursing

A fifth major area of responsibility for the RN as a member of the discipline of nursing is professional stewardship and supporting the advancement of nursing. Chapter 4 provides an in-depth discussion on the transitions that have occurred in nursing.

Through the efforts of individual nurse leaders, nursing as a profession continues to grow in its knowledge and practice base. As you transition to the RN level of practice, your involvement as a member of the profession will be essential in the areas of governance and decision making, participation in professional organizations, and recruiting and mentoring new nurses entering the profession.

### Governance and Decision Making

Increasing opportunities exist for the RN in decision making in the healthcare industry. Many agencies have established shared governance councils among nursing, medicine, and healthcare administrators. Staff nurses are assuming a greater role in hiring practices, peer review processes, committees for policy making, and the development of standards of practice. In addition, at the unit level, staff nurses have increased their involvement in scheduling, staffing, and other decision-making processes traditionally done by the charge nurse.

On the state and national levels, nurses participate in decision making by joining and being active in professional organizations. Technologic advances have created new opportunities for nurses to have dialogue about issues important to nursing and participate in decision making by satellite conferencing and the worldwide web. Newer technologies enable nurses to communicate more easily and enhance nurses' ability to speak with one voice.

### Providing Leadership Through Professional Organizations

Another responsibility you will have as an RN is to provide leadership for the discipline of nursing through membership and active participation in professional organizations at the state or national level. Such RN involvement generates rich dialogue and discussions about issues important to nurses. Professional organizations provide a forum for expressing viewpoints from a variety of perspectives, establishing position papers and standards to guide the profession and assist it to speak with one voice, and engaging in cooperative efforts to identify and achieve common goals.

> ### ▶ Thinking Critically
>
> Review the content on critical thinking presented in Chapter 8. How can you put your critical thinking skills to work through active participation in a professional organization to provide leadership for the nursing profession?

Chapter 4 provides an in-depth review of the ANA and the NLN. Both the ANA and the NLN are organized at the state level; for example, in California, nurses can join the California Nurses Association or the California League for Nursing and the national organization.

Participating in professional organizations provides the nurse with valuable information on advancements in nursing and the profession's interdependent and collaborative efforts with medicine and other professions. The ANA's (1995) *Nursing: A Social Policy Statement* (see Display 7-3) clarifies the definition of nursing as a discipline, identifying it as an entity discrete from medicine with its own unique purpose and autonomous practice. Nursing's professional organizations play a key role in further defining the discipline, identifying entry-level competencies, and establishing professional standards of practice. Chapter 7 also discusses the difference between LPN/LVN and RN scopes of practice in their respective nurse practice acts. Professional organizations provide guidance and practice standards for RNs, who practice autonomously and in collaboration with other professionals. Such activity is critical for professional stewardship and the advancement of nursing.

## Recruiting and Mentoring New Nurses

As you transition to the RN level, you become an important contributor to the advancement of nursing through your efforts in recruiting and mentoring new nurses. Earlier in this chapter, you examined the impact of your comments and behaviors on the image of nursing.

### RECRUITMENT

Nursing continues to strive for diversity in an effort to meet the needs of clients. In particular, more men and under-represented (minority) members are needed in the profession. In addition, as nursing competes with professions such as business, medicine, and law for the best and brightest, the challenge for each RN as a member of the profession is to seek methods to attract these individuals.

### MENTORING

Nurses also play a role in mentoring new nurses entering the profession. As you begin your practice at the RN level, you will find it helpful to confer with more experienced RNs. This is especially true in expanded scope of practice areas, such as the manager of care role and aspects of the care provider role (e.g., client education, referrals, responsibilities related to nursing process). Chapter 7 compares and contrasts LPN/LVN and RN knowledge, roles, and competencies. Chapter 8 discusses the independent (autonomous) and collaborative practice components at the RN level and provides more information in the area of nursing process, describing the use of clinical judgment to formulate nursing diagnoses. A review of these chapters will assist you in identifying areas in which you may need a mentor.

Carpenito (2002) and others have done extensive work in the area of nursing diagnosis, its application, and the formulation of collaborative problems. As you transition to the RN level, this new practice expectation may cause you some difficulty. Benner (2001) notes that the ability to cluster data intuitively, identify patterns, and thereby exercise clinical judgment in formulating nursing diagnostic statements increases with experience. By conferring with other more experienced nurses who serve as your mentors, you will develop this intuitive experiential knowledge to move from novice to expert.

> ### Thinking Critically
>
> Reflect on your own practice in nursing and the competencies you anticipate acquiring as you transition to the RN level. In what areas are you experienced and can offer to mentor others? In what areas might you seek a mentor to assist you?

As nurses gain expertise in assessment, clinical judgment, nursing diagnosis, client education, and management of care they have a responsibility as members of the profession in a leadership role to model these competencies and serve as mentors (and preceptors) to student and novice nurses entering the profession.

# Client Advocacy

A sixth area of responsibility for the RN is that of client advocacy. Client advocacy means speaking for the client or representing the client's point of view. This may involve speaking for the client because he or she is unable to do so alone, or it may involve translating or articulating the client's intent when, in the nurse's view, it is not being heard, perceived, or understood accurately or consistently with the client's original thinking. As an LPN/LVN, you played a role in client advocacy. However, at the RN level, you will have ultimate accountability in advocating for the client and ensuring the client's desires are understood and his or her rights (and freedom of choice) protected.

## Speaking for the Client

At times the client needs assistance communicating his or her desires. Respiratory devices, lowered states of consciousness, or other physical impairments may impede or limit the client's ability to express herself or himself. Language or cultural barriers may be present. The client may be illiterate, mentally or learning disabled, or unable to read, comprehend, or communicate adequately. The client may simply not grasp the concept of what is being explained. The RN's educational preparation in communication skills and his or her assessment skills will assist the nurse in ascertaining the client's needs and serving as a spokesperson and client advocate.

## NCLEX–RN Might Ask 14-2

The nurse is interceding for a client who has refused radiation treatment for a slow-growing malignant tumor. In this role, the nurse is acting as

A. teacher.
B. benefactor.
C. advocate.
D. proxy.

- *See Appendix A for correct answer and rationale.*

## Informed Decision Making

It is the RN's responsibility to ensure that clients are well informed to make choices and decisions about their care. Information should be provided verbally and in writing and should not be rushed. The nurse uses her or his knowledge and application of effective communication skills to ensure that the client has not only been provided with the information, but also has comprehended it. The client should be able to describe to the nurse what procedure or treatment is to be done or his or her understanding of the information given and the consequences of such (both positive and negative). When more than one alternative exists, the nurse ensures that all alternatives are understood. The nurse communicates in a nonjudgmental manner; when uncertainty is apparent, the nurse helps the client to acquire more information or to obtain a second medical opinion, or otherwise works to remove the client's uncertainty. Informed consent and the nurse's role related to advance directions (such as living wills) are discussed in Chapter 15.

## Referral

In addition to assisting the client in gaining more information and second medical opinions, the RN also is the client's advocate in making referrals. In transitioning from the LPN/LVN to the RN role, your scope of practice will include the need to make referrals. Referrals are indicated when information or intervention needed by the client is outside the scope of RN practice or when that intervention will take place under another nurse's care (such as in the transfer from acute to ambulatory care). Referrals generally are within the healthcare provider environment but occasionally are to other entities, such as behavioral scientists. Referrals are written to convey the client's needs and desires and to speak for the client as an advocate. Sometimes referrals by RNs are made in-house to other RNs with specialized expertise, such as enterostomal therapy nurses, lactation nurse specialists, special procedures nurses, oncology nurses, or diabetes education nurses.

## Protection of Rights

Finally, in the area of client advocacy, the RN ensures that each client's rights are protected. Chapter 12 discusses the nurse's role in managing diverse and sensitive human situations and systems. The client is viewed as a member of a cultural group, a social being, a sexual being, and a spiritual being. The importance of respecting and protecting each client's individual preferences is emphasized. Client advocacy means supporting the client in exercising individual preferences and exploring intervention strategies that will promote health within the client's belief system. At times, this means serving as an advocate for the client's right to refuse intervention, even if it means a decline in health.

# Legal and Ethical Practice

The seventh and final area of responsibility for the RN as a member of the discipline of nursing is legal and ethical practice. Both the ANA (2001) in *Code of Ethics for Nurses*

---

**TABLE 14-1**
**ANA CODE FOR NURSES STATEMENTS RELATED TO AREAS OF RESPONSIBILITY FOR REGISTERED NURSES (RNs) AS MEMBERS OF THE DISCIPLINE OF NURSING**

| RN as Member of Discipline Seven Areas of Responsibility | ANA Code for Nurses Statements |
| --- | --- |
| 1. Modeling and valuing nursing | The nurse participates in the profession's efforts to protect the public from misinformation and misrepresentation and to maintain the integrity of nursing. |
| 2. Making a commitment to ongoing professional growth | The nurse maintains competence in nursing. |
| 3. Ensuring that high standards of nursing are practiced | The nurse acts to safeguard the client and the public when health care and safety are affected by the incompetent, unethical, or illegal practice of any person. The nurse assumes responsibility and accountability for individual nursing judgments and actions. The nurse exercises informed judgment and uses individual competence and qualifications as criteria when seeking consultation, accepting responsibilities, and delegating nursing activities to others. |
| 4. Contributing to and using nursing research in practice | The nurse participates in the profession's efforts to establish and maintain conditions of employment conducive to high-quality nursing care. |
| 5. Practicing professional stewardship to support the advancement of nursing | The nurse participates in activities that contribute to the ongoing development of the profession's body of knowledge. |
| 6. Serving as a client advocate | The nurse provides services with respect for human dignity and the uniqueness of the client unrestricted by considerations of social or economic status, personal attributes, or the nature of health problems. The nurse collaborates with members of health professions and other citizens in promoting community and national efforts to meet the health needs of the public. |
| 7. Practicing within the legal boundaries and ethical framework of nursing | The nurse safeguards the client's right to privacy by judiciously protecting information of a confidential nature. |

*with Interpretive Statements* and the NLN (2000) in its delineation of competencies for the ADN graduate emphasize the importance of practicing within the legal boundaries and ethical framework of nursing. Through these mechanisms, nursing maintains its accountability to society. Legal and ethical issues are explored in Chapters 15 and 16, as is the role of the RN in regard to these issues.

# Conclusion

This chapter examines the professional responsibilities of the RN, including those related to nursing research and stewardship of the profession. Roles of the LPN/LVN and RN as members of the discipline of nursing are compared and contrasted, highlighting competencies identified by the NLN.

Seven major areas of responsibility for the RN are examined. As you complete this chapter and prepare for Chapters 15 and 16 and their focus on legal and ethical issues, respectively, you may find it helpful to reflect on these seven areas of responsibility and their relation to the ANA's (1985) *A Code for Nurses*. This relation is provided for you in **Table 14-1**.

## Student Exercises

1. Observe a practicing RN in the clinical setting for several hours.
   a. Cite statements made by the nurse or behaviors displayed by the nurse that tell you the degree to which she or he values (or does not value) nursing as a profession.
   b. Who was present at the time of these statements (e.g., patients, visitors, students, other healthcare workers)? How might these observers' perceptions of nursing be influenced (positively or negatively) by what they observed?
   c. How might these perceptions contribute to the evolving image of nursing and progress of the profession?

2. Imagine you have just completed the associate degree nursing program and are beginning your career in registered nursing. Design a professional growth plan for yourself by completing the outline below, identifying your strategies for maintaining competence during your first few years of nursing practice.
   a. Maintaining a current knowledge base
   b. Remaining technologically current
   c. Applying current research to practice
   d. Participating in professional organizations
   e. Responding to societal changes and needs

3. Reflect on who might be your mentor as you transition to the RN role. List individuals, and describe why you have selected them.

# References

American Nurses Association (ANA). (2001). *Code of ethics for nurses with interpretive statements.* Washington, D.C: American Nurses Publishing.

American Nurses Association (ANA). (1995). *Nursing: A social policy statement.* Kansas City, MO: Author.

Benner, P. (2001). From novice to expert: Excellence and power in clinical nursing practice (Commemorative ed.). Upper Saddle River, NJ: Prentice-Hall Health.

Carpenito, L. J. (2002). *Handbook of nursing diagnoses* (9th ed.). Philadelphia: Lippincott Williams & Wilkins.

Craven, R. F., & Hirnle, C. J. (2003). *Fundamentals of nursing: Human health and function* (4th ed.). Philadelphia: Lippincott Williams & Wilkins.

Heller, B. R., Oros, M. T., & Durney-Crowley, J. (2002). The future of nursing education: Ten trends to watch. Retrieved February 16, 2002, from *www.nln.org/nlnjournal/infotrends.htm.*

Kalisch, P. A., & Kalisch, B. J. (1982a). Nurses on prime-time television. *American Journal of Nursing, 82*(2), 264.

Kalisch, P. A., & Kalisch, B. J. (1995). *The advance of American nursing* (3rd ed.). Philadelphia: J.B. Lippincott.

Kalisch, P. A., Kalisch, B. J., & Scobey, M. (1981). Reflections on a TV image. *Nursing and Health Care, 5*(5), 248–255.

Leddy, S., & Pepper, J. M. (1998). *Conceptual basis of professional nursing* (4th ed.). Philadelphia: Lippincott-Raven Publishers.

Messias, D. K. (2001). Globalization, nursing, and health for all. *Journal of Nursing Scholarship, 33*(1), 9–11.

Muff, J. (1982). *Socialization, sexism, and stereotyping.* St. Louis: CV Mosby.

National League for Nursing (NLN). (2000). *Educational competencies for graduates of associate degree nursing programs.* Boston: Jones and Bartlett Publishers.

# Suggested Reading

Alfaro-LeFevre, R. (2002). *Applying nursing process: A step-by-step guide* (5th ed.). Philadelphia: Lippincott Williams & Wilkins.

Brown, S. (1999). *Knowledge for health care practice: A guide to using research evidence.* Philadelphia: WB Saunders.

Ellis, J. R., & Hartley, C. L. (2000). *Managing and coordinating nursing care* (3rd ed.). Philadelphia: Lippincott Williams & Wilkins.

Ellis, J. R., & Hartley, C. L. (2001). *Nursing in today's world: Challenges, issues, and trends* (7th ed.). Philadelphia: Lippincott Williams & Wilkins.

Gebbie, K., Wakefield, M., and Kerfoot, K. (2000). Nursing and health policy. *Journal of Nursing Scholarship, 32*(3), 307–315.

Grant, A. B. (1994). *The professional nurse: Issues and actions.* Springhouse, PA: Springhouse.

Kelly, L. Y. (1992). *The nursing experience: Trends, challenges, and transitions.* New York: McGraw-Hill.

Marion, J. (1995). Understanding the seven stages of change. *American Journal of Nursing, 95*(4), 41–43.

Mullem, C., Burke, L., & Dobmeyer, K. (1999). Strategic planning for research use in nursing practice. *The Journal of Nursing Administration, 29*(12), 38–49.

National League for Nursing (NLN). (1999). *Entry-level competencies of graduates of educational programs in practical nursing.* New York: Author.

Polit, D. F., Beck, C.T., & Hungler, B. P. (2001). *Nursing research: Methods, appraisal and utilization* (5th ed.). Philadelphia: Lippincott Williams & Wilkins.

Russwurm, M., & Larrabee, J. (1999). A model for change to evidence-based practice. *Image, 31*(4), 318.

Roy, C. (1995). Developing nursing knowledge. Practice issues raised from four philosophical perspectives. *Nursing Science Quarterly, 8*(2), 79–85.

Tanner, C. A., & Lindeman, C. A. (1989). *Using nursing research*. New York: National League for Nursing.

Taylor, C., Lillis, C., & LeMone, P. (2001). *Fundamentals of nursing: The art and science of nursing care* (4th ed.). Philadelphia: Lippincott Williams & Wilkins.

Trossman, S. (1999). Nurse researchers open doors. *American Journal of Nursing, 99*(9), 68, 70.

Zerwekh, J., & Claborn, J. C. (1997). *Nursing today: Transition and trends* (2nd ed.). Philadelphia: WB Saunders.

*On the Web* · · · · · · · · · · · · · · · · · · · · · · · · · · · · · · · · · · · · · · ·

*www.evidencebasednursing.com*: Evidence-based nursing

# CHAPTER 15

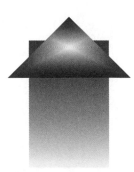

# Legal Accountability

## LEARNING OBJECTIVES

*By the end of this chapter, the student will be able to:*

1. Describe the origins of United States law.
2. List the differences among public, private, and nursing law.
3. Identify the components of accountability and the impact for nursing.
4. Identify the nurse's role in delegation.
5. Define negligence, malpractice, and liability.
6. Discuss methods to avoid litigation.
7. Identify legal issues that affect nursing practice.
8. Differentiate between the role of the licensed practical/vocational nurse (LPN/LVN) and registered nurse (RN) in relation to legal responsibilities.

## KEY TERMS

advance directive
civil law
common law
contract law
documentation
durable power of attorney
incident report
informed consent

liability
living will
malpractice
negligence
risk management
standards of care/practice
statutory law
tort

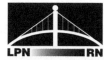

**VIGNETTE**

Cal Thomas is returning to school after working as an LPN at busy Willow Glen Medical Center. Cal is in his first semester and is halfway through his first nursing course. Cal is talking to his nurse manager, Joann Francheski. Joann has been a practicing nurse for more than 20 years; she too started out as an LPN.

**Cal:** I never really gave much though to the responsibilities RNs have until recently. The RN is not only accountable for what she does, but she is also accountable for those who work with and for her, especially when she is in charge. It was so comfortable doing and being what I am before I started school. Now, I'm not so sure I can live up to this kind of responsibility and accountability.

**Joann:** Yes. You will be functioning on a level that is much different from how you have practiced in the past. I found the role transition from an LPN to RN tough, and the staff will also have to deal with you in your new role. However challenging, it is a very rewarding step in your growth as a professional. Come, let's talk about what your responsibilities will be and how you can adjust into that role and grow. I have lots of success stories to tell you about my own and others doing what you are almost ready to do.

The healthcare delivery system is extremely complex. Health maintenance and healthcare provision are the primary functions of the healthcare delivery system. However, the system is not isolated from society, so it affects and is affected by societal values and beliefs. It also is accountable for maintaining legal and ethical standards established by society, healthcare providers, and healthcare consumers. In the Vignette, Cal is realizing the change in this role function as an LPN/LVN and the increased responsibility and accountability he has in fulfilling his new role. In this role, Cal will be even more immersed in legal and ethical decisions that affect his clients and his practice. "A wise nurse considers legal issues before a crisis arises and uses sound information to help guide action in situations where questions arise" (Ellis & Hartley, 2001, p. 297.) This chapter concentrates on how law affects nursing.

Laws are simply defined as rules for conduct and actions within a society and are binding for all citizens. Laws are developed by the people of that society and are enforced by a particular authority. Within the United States, laws are created by local, state, and national governments and courts and are enforced by officers and agencies of the government and courts.

The law influences many decisions made by nurses. As nursing has evolved to a more independent level, nurses are more responsible for their actions and decisions. Many situations faced by nurses today involve concerns about protecting client rights, carrying out accepted modes of treatment, and maintaining practice standards. Issues related to competence, safety, and optimal care can pose difficult dilemmas for nurses. The legal aspects of healthcare are closely aligned with ethical concerns. Because societal values and views change before law, law enforcement is the carrying out of ethical "shoulds." Frequently conflicts in the law can arise from an ethical problem (see Chapter 16).

In the following pages, you are introduced to general concepts of law. There are opportunities for you to consider legal implications for your own practice. Although you will not emerge as an expert in legal issues, you will have greater understanding of the concepts and a better appreciation of these principles for your own practice. You also will have an increased appreciation for the role transition that you are making in terms of legal responsibilities.

# Legal Considerations

This portion of the chapter provides brief explanations of legal terminology and introduces you to legal concepts that are important in your nursing practice. The expanded work role of the nurse necessitates that each nurse remain informed of current laws and regulations that affect the healthcare system. Origins and classifications of law in the United States are discussed. In addition, issues related to accountability, contracts, negligence, malpractice, and liability are introduced. An important part of this section is a brief examination of legal issues and public policies that affect nursing practice. You have an opportunity to consider several legal issues and their impact in your work world. Critical thinking activities provide an opportunity to apply legal concepts to the practice world.

# Sources of Law

The healthcare system is affected by several sources of law. In the United States, there are four sources.

## Constitutional Law

The US Constitution guarantees particular fundamental freedoms to all people in the United States. Constitutional law affects nurses in that their basic rights are protected. For example, freedoms of speech and the right to privacy are rights that nurses have as US citizens.

## Statutory Law

Legislative bodies at the local, state, and federal levels enact laws that are formalized, written, and voted on by the appropriate legislators. These laws can have a major impact on healthcare practitioners. For example, the diagnosis-related group (DRG) law enacted in 1983 decreed that hospitals in the United States that were reimbursed by Medicare could use the prospective reimbursement system for identified DRGs. The implementation of DRGs has had a profound effect on nursing and healthcare. Examples of state statutory laws are nurse practice acts. To change statutory law, amendments or repeals must be agreed on by the assigned legislators.

## Common Law

This type of law also is referred to as "judicial law" because it is based on court judgments, decisions, and decrees. Common law is based on earlier court decisions and precedents for interpretations of laws. The principle of *stare decisis* ("let the decision stand") evolved when courts began to present written decisions based on prior court cases; the same rules and principles are applied. In other words, if one court has previously made a decision for a particular case and another court has a similar case, the same decision will be made, citing the precedent of the earlier case. New rules will be made if the precedent is no longer applicable or is outdated. Although the decisions are considered binding within the court's jurisdiction, they are guidelines for other jurisdictions.

According to Taylor, Lillis, and LeMone (2001), "Common law helps prevent one set of rules from becoming used to judge one person and another set to judge another person in similar circumstances" (p. 100).

## Administrative Law

These laws are created by administrative agencies directed by the executive portion of the government. For example, nurse practice acts are formed by statutory law, but the authority to regulate that act is given to an administrative agency overseen by the governor. Regulations developed and approved by that agency are considered to be administrative laws.

## Classifications of Law

There are various ways to classify laws. For purposes of this text, the types of law presented are those that have direct implications for nursing practice. Two types of laws are presented: civil law and contract law.

### Civil Law

Civil law is the protection of individual rights and the governance of conduct between individuals and private organizations. A violation of civil law is called a **tort**. Nurses and other healthcare workers are affected by civil law in that malpractice and negligence cases fall within civil law. An intentional tort is one in which there was a conscious intent of harm (e.g., assault or false imprisonment). Unintentional tort is one in which there was no intent to cause harm. **Display 15-1** gives examples of intentional and unintentional torts that could be levied against the professional nurse.

### Contract Law

Contract law is about the agreements that are formed between two parties in which there is a duty or an obligation involved. Contracts are written or oral, and particular duties may be clearly stated or less definitively implied. Nurses generally become involved with contract law with employee and employer agreements. In the past 20 years, amendments to the original Labor Relation's Act have allowed nurses to form collective bargaining units. In the bargaining process, the employer and employees agree on a contract that is legally binding for both parties. The collective bargaining

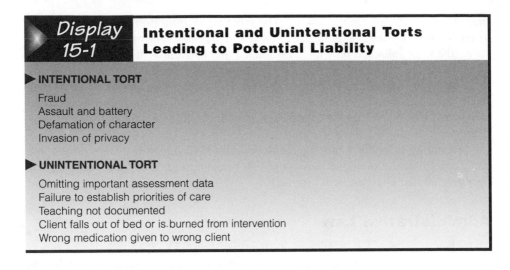

**Display 15-1**

# Intentional and Unintentional Torts Leading to Potential Liability

▶ **INTENTIONAL TORT**

Fraud
Assault and battery
Defamation of character
Invasion of privacy

▶ **UNINTENTIONAL TORT**

Omitting important assessment data
Failure to establish priorities of care
Teaching not documented
Client falls out of bed or is burned from intervention
Wrong medication given to wrong client

process is complex. If you are employed in a setting that has a union contract, it is essential that you seek the information needed for you to make informed decisions.

# Accountability

The term *accountability* has become a primary focus for nurses as they have moved to greater professionalization and independence. Accountability means that the nurse accepts responsibility for her or his own actions or behaviors. According to the American Nurses Association standards and the state nurse practice acts, nurses are responsible to demonstrate competence, sound judgment, and critical thinking in their role as caregiver. In addition, as a supervisor of LPN/LVNs and unlicensed assistive personnel (UAPs), the nurse must ensure safe care by delegating only routine care and evaluating the results of the delegated care **(Display 15-2)**. A nurse can delegate tasks, but she/he cannot delegate any aspect of professional judgment or decision-making about the client's needs. If a nurse delegates a task a UAP isn't competent to perform, the nurse may be liable if harm befalls the client. However, if the UAP does a task on his/her own

# NCLEX–RN Might Ask 15-1

A nurse accidentally administers an incorrect dose of morphine sulfate to a client. Which source of law *best* addresses this situation?

    A. Civil law
    B. Criminal law
    C. Common law
    D. Administrative law

• *See Appendix A for correct answer and rationale.*

---

| **Display 15-2** | **Guidelines for Delegating to Other Healthcare Personnel** |
|---|---|

- Is the task delegated "routine care?"
- Do agency policies cover the task delegated?
- Is the person delegated to competent to perform the care?
- Will the delegated individual be able to perform the task in a timely manner?
- Are you available to provide assistance to the person if needed?
- Does the task require assessment, planning, and evaluation? If so, the nurse should assume the task.

---

without consulting the nurse and the task is beyond her/his scope of training, the UAP, and not the nurse, would be liable.

As a student nurse, you also are accountable. You should do only skills you are competent to do, and you should never attempt anything invasive without the direction/presence of your instructor. The standard of care you are held to is that of a professional nurse, not a student and not an LPN/LVN. Before you perform any skill, ask your clinical supervisor if you are unclear about what to do. Client safety is the most important issue and supersedes your learning experiences.

## Documentation

A major factor in accountability is the requirement of documentation. Nurses increasingly are held responsible or liable for information that is either included or not included in reports and documentation. The work setting does not change the need for accurate and complete documentation. Generally the nurse remains responsible for a major portion of the client record. Accurate, descriptive, and impeccable documentation provides and ensures that the nurse has met the standard of care. "Without a complete and legible medical record, nursing staff members may be unable to defend themselves successfully against allegations of improper care" (*ChartSmart*, 2002, p. ix).

To cut down on the time required to chart, many agencies are adopting flow sheets that cover the normal standards of care. Coupled with charting by exception, where only abnormal results and ongoing problems need be addressed, such flow sheets maintain the legal requirements and standards, but the time required to complete them is more in tune with the nurse's busy day. Computerized documentation is also reducing time spent away from the bedside.

## Standards of Practice

Another aspect of accountability is the need for a profession to determine the aspects for which its members are accountable. The American Nurses Association (ANA) has developed standards of nursing practice, service, and education. These standards provide the means to assess the competency of the nurse members. In general, standards of practice have a common reasonable person rule. This rule assumes that the expectation for a nurse is that a reasonable level of knowledge, skills, and care will be held by other nurses with similar education and experience (Zerwekh & Claborn, 1997).

# Liability, Negligence, Malpractice ▬▬▬▬▬▬▬

The expanded roles of nurses and the increased need for nurses to have education and to demonstrate competence and technical ability have increased the responsibility of the nurse. However, with increased responsibility, nurses also are more likely to encounter issues of liability. In this section, definitions for the terms *liability*, *negligence*, *malpractice*, and *risk management* are provided. In addition, issues related to risk management and avoiding litigation are presented. You also have the opportunity to differentiate the role of the LPN/LVN and the RN in situations related to liability.

## Liability

Liability and legal responsibility are essentially synonymous terms. As a nurse, you are responsible for maintaining **standards of care**. If an action or lack of an action fails to maintain a standard and results in harm to the client, the nurse is liable or legally responsible. For example, the nurse is expected to administer medications safely and on time. If a client receives the wrong medication and is harmed as a result, that nurse is liable.

## Negligence

Negligence is a term closely related to liability. "Negligence has been defined as the omission to do something that a reasonable person, guided by the considerations that ordinarily regulate human affairs, would do or as doing something that a reasonable and prudent person would not do" (Marquis & Huston, 2000, p. 511). In other words, the actions of an individual thought to have made a mistake would be compared with those of a person with similar training to determine if the actions taken were reasonable and prudent or negligent.

## Malpractice

Malpractice also is called professional negligence/malpractice. In other words, professionals are expected to maintain a reasonable standard that has been defined by the specific profession. A professional is held liable for malpractice when she or he does not practice as his or her professional colleagues with similar knowledge and education would have in a similar circumstance. A negligent act is considered malpractice only if it is done by a professional conducting professional responsibilities. For example, a nurse involved in a car accident is held only to a negligence standard, not to a higher malpractice standard. However, if a nurse infuses intravenous solution into an infant at the rate used for an adult and the action causes brain damage in the infant, the nurse is

**Display 15-3** | **Definitions of Liability, Negligence, and Malpractice**

**Liability:** Legal responsibility for actions that do not reflect the standard of care and cause harm, or a failure to act to prevent harm
**Negligence:** An unreasonable or careless act or the failure to act in a reasonable and prudent manner that results in harm to an individual or group
**Malpractice:** Professional negligence; an act or failure to act by a professional in a reasonable and prudent manner in conducting professional duties as defined by members of the profession

held to the malpractice standard. **Display 15-3** provides definitions of the terms **liability, negligence,** and **malpractice**. For a plaintiff (party with the complaint) to be awarded **damages**, the lawyer must prove that the defendant (the nurse) had a **duty** to the plaintiff, and that there was a **breach of duty** and **direct causation**. **Display 15-4** gives a brief explanation of these terms.

Often the terms described in the preceding paragraphs strike a chord of fear in nurses. Although the following information may not remove the fear, it may assist you to reduce the possibility of litigation proceedings (lawsuits). As an LPN/LVN moving into the RN role, it is important to differentiate responsibility.

## Risk Management

Risk management is a term that was developed by insurance agencies. It refers to the process of identifying the cost of anticipated losses and then reducing the occurrence of such losses. Healthcare institutions now use this term; you are probably familiar with it at some level. Many healthcare agencies employ a person identified as the risk management officer or some similar title. This person has the responsibility of reviewing all the problems that occur at the place of employment, identifying common elements of the problems, and developing methods to reduce the risk of their recurrence.

One of the primary tools to review problems is the **incident report**. When an error is made or discovered or something out of the ordinary occurs that results in harm, an incident report is completed. This report identifies the nature of the incident, who was involved, and what steps were taken to remedy the situation. The incident report was

**Display 15-4** | **The Four Ds of a Successful Lawsuit**

**Duty:** The nurse has a duty to the client (usually found on assignment sheet or chart).
**Dereliction of Duty:** A standard of care was violated.
**Direct Cause:** The nurse's actions caused harm (usually hardest to prove by the defense).
**Damages:** A money amount to be awarded to the client because of pain/suffering.

In order for the plaintiff (person charging the complaint) to be awarded damages, the plaintiff must prove duty, dereliction of duty, and direct cause.

---

## NCLEX–RN Might Ask 15-2

The scope of nursing practice is legally defined by

    A. state nurse practice acts.
    B. professional nursing organizations.
    C. hospital policy and procedure manuals.
    D. physicians in the employing institutions.

• *See Appendix A for correct answer and rationale.*

---

not designed to be a punitive tool against employees but is a means to study a problem or series of problems and take steps to prevent the recurrence of such problems. Information should be as factual and complete as possible, and excuses for behaviors or actions should not be included. In addition, the incident should be documented in the medical record if a client was involved, although it does not need to be documented that an incident report was completed (most authorities recommend that the incident report should not be mentioned).

Risk management also can be applied to the individual employee. Although nurses do not generally call themselves risk managers, many of the procedures and steps that nurses use are methods to reduce harm to clients or employees and reduce the possibility of litigation. As an LPN/LVN, you are aware of the importance of following procedures, documenting your observations, and reporting to the appropriate people. All of these methods not only ensure proper care of your clients, but also reduce the risk of injury to your clients and others, including yourself. As an RN, this will not change, but the responsibility for care that clients receive will be greater. You are a care provider and a manager of care (refer to Chapter 14). This role necessitates that you are managing care for a group of clients but are not necessarily in direct supervision of that care. That also means that it is up to you to ensure that procedures and policies are followed and that client needs are being met.

As you move into the RN role, part of being a risk manager will involve identifying common problems and developing solutions to eliminate or reduce the incidence of particular situations. This should sound familiar on two levels. First, the nursing process uses the method of assessment, diagnosis, planning, implementation, and evaluation. In essence, when a nurse is looking for solutions to common problems, she or he is using a problem-solving method. Second, you may be familiar or involved with some form of quality assurance or quality improvement in your place of employment. This system is used by healthcare agencies to monitor and identify methods to improve services to the consumer. In that many of the consumer services are care related, RNs are heavily involved in quality assurance or improvement programs. As you progress through your associate degree nursing program, you will become more aware of the need to be a consumer advocate and to be involved in the assurance of quality care to clients. You may be asked to identify and implement an in-service or a procedure for a group of employees. For example, you may have observed that certified nurses aides are unfamiliar with the potential risk in transferring clients without a walker after they

> ### Display 15-5
> ### Risk Management Tips to Avoid Legal Ramifications
>
> 1. Listen to patients and families; they usually sue because they are angry.
> 2. Stay within the scope of your nursing practice acts and your professional competency level.
> 3. Act with the client's safety foremost in mind.
> 4. Know your agency's policies/standards/procedures.
> 5. Seek continuing education opportunities to increase cognitive, psychomotor, and affective skills.
> 6. Maintain and understand your professional liability insurance.

have undergone total hip replacement. To provide a constructive remedy, you could develop a procedure/policy or conduct an in-service. As an RN, it will be essential for you to be involved in risk management methods for yourself and for your colleagues. **Display 15-5** provides some tips on using risk management techniques to avoid legal ramifications.

### Thinking Critically

You have been assigned by your nurse manager to do an in-service for LPNs and UAPs regarding the legal implications of documentation. In your role as an RN, what would you include in this in-service? What is essential to include? What might you use to assist you in illustrating the key points?

## Legal Issues That Affect Nursing

A variety of issues within healthcare today can have a great impact on nursing. The technical advances in medicine and the increased knowledge of consumers have undoubtedly increased the legal implications for nursing. This section addresses a few of the issues that have an impact on nursing. It is not meant to be a complete list but to represent some of the issues.

### Advance Directives

Advance directives are documents that competent people execute to have control over their future healthcare. Examples of these documents are living wills and durable power of attorney. A **living will**, signed by an individual, indicates that her or his life is not to be sustained by extraordinary measures. Although this document is not always considered legally binding, it does provide information about the wishes of that individual. Individuals also use **durable power of attorney** for future healthcare decisions. With this type of agreement, a person assigns another individual to make healthcare decisions in the event that the person cannot do it for herself or himself. Generally, if the document is signed and notarized, it is considered binding. However, it is best to have the advice of a lawyer and to ensure that family members are aware of the document.

Advance directives can affect nursing in several ways. The first is that the RN must be aware of agency policies regarding advance directives. For example, some hospitals require that nurses ask clients or families about advance directives as part of the admission assessment. It also is the nurse's responsibility to inform physicians about client wishes regarding a living will or if the family is experiencing conflict about the wishes expressed in the document of durable power of attorney. Another responsibility is to provide support for decisions that the client and family have made. Making end-of-life decisions is painful at best. Although advance directives have not solved all of the issues related to these decisions, they are at least a legal method to ease the decision-making process.

## Informed Consent

Another issue that has many legal ramifications is informed consent. By definition, this means that a client must be provided with information about a procedure or treatment that informs the client of the benefits, risks, and all alternatives. In this way, the client is able to make an informed decision about the procedure or treatment. Consent is given voluntarily and may be withdrawn if the client has a change of heart. Clients also may refuse a particular treatment, although there have been incidents in which courts overruled the wishes of a parent or legal guardian. If a client does not believe procedures for obtaining informed consent were followed, he or she may sue for assault and battery (see **Display 15-6** for definitions of these terms) or for negligence in failing to obtain informed consent.

The nurse's responsibility in informed consent may be to witness the signature of a client when signing the consent form. The nurse's signature indicates the client has signed the form. The responsibility for providing information to the client rests with the physician. Before a nurse witnesses a client's signature, she or he should ask the client if the physician has provided an explanation of the procedure, its risks, benefits, and alternatives. At this time, the nurse may reinforce information given by the physician or inform the physician if the client has any questions or concerns. The nurse also can document the client's understanding of the procedure as related by the client. It also is important for RNs to be familiar with their particular state's laws regarding informed consent and each agency's policies so that RNs can be in compliance with all regulations.

---

> *Display 15-6* **Definitions of Assault and Battery**

**Assault:** An intentional act of one person that causes another person to fear that she or he will be injured or touched in an offensive way; touching does not actually need to occur.
**Battery:** If the act of touching or injuring actually takes place, the act is called battery. Medical treatments and procedures done without prior consent may be considered assault and battery, with exceptions made for emergency treatment.

## NCLEX–RN Might Ask 15-3

The physician approaches the client for permission to perform open heart surgery. For the client to give informed consent,

    A. the nurse must leave the room.
    B. the client must realize that any information gained from the procedure may be used for research.
    C. the client must be informed about the benefits and risks of the procedure, as well as alternatives to the procedure.
    D. the patient may not withdraw consent once it is given.

• *See Appendix A for correct answer and rationale.*

## Defamation

A final example of a legal issue that can affect nursing practice is defamation. An individual may be held liable for sharing information that is considered damaging to that person's reputation. Libel is written defamation, and slander is the term for oral defamation. Nurses traditionally have difficulties with defamation issues in relation to client confidentiality. For example, a client is admitted with a medical diagnosis of pneumonia. The medical record reveals the client has the human immunodeficiency virus. Nurses with access to that record tell various people the client has acquired immunodeficiency syndrome. The client later claims her business, a beauty salon, endured economic losses as a result of the disclosures by the nursing staff, and the client sues for slander.

Defamation of character may also be charged by a healthcare provider who believes that statements made by another professional are false, malicious, and have caused harm. There are accepted mechanisms for confidentially reporting inappropriate care or errors, and these should be used, rather than making statements to uninvolved third parties (Ellis & Hartley, 2001).

Defamation issues are often considered by participants to be innocent and harmless but may be injurious to a person's reputation. As an RN, it is essential that you recognize potentially harmful defamation and be alert to issues in which other employees are engaged. You may find it necessary to plan appropriate in-services or to speak with employees you are supervising.

### ▶ Thinking Critically

Research a current legal–medical issue that has relevance for nursing practice. For example, examine recent articles about assisted suicide, right to life, medical guardianship, or nurse negligence. Analyze these articles in class with attention to RN role and responsibility.

# Conclusion

This chapter emphasizes that nurses have legal responsibilities. Many issues that nurses face require legal knowledge. Legal responsibilities are pertinent to everything a nurse does. Standards of care, licensure laws, negligence and malpractice, and other issues related to liability determine the nurse's responsibilities. Methods such as accuracy in documentation or the performance of a procedure provide the nurse with the ability to demonstrate professional accountability and responsibility.

When making the transition from LPN/LVN to RN, students begin to recognize that there are legal consequences for the work nurses do. If a nurse does not practice as defined by legal standards and the client is harmed, the nurse is liable. The most important concern for nurses is the rights of clients, followed by the rights and responsibilities of the nurses' colleagues.

The nursing profession will continue to be challenged by changes in legal issues. Society will be faced with dilemmas that have no answers. The role of government in determining legal answers for ethical questions will bring forth other issues for nurses. Awareness of your personal and professional values will assist you in clarifying legal issues. Continuing self-growth and development will enhance your ability to deal with legal dilemmas. Although you may hope you are never placed in a situation of conflict, it is likely to happen. Be informed. Be prepared. Be knowledgeable.

## Student Exercises

As an RN, you have been hired to be the evening supervisor in a 50-bed long-term care facility. After an orientation to the role and responsibilities, you are officially the evening charge nurse. There are two units in this agency; one unit is designated for clients with Alzheimer's disease. On each unit is one LPN/LVN to be the charge person, one certified nurse's aide (CNA) with advanced training to administer oral medications, and three CNAs to provide basic care to the clients.

1. As the RN supervisor, what do you need to know from a legal perspective to do your job? Think in terms of delegating, competencies of other personnel, and your responsibility for the care that clients receive.

2. From a legal perspective, what is your responsibility if an employee practices unsafely?

## References

*ChartSmart: The A-to-Z guide to better nursing documentation.* (2002). Springhouse, PA: Lippincott Williams & Wilkins.

Ellis, J., & Hartley, C. (2001). *Nursing in today's world: Challenges, issues and trends* (7th ed.). Philadelphia: Lippincott Williams & Wilkins.

Marquis, B., & Huston, C. (2000). *Leadership roles and management functions in nursing: Theory and application* (3rd ed.). Philadelphia: Lippincott Williams & Wilkins.

Taylor, C., Lillis, C., & LeMone, P. (2001). *Fundamentals of nursing: The art and science of nursing care* (4th ed.). Philadelphia: Lippincott Williams & Wilkins.

Zerwekh, J., & Claborn, J. (1997). *Nursing today: Transitions and trends* (2nd ed.). Philadelphia: WB
Saunders.

## Suggested Reading

Brown, S. (1999). Good Samaritan laws: Protections and limits. *RN, 62*(11), 65–68.
Dunn, D. (1999). Exploring the gray areas of informed consent. *Nursing '99, 99*(6), 41–44.
Infante, M. (2000). Malpractice may not be your biggest legal risk. *RN, 63*(7), 67–73.
Laboy, A. (2001). How to survive a lawsuit. *Nursing Spectrum, 10*(18), 19.
Maltz, A. (2001). Keeping pace with new patient privacy rules. *RN, 64*(9), 71–74.
Mantel, D. (1999). Off-duty doesn't mean off the hook. *RN, 62*(10), 71–74.
National Council of State Boards of Nursing. (1995). *Delegation: Concepts and decision-making process.*
Chicago: Author.
*Nurse's legal handbook* (4th ed.). (2002). Springhouse Corporation. Springhouse, PA: Author.
Polston, M. (1999). Whistleblowing: Does the law protect you? *American Journal of Nursing, 99*(1), 26–31.
Sheehan, J. (2001). Delegating to UAPs: A practical guide. *RN, 64*(11), 65–66.

*On the Web*  · · · · · · · · · · · · · · · · · · · · · · · · · · · · · · · · ·

*www.ncsbn.org/public/regulation/delegation/htm:* National Council of State Boards
of Nursing

*www.npg.com/npg/cases.htm:* The Nurses Protection Group

*www.ahima.org:* American Health Information Management Association (Patient
Confidentiality)

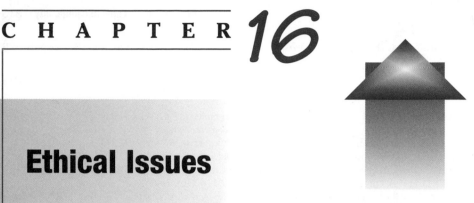

# CHAPTER 16

# Ethical Issues

## LEARNING OBJECTIVES

*By the end of the chapter the student will be able to:*

1 Explain the differences between law and ethics.
2 Describe the differences among ethics, bioethics, and nursing ethics.
3 Identify common ethical dilemmas a nurse might face.
4 Describe two common ethical theories.
5 List factors that influence ethical decision making.
6 Apply the nursing process as a decision-making model in analyzing an ethical dilemma.
7 Differentiate between the role of the RN and LPN/LVN in the decision-making process.

## KEY TERMS

advocate
ANA Code of Ethics
  for Nurses
autonomy
beneficence
bioethics
deontology
ethical dilemma
ethics

fidelity
justice
nonmaleficence
nursing ethics
standards of nursing
teleology
utilitarianism
values
veracity

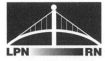

## VIGNETTE

Janet Bieber calls her nurse manager, Jean Close, to report a situation in the surgical intensive care unit.

**Janet:** I called to let you know that Dr. Brown, the cardiothoracic surgeon, will be calling you soon.

**Jean:** Oh. What about?

**Janet:** We refused to medicate Mr. Swartz. He is supposed to be going for triple bypass grafts in 1 hour, and we don't think he knows fully what is going to happen to him.

Would you as the charge nurse have the strength to stand up to Dr. Brown? Could you be the **advocate** for the client if he didn't understand the full implications of the surgery he is about to undergo?

# Ethics and Bioethics ▪▬▬▬▬

In the previous chapter, the laws and their relationship to nursing were explored. Ethics transcends the law. Changes in the law are actually a result of changes in the values of society. **Table 16-1** differentiates law and ethics.

According to the *Nurse's Legal Handbook,* 4th edition (Springhouse Corporation, 2000, p. 278), "**Ethics** is the area of philosophical study that examines values, actions and choices to determine right and wrong." Marquis and Huston (2000) define ethics as

> the systematic study of what a person's conduct ought to be with regard to him or herself, other human beings and the environment; it is the justification of what is right or good and the study of what a person's life and relationships ought to be, not necessarily what they are. (p. 479)

The study of how recent advances in medical technology affect decisions about right and wrong is called **bioethics**. In the nurse's daily practice, ethical decisions about right and wrong are made frequently. An **ethical dilemma** occurs when a nurse's view-

**TABLE 16-1**
LAW VERSUS ETHICS

| Law | Ethics |
|---|---|
| Rules of conduct are clear | Unclear, ambiguity exists |
| Impartial | Individual |
| Black and white | Gray areas |
| Courts decide | Individuals decide |
| Do not keep pace with society | Change with societal attitude changes |
| Doing things right | The right things to do |
| Legal counsel | Ethics committee |
| Regulated by authorized organizations and law officers | Ethical guidelines do not have a formal enforcement system |

| Display 16-1 | Common Ethical Problems |
|---|---|

Client's refusal of treatment/medications
Truth telling
Futile care
Participation in research protocols
Breaches in confidentiality
Incompetent or unethical practices by colleagues

point differs from that of a patient, family, physician, or other healthcare worker. For example, when the nurse observes activities such as cost-cutting strategies that are not within the standard of care, an ethical dilemma occurs. **Display 16-1** lists common ethical problems.

## Nursing Ethics

Nursing ethics is a part of bioethics **(Figure 16-1)**. Nursing ethics has evolved as nurses have become more involved as client advocates. The decisions a nurse makes are far from the same in each case and are not black and white. No two situations about client care are clear and exactly alike. The nurse needs to make ethical decisions based on professional standards and the American Nurses Association's (2001) *Code of Ethics for Nurses with Interpretive Statements*. In nursing education, nurses learn the technical skills needed to deliver competent care, but a "balance between morality and science must be sought and understood" (Cherry & Jacob, 2002, p. 203).

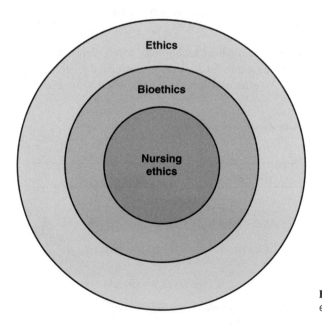

**FIGURE 16–1 ▼** Model of ethics.

> ### Display 16-2    **Definitions Related to Ethics**

**Ethics:** Decisions regarding what is right and wrong; often a system that is used to protect the rights of individuals or groups
**Code of ethics:** Standards of conduct and values as defined by a profession; forms the basis for ethical decision making by a profession
**Values:** The ideals and beliefs held by an individual or group; usually influenced by family, society, and religion; have a great impact on behavior
**Morals:** An individual's standards of right and wrong; formed in childhood (see Chap. 2); also influenced by family, society, and religion
**Bioethics:** Ethical questions surrounding life and death; questions and concerns regarding quality of life as it relates to advanced technology
**Ethical dilemma:** A situation in which an individual must choose between two alternatives that are not desirable; often involves examining rights and obligations of particular individuals; choice frequently defended

In the following pages, you are introduced to theories and systems of ethics that have influenced the development of nursing ethics and factors that affect ethical decision making. **Display 16-2** outlines terms relevant to nursing ethics.

# Ethical Theories

Ethical theory is a complex philosophical endeavor. The purpose of this section is not to provide an in-depth examination of various ethical theories but to briefly present the primary ethical theories used for ethical decision making in nursing. In general, an ethical theory is used for the purpose of determining the rightness or wrongness of a particular situation. In nursing ethics, two systems or theories are predominant: teleology and deontology.

## Teleology

Teleology has evolved from a humanistic and outcome-oriented approach to decision making. This system of teleology also is called **utilitarianism** theory (which refers to the end or outcome). Teleology has two principles: The greatest good for the greatest number, and the end justifies the means. These principles are probably familiar to you, but in terms of ethical decision making, they need further examination. Teleology implies that the consequences of actions must be considered—that is, the benefits to many will outweigh the harm to a few. For instance, the allocation of funds may be determined by the number of individuals who benefit from a particular service. Ellis and Hartley (2001) demonstrate this with an example about a decision to provide funds for the vaccines for many children as opposed to the funding of an organ donation for one person; the money would be allocated for the greater good.

The advantage of using teleology is that the needs of the majority are considered. In this way, research is promoted when it involves finding the causes of a disease with which many are afflicted, or finding treatments that will help many people and are of benefit to a particular company or research institute. The drawback of teleology is that the rights of individuals are not considered. The institution may have greater claim to conducting procedures or treatments without an individual being aware of alternatives; the premise is that the end justifies the means.

## Deontology

The second theory that is often used for ethical decision making is called deontology. This system is based on moral principles and obligations and has evolved from Judeo-Christian origins, in which duty to and respect of others are the primary considerations. Zerwekh and Claborn (1997) state the following:

> As a result of the rules and duties that the deontological approach outlines, the individual has clear direction about how to act in all situations. Right or wrong is based on one's duty or obligation to act, not on consequences of one's actions. Abortion and euthanasia are not acceptable actions because they violate the duty to respect life. Lying is never acceptable because it violates the duty to tell the truth. (p.357)

One advantage of using the deontologic approach is that the rights of each person are considered. A second advantage is that the obligation to duty and moral thinking is foremost, so the decisions are the same for similar situations. However, it may become difficult to apply the deontologic method when the consequence of the decision can be harmful to an individual. For example, the decision to maintain life for all infants regardless of the outcome may be difficult when the infant is severely deformed and will require many invasive and expensive procedures to survive in a vegetative state.

### ▶ Thinking Critically

The physician has ordered a placebo for a client who reports chronic pain. The RN assigned to this client is uncertain about the use of a placebo to treat pain. Using the ethics theories described in the preceding pages, list the advantages and disadvantages of applying the system of teleology and deontology to this situation when making a decision. Be specific regarding the impact on the client and the nurse.

Theoretically, selecting a system for ethical decision making should simplify the process. However, most of us do not necessarily use a particular theory to make an ethical decision and are influenced by many factors, not just a knowledge of ethical theory. The next part of this chapter examines factors that influence ethical decision making, and then moves to a framework for ethical decision making that incorporates the use of ethical theory and recognition of various influences.

# Factors That Influence Decision Making ▬▬▬

As you begin the process of studying ethical issues, you must recognize that many factors affect the way you think about something. Often these factors overlap or are interdependent. They also may be dynamic because in a particular situation, circumstances will influence the decision you make. The following section examines the factors that can influence ethical decision making.

## Legislative and Judicial Factors

The impact of societal thinking and the resulting legislative and judicial decisions have an obvious impact on the ethical decision making process. For example, the issue of declaring death has been a dilemma in relation to technologic advances. Formerly, the loss of cardiac and respiratory function was the deciding determinant for death. However, with greater abilities to maintain cardiac and respiratory function, medicine and society were compelled to redefine death. This resulted in the concept of brain death, which includes unreceptivity and unresponsiveness, a lack of movements or breathing, no reflexes, and a flat electroencephalogram reading. This definition is widely accepted by most states. The ethical issue for many nurses are related to their own beliefs about the dignity of life, the harvesting of donor organs from an individual who is brain dead, and supporting the family who may be asked to make decisions. The legality of brain death issues has removed some of the uncertainties for nurses regarding ethical considerations.

## Science and Technologic Advances

In the preceding paragraph, the effect of technologic advances on ethical decisions is described. The developments in science and technology have created ethical issues that were unheard of even 10 years ago. For example, the ability to artificially impregnate a woman who is past menopause has caused some governments to consider age limitations for women to bear children. Genetic engineering is a modern phenomenon that has the potential to harm humans by genetic alteration. Fears related to this issue were only the stuff of science fiction a few years ago. These dilemmas created by science and technologies contribute to issues with which nurses are or will be involved. Often the duty to the client is obscured by the need to promote science and progress.

## Societal Influences

Chapter 2 discusses the development of moral reasoning, as theorized by Kohlberg and by Gilligan. The development of morals and values is influenced by the expectations of society. Changes in societal thinking affect a person's view of what is right and wrong. As an example, the women's movement, the gay rights movement, and the increasing call for an end to sexual harassment have had a great impact on behavior and society's views of what is acceptable. The rights of individuals have become more important; the demand for a say in a person's own care is seen as a right. Nurses and other healthcare providers are compelled to provide individualized and safe, competent care at all times. Situations that require an ethical decision may no longer seem as clear-cut as they once did.

## Healthcare Reform

The increased emphasis on cost control, shorter hospital stays, increase in client acuity, exploration of alternative healthcare provision, managed care, and other factors that are changing healthcare delivery have and will have a direct impact on ethical decision making. The discharge of clients to their homes when they are sicker and more vulnerable is of great concern. Issues related to the allocation of healthcare funds to those who need it most or who have the greatest potential to have a positive outcome also are ethically challenging. Nurses will continually face questions that make them examine their own values as they relate to providing quality care to clients and families.

## Professional Values Versus Client Values

**Values** are the beliefs and concepts that individuals and groups hold as the most meaningful in their lives. These values have their origins in family, religious, and community ideals to which one is exposed early in life. Most of us can list what we feel is most important in our lives and what principles we use to make decisions.

Professional values are beliefs in relation to the work that a person does. Some of those values do not differ from personal values, and some may derive from a person's education for a particular profession. Several values guide the decisions that nurses make. These values are also called principles of nursing ethics **(Display 16-3)**.

1. **Beneficence** is the duty to do good for the clients assigned to the nurse's care. This good includes technical competence and a humanistic and holistic approach. There may be a conflict when the nurse and the client differ about what is "good."
2. **Nonmaleficenc**e is the duty to do no intentional or unintentional harm to the client. It is difficult to discuss nonmaleficence without beneficence because the choice of treatment for a client may initially cause harm, although the outcome is potentially good. For example, a client with colon cancer undergoes a colostomy and endures the pain of surgery and the reality of a change in body image. In

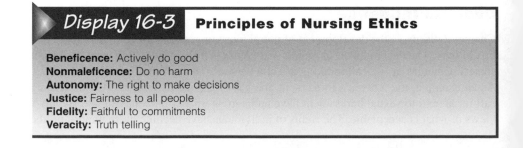

**Display 16-3** | **Principles of Nursing Ethics**

**Beneficence:** Actively do good
**Nonmaleficence:** Do no harm
**Autonomy:** The right to make decisions
**Justice:** Fairness to all people
**Fidelity:** Faithful to commitments
**Veracity:** Truth telling

addition, she agrees to have chemotherapy and radiation therapy. Although harmed in many ways, the ultimate goal is for her to be cancer free. In some instances, this may be a difficult choice if the outcome is likely to be poor despite the treatment.

3. **Autonomy** is a client's right of self-determination or a freedom to make choices and decisions without opposition. Nurses must respect the client to have this right, even if the client's decision is in direct conflict with the nurse's.

4. **Justice** is the duty to be fair to all people, regardless of their age, gender, race, or other factors. You may recall that this is the first statement in the ANA's (2001) *Code of Ethics for Nurses* (Chapter 4). A conflict may occur if there are limited healthcare resources or when fairness to one means discrimination to another.

5. **Fidelity** is the duty to maintain commitments of the professional obligations and responsibilities. This generally is defined by nurse practice acts and requires that the nurse be faithful to role constraints.

6. **Veracity** is the duty to tell the truth. The nurse is obligated to provide factual information to the client so that she or he may have autonomy. There are potential conflicts if the family or the physician withholds information from the client. The issues of beneficence and nonmaleficence can enter into this ethical conflict.

The values described previously are some of the principles that guide the decisions that nurses make. A client's values may differ totally from the RN's values. There is not necessarily a right or a wrong decision but a recognition that the client has a different value system. There also can be conflict if the client's decision will be harmful.

## Thinking Critically

Review the ANA's *Code of Ethics for Nurses* in Chapter 4. Determine the value (described in the preceding paragraphs) that is addressed by each statement. Examine the recent additions to the *Code of Ethics for Nurses* (Display 16-4). What is the impact of these new additions? Are any values not addressed? Do you feel that any should be added? Discuss this with a group of your classmates and determine if these values are the same or different for LPN/LVNs.

## NCLEX–RN Might Ask 16-1  ❓ ❓ ❓

The nurse is caring for a client with terminal cancer. The client is ready to know the truth about the prognosis of the disease, but her husband wants all healthcare workers involved to avoid talking about this illness. The nurse's duty to tell the truth in this situation is the principle of nursing ethics called

    A. nonmaleficence.
    B. beneficence.
    C. veracity.
    D. justice.

• *See Appendix A for correct answer and rationale.*

The preceding material has described some of the influences involved in ethical decision making. The awareness that many factors are involved in an ethical decision should assist you to examine ethical issues more broadly and with less bias for a particular way of thinking. Letting go of former ways of thinking and not personalizing every issue is particularly difficult. In your role transition from LPN/LVN you are increasing your responsibility and obligation to be a client advocate. The increased responsibility requires that you demonstrate a greater understanding of ethical decision making. In the next section, you have the opportunity to do some group work with ethical decision making. Use the information you have learned in the preceding pages to examine ethical dilemmas and develop strategies to make ethical decisions.

# Ethical Decision Making ▬▬▬▬▬▬▬▬▬▬▬▬▬

As implied, using ethical theories to make decisions will probably be somewhat abstract for many nurses. However, using the theories does assist in eliminating emotions from the decision-making process. Nurses have always used a problem-solving approach to provide care to clients. In the same way, a problem-solving approach can be used for ethical dilemmas and will incorporate the ethical theories described previously.

The method used to make ethical decisions generally involves the nursing process in the following steps:

1. *Assessment:* Identify the problem, and describe it. Determine what values are involved, who is involved, and who will be affected by the decision. Are there legal ramifications? Obtain as much information as possible to understand the situation.
2. *Diagnosis:* A statement of the dilemma (after looking at all the data) will assist you to see the issue as concisely as possible.
3. *Planning:* List all the possible options for solving the dilemma; do not get involved with determining the consequences at this point. This process is referred to as brainstorming. Identify any time constraints and your relationship to the situation. Examine the advantages and disadvantages of each option. Look at each option with an awareness of a teleological or deontological approach. Consider the effects on individuals for each option. Consultation with a more experienced nurse, nurse manager, or ethics committee may take place at this point. Evaluate similar cases.
4. *Implementation:* Make the decision and follow through on it.
5. *Evaluation:* Evaluate the decision in terms of effects and results. Evaluate your comfort with the decision.

Using a methodology for solving ethical dilemmas may at first be awkward for you. The following situation provides some practice for you to apply the decision-making process.

## EXAMPLE
■ Early on a Saturday evening, Patty L., a 25-year-old RN, was on her way to work a 12-hour shift at the local hospital. As she drove down a road about 2 miles from the hospital, a car came rapidly toward her, weaving from side

## NCLEX–RN Might Ask 16-2

The RN is reviewing the results of a decision-making process involving removing life support for a brain-dead child. The nurse is using the _____ step of the ethical decision-making process.

    A. assessment
    B. diagnosis
    C. planning
    D. evaluation

• *See Appendix A for correct answer and rationale.*

to side. The road was narrow and not well lit. Patty apparently tried to avoid the car, but the other driver was going very fast and was generally out of control, with his car on the wrong side of the road. The other car hit Patty's car on the driver's side, and then her car struck a telephone pole. She was killed as a result of the two impacts. The driver of the other vehicle (Billy K.) was not fatally injured but did sustain multiple orthopedic injuries and a closed head fracture and was taken to the local hospital. Blood levels revealed that he was intoxicated at the time of the accident. Local police also stated that Billy was driving without a driver's license; it had been suspended for other charges of driving while under the influence of alcohol.

Both Patty and Billy had been brought to the local emergency room. Billy was taken to surgery and then admitted to the intensive care unit. Patty's body was identified by her roommate, also a nurse, who had been working on the maternity unit. She notified Patty's family and helped to make initial arrangements for Patty's body to be moved to a funeral home in Patty's hometown. Employees at the hospital were shocked and grief stricken; even those who had not known Patty were in anguish.

Two weeks later, Billy was moved to a step-down unit on the orthopedic unit. When Brian M., RN, arrived to work for the 11 PM to 7 AM shift, he was assigned to work in the step-down unit. When he realized that he was assigned to Billy, he told the charge nurse that he refused to care for him: "I will not take care of a lousy drunk who killed a friend of mine; why did he live and she die? He should be taken out behind the hospital and shot." Brian was unaware that Billy's sister was near the telephone and heard the entire conversation. ■

You are the charge nurse. What is the best way to deal with this situation? You had assigned Brian to the care of Billy because of his expertise and because the other most experienced nurse had called in sick.

• Use the steps described for making an ethical decision.
• Write a statement for the ethical dilemma after you have identified the relevant facts for this situation. Do you need other information?

- Determine possible actions for this dilemma. Examine these choices in relation to teleology and deontology.
- What are the consequences of each action?
- What decision did you choose?
- What effect does this decision have on Billy, his sister, or the other nursing staff?
- In reviewing the ANA's (2001) *Code of Ethics for Nurses*, are there times when nurses may refuse an assignment?

There will be many ethical issues with which you as an RN may have to contend. Ellis and Hartley (2001) have categorized issues that they think are relevant to RNs in their respective practices: those that are related to commitment to the client, commitment to personal excellence, and commitment to the nursing profession as a whole (**Display 16-4**). Dealing with ethical issues is never an easy task.

> The ongoing challenge for all of us, grounded in history and tradition, is how everyday working relationships in complex health care systems can be shaped and influenced for effective and compassionate delivery of patient care and for respectful treatment of staff and employees. Respect for all persons as responsible, self-determining moral agents who are interconnected and interdependent citizens of the moral community of health care at a given point in time is fundamental. *(Aroskar, 1998, p. 323)*

## ▶ Thinking Critically

Consider other ethical issues with which you may have to deal: observing inadequate care of a client, recognizing that you lack certain skills or knowledge for the job to which you are assigned, observing a fellow nurse refusing to care for a client because that client is of a different race. Develop your own scenarios and then use the framework for ethical decision making to make a decision and carry it out. Draw on your experiences as an LPN/LVN; dilemmas that you have faced in those roles will have a different impact as you move into the RN role.

## Conclusion

This chapter emphasizes that nurses have ethical responsibilities and need to acquire ethical knowledge. Ethical issues have a direct impact on the work nurses do. The decisions are not easy and promise to get more difficult as science and technology continue

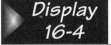

**Display 16-4** | **Additions to the Code of Ethics for Nurses**

- The nurse must be focused on the client.
- The nurse has a duty to her/himself.
- The nurse must commit to work on public policy.

to advance. Having knowledge of an ethical framework for decision making assists the nurse to make decisions and carry out actions that are acceptable personally and professionally.

When making the transition from LPN/LVN to RN, students will begin to recognize that there are ethical consequences for the work that nurses do. If the nurse practices in an unethical manner, the issues are more relevant to what is right or wrong in particular situations. The most important concern for a nurse is the rights of clients, followed by the rights and responsibilities of the nurse's colleagues.

The nursing profession will continue to be challenged by changes in ethical issues. Society will be faced with dilemmas that have no answers. The role of government in determining legal answers for ethical questions will bring forth other issues for nurses. Awareness of your personal and professional values will assist you in clarifying ethical issues. Continuing self-growth and development will further enhance your ability to deal with and to consider ethical dilemmas. Although you may hope you are never placed in a situation of conflict, it is likely to happen. Be informed. Be prepared. Be knowledgeable.

## Student Exercises

As an RN, you have been hired to be the evening supervisor in a 50-bed long-term care facility. After an orientation to the role and responsibilities, you are officially the evening charge nurse. There are two units in this agency; one unit is designated for clients with Alzheimer's disease. On each unit is one LPN/LVN to be the charge person, one certified nurse's aide (CNA) with advanced training to administer oral medications, and three CNAs to provide basic care to the clients.

1. As the RN supervisor, what do you need to know from a legal perspective to do your job? Think in terms of delegating, competencies of other personnel, and your responsibility for the care that clients receive.

2. From a legal perspective, what is your responsibility if an employee practices unsafely?

3. From an ethical perspective, what is your responsibility if an employee practices unsafely?

## References

American Nurses Association (ANA). (2001). *Code of ethics for nurses with interpretive statements.* Washington, D.C.: American Nurses Publishing.

Aroskar, M. A. (1998). Ethical working relationships in patient care: Challenges and possibilities. *Nursing Clinics of North America, 33*(2), 313–324.

Cherry, B., & Jacob, S. (2002). *Contemporary nursing: Issues, trends and management* (2nd ed.). Philadelphia: Mosby.

Ellis, J. R., & Hartley, C. L. (2001). *Nursing in today's world: Challenges, issues, and trends* (7th ed.). Philadelphia: Lippincott Williams & Wilkins.

Marquis, B., & Huston, C. (2000). *Leadership roles and management functions in nursing* (3rd ed.). Philadelphia: Lippincott Williams & Wilkins.

*Nurse's legal handbook* (4th ed.). (2000). Springhouse, PA: Springhouse Corporation.

Zerwekh, J., & Claborn, J. C. (1997). *Nursing today: Transitions and trends* (2nd ed.). Philadelphia: WB Saunders.

## Suggested Reading

Burns, N., & Grove, S. (2001). *The practice of nursing research: Conduct, critique and utilization* (4th ed.). Philadelphia: WB Saunders.

Chinn, A. (1999). Legalized physician-assisted suicide in Oregon: The first year's experience. *New England Journal of Medicine, 340*(7), 557–583.

Creasia, J. L., & Parker, B. (2001). *Conceptual foundations of professional nursing practice: The bridge to professional nursing practice* (3rd ed.). St. Louis: Mosby.

Davis, A., Aroskar, M., Liaschenko, J., & Drought, T. (1997). *Ethical dilemmas & nursing practice* (4th ed.). Stamford, CT: Appleton & Lange.

DeLaune, S. C., & Ladner, P. (2002). *Fundamentals of nursing: Standards and practice* (2nd ed.). Albany, NY: Delmar Thomson Learning.

Fowler, M. (1999). Relic or resource? The Code for Nurses. *American Journal of Nurses, 99*(3), 56–57.

Fowler, M., & Benner, P. (2001). Implementing the new Code of Ethics for Nurses: An interview with Marsha Fowler. *American Journal of Critical Care, 10*(6), 434–437.

Judson, K., & Hicks, S. (1999). *Law and ethics for medical careers* (2nd ed.). New York: Glencoe McGraw-Hill.

Hinderer, D., & Hinderer, S. (2001). *A multidisciplinary approach to health care ethics.* Mountain View, CA: Mayfield Publishing Company.

Kinsella, L. (2001). Truth telling in patient care: Resolving ethical issues. *Nursing 2001, 31*(12), 52–55.

Schwartz, J. K. (2000). Have we forgotten the patient? Evaluating the ethical dimensions for the long term. *American Journal of Nursing, 100*(2), 61–64.

Turkoski, B. (2001). Ethics in the absence of truth. *Home Healthcare Nurse, 19*(4), 218–222.

Wolfe, S. (1999). Quality vs cost. *RN, 62*(1), 28–34.

*On the Web* • • • • • • • • • • • • • • • • • • • • • • • • • • • • • • • •

*www.nora.edu*: Biomedical ethics resources

*www.acusd.edu*: Ethics of reproductive technology

*www.thehastingscenter.org*: The Hastings Center for Bioethics

*www.georgetown.edu*: Kennedy Institute of Ethics

*www.ethics.acusd.edu*: Reproductive technology, cloning, bioethics, ethics

*www.midbio.org*: Midwest Bioethics Center

*www.ccf.org/ed/bioethic/*: Cleveland Clinic Foundation on xenotransplantation

*www.advancefornurses.com/CE_Tests?ClinEthics/html*: Good article on ethical decision making

# APPENDIX A

# ANSWERS TO "NCLEX-RN MIGHT ASK" QUESTIONS

## CHAPTER 1
### NCLEX-RN Might Ask 1-1

Choice **B** is correct. *Rationale*: This is part of the conflict stage after the bliss of the honeymoon stage. Reintegration is characterized by hostility, withdrawal, and negative feelings. Resolution has four possible phases.

## CHAPTER 2
### NCLEX-RN Might Ask 2-1

Choice **C** is correct. *Rationale:* The child's identification with her peer group is making adhering to a diet difficult. Trust vs. mistrust is found in ages birth to 18 months. Industry vs. inferiority is found in the 6- to 12-year age group and involves development of motor tasks and coping skills. Intimacy vs. isolation is a job of the early adult who is developing intimate relationships.

### NCLEX-RN Might Ask 2-2

The *incorrect* choice is **D**. *Rationale:* Be careful reading this because the stem (question) is asking for an incorrect answer. The professional role is merged with both personal and professional ideas. Choices A, B, and C are acceptable according to Cohen's theory.

## CHAPTER 3
### NCLEX-RN Might Ask 3-1

Choice **B** is correct. *Rationale:* A transformational change refers to a radical difference in how a group is handled as a result of the change. This is a planned change, so C and D are incorrect. There has been no mutual agreement by the stakeholders, so A is incorrect.

### NCLEX-RN Might Ask 3-2

Choice **B** is correct. *Rationale:* A slight increase in vital signs and blood sugar are characteristic of stimulation of the sympathetic nervous system found in the alarm reaction stage. The changes are not normal and do not indicate those seen in resistance or exhaustion (which can lead to death).

### NCLEX-RN Might Ask 3-3

Choice **B** is correct. *Rationale:* Refusing to look at the site and be involved in the dressings is the BEST answer. If the client had accepted the mastectomy, she would be able to be involved in her care. Bargaining would be indicated by the client saying something like "If only I would have stopped smoking." Depression would be indicated by withdrawal behaviors.

## CHAPTER 4

### NCLEX-RN Might Ask 4-1

Choice **C** is correct. *Rationale:* Discipline, devotion, and obedience in nursing do not have ancient or religious origins.

### NCLEX-RN Might Ask 4-2

Choice **C** is correct. *Rationale:* The NLN is the only nursing association challenged with accrediting schools of nursing. The AMA is a governing body for physicians; the NSNA is a governing body for student nurses; the ANA is involved with advanced certification and continuing education credits.

## CHAPTER 5

### NCLEX-RN Might Ask 5-1

Choice **B** is correct. *Rationale:* Teaching a client how to irrigate his ostomy involves manipulating and practicing a new skill. Cognitive skills would be more about how and why the stoma functions. Affective learning would explore how the client feels about having the device and how it affects his lifestyle. Communication is not a learning domain.

### NCLEX-RN Might Ask 5-2

Choice **D** is correct. *Rationale:* Because the LPN is a student studying to be an RN, she/he is held to the level of an RN.

## CHAPTER 7

### NCLEX-RN Might Ask 7-1

Choice **A** is correct. *Rationale*: The nurse practice acts are regulations, legislated by state law. They do include permissive language. Policies and standards are proclaimed from national nursing organizations.

### NCLEX-RN Might Ask 7-2

Choice **D** is correct. *Rationale:* When the RN is working with others, she is collaborating for client care. Independence and autonomy are working and making decisions alone. In the advocacy role, the RN would be working for the client.

### NCLEX-RN Might Ask 7-3

Choice **D** is correct. *Rationale:* Only minimal safety and competency levels are demonstrated by the RN candidate when the NCLEX-RN test is successfully completed. Average, specialty, and excellent practice levels are not demonstrated by passing this examination.

## CHAPTER 8

### NCLEX-RN Might Ask 8-1

Choice **A** is the *incorrect* statement. *Rationale:* Be careful; this is asking you to identify the *wrong* answer. Critical thinking involves recognizing and overcoming feelings as a basis for decisions. It also involves exploring options, problem solving, and not letting age, culture, or personal background influence decisions.

### NCLEX-RN Might Ask 8-2

Choice **C** is correct. *Rationale:* Choice C demonstrates the student needs additional clarification. Critical thinking is based on facts and evidence and not how the student feels about a given situation.

## CHAPTER 9

### NCLEX-RN Might Ask 9-1

Choice **A** is correct. *Rationale*: You are looking for the only WRONG answer to this question. If the new nurse states that the nursing process is an extension of the medical plan, she/he needs additional help in understanding that the nursing process is independent of the medical plan. The other choices are correct and are characteristics of the nursing process.

### NCLEX-RN Might Ask 9-2

Choice **C** is correct. *Rationale:* Sleep pattern disturbance is the NANDA stem. Death of spouse is the cause, and the last two parts are sign/symptoms of a sleep pattern disturbance. Choice A has only two parts. B is correctly written but is not an actual diagnosis. D has only two parts and needs a third part that includes signs/symptoms.

### NCLEX-RN Might Ask 9-3

Choice **D** is correct. *Rationale:* Airway problems always take top priority. Choice C indicates a "risk for" diagnosis; it can wait. Choices A and B are lower in Maslow's hierarchy.

### NCLEX-RN Might Ask 9-4

Choice **B** is correct. *Rationale*: This goal stresses the immediate needs of the client in that this it is potential airway problem and needs to be corrected immediately. Choice A does not relate to the nursing diagnosis and does not have a target date. C has a target date and would be a goal, but it doesn't relate to the emergency need indicated by this client's signs and symptoms. D is an ongoing assessment for the client with this nursing diagnosis.

## CHAPTER 10

### NCLEX-RN Might Ask 10-1

Choice **D** is correct. *Rationale:* Therapeutic interaction is done for the purpose of providing safe, effective nursing care. C is only part of the reason nurses use therapeutic techniques. B may not be necessary in a professional association. One of the goals for communication is to get the client to become more independent.

### NCLEX-RN Might Ask 10-2

Choice **B** is correct. *Rationale:* Active listening techniques let the client know the nurse is interested in what the client says and in the client as an individual. Choices A and C are useful techniques for leading an interaction. Choice D is incorrect: a nurse can be professional in appearance but can be cold and uncaring.

## CHAPTER 11

### NCLEX-RN Might Ask 11-1

Choice **A** is correct. *Rationale:* Severe pain can block a client's concentration and decrease learning ability. B, C, and D are usually thought of as positive factors for effective learning.

### NCLEX-RN Might Ask 11-2

Choice **B** is correct. *Rationale:* B is the correct answer and the easiest to do in the home setting. Choice A isn't practical, costs money, and may be demeaning to the client. C and D may also make the client feel inferior.

### NCLEX-RN Might Ask 11-3

Choice **B** is correct. *Rationale:* The cause of the impaired communication is related to the client's learning need. Choices A, C, and D are correct for the nursing diagnosis but do not clearly state a learning need.

## CHAPTER 12

### NCLEX-RN Might Ask 12-1

Choice **B** is correct. *Rationale:* Choice B is more global than Choice A. Choice A is only partly right. C ignores the problem and doesn't help the nurse. D shows the nurse lacks cultural sensitivity.

### NCLEX-RN Might Ask 12-2

Choice **D** is correct. *Rationale:* Enculturation is assimilating something outside one's culture. Choices A and C are the opposite of cultural relativism.

### NCLEX-RN Might Ask 12-3

Choice **B** is correct. *Rationale:* The client speaks only Chinese. There are no data to support the etiologies of the other nursing diagnoses in this scenario.

## CHAPTER 13

### NCLEX-RN Might Ask 13-1

Choice **B** is correct. *Rationale:* The first step in any decision-making process is assessment. A is incorrect because monitoring and assessing outside the normal is not the sole responsibility of the RN. C is incorrect because the nurse needs to trust members of the healthcare team. D is incorrect because the nurse cannot assume a task is completed. He/she is responsible for the level of care.

### NCLEX-RN Might Ask 13-2

Choice **A** is correct. *Rationale:* B and C are strategies that make the nurse more efficient.

### NCLEX-RN Might Ask 13-3

Choice **B** is correct. *Rationale:* This is a problem with interpretation of the RN's assignment. There are no data to support any of the other answers.

## CHAPTER 14

### NCLEX-RN Might Ask 14-1

Choice **B** is correct. *Rationale*: This is the only answer that encompasses Leddy and Pepper's (1998) characteristics of a professional. Although traditions are important, the RN must be willing to part with them if scientific research proves that traditional practices detract from client care.

### NCLEX-RN Might Ask 14-2

Choice **C** is correct. *Rationale*: When a nurse tries to explain what the client's wishes are, she or he is acting in the role of an advocate.

## CHAPTER 15

### NCLEX-RN Might Ask 15-1

Choice **C** is correct. *Rationale*: This is an unintentional tort because it is an accident, so it would fall under common law.

### NCLEX-RN Might Ask 15-2

Choice **A** is correct. *Rationale*: The state nurse practice acts define the scope of nursing practice. Professional organizations develop standards. Hospitals and physicians need to adhere to the practice acts and standards.

### NCLEX-RN Might Ask 15-3

Choice **C** is correct. *Rationale*: To be informed comprehensively, the client needs to be informed about alternatives and about risks and benefits associated with the procedure the physician wishes to perform. A client may withdraw consent at any time. The nurse has an ethical responsibility to the client to ensure that he or she understands the physician's explanations. Not all information gained from a client involves research. A research study would require special permission from the client.

## CHAPTER 16

### NCLEX-RN Might Ask 16-1

Choice **C** is correct. *Rationale*: The nurse must tell the truth. The prognosis is something the client probably knows already but is attempting to confirm; she is ready to know if she asks. Nonmaleficence is the duty to do no harm, and beneficence is the duty to do good. Justice is fairness to all patients.

### NCLEX-RN Might Ask 16-2

Choice **D** is correct. *Rationale*: The nurse is using evaluation in reviewing results. Assessment gathers information about the problem. Diagnosis states the ethical dilemma once fact finding is completed. Planning involves looking at alternatives and deciding on choices.

# ANSWERS TO "THINKING CRITICALLY" QUESTIONS

### CHAPTER 9, PAGE 195

Review the database for Bill Akins in Display 9-3, and write actual, possible, and potential (risk) nursing diagnoses using the PES format.

1. Actual Nursing Diagnosis: Constipation *[NANDA stem]* related to bed rest *[etiology]* as manifested by abdominal cramping and absence of bowel movement in 3 days *[signs/symptoms]*
2. Possible Nursing Diagnosis: Possible Ineffective Coping (unknown etiology)
3. Potential Nursing Diagnosis: Risk for Decreased Cardiac Output *[NANDA stem]* related to decreased blood supply to the myocardium *[etiology]*

### CHAPTER 9, PAGE 199

Write goal or client outcome statements for the nursing diagnoses you developed for Bill Akins in the previous Thinking Critically activity

*Constipation:* The client will have a bowel movement within 1 day.
*Possible Ineffective Coping:* Before being discharged, the client will state three ways to decrease his stress level.
*Risk for Decreased Cardiac Output:* Within 2 days, the client will list five foods he has consumed that are high in cholesterol.

### CHAPTER 9, PAGE 201

Write nursing orders for the outcome criteria you developed for Bill Akins in the previous Thinking Critically activity. Be sure to include interventions appropriate for reassessing, doing, and teaching activities of nursing care.

*Constipation:* The client will have a bowel movement within 1 day.

**Interventions**

*Assessments:*
• Reassess the client's bowel sounds every shift.

*Measures:*
• Get client out of bed as soon as possible.
• Give client stool softener or laxative as prescribed.

*Teaching:*
• Teach client to increase fiber in diet.
• Teach client to increase fluid intake to 2 to 3 L/day.

# APPENDIX C

## NANDA NURSING DIAGNOSES 2001-2002

Activity Intolerance
Activity Intolerance, Risk for
Adjustment, Impaired
Airway Clearance, Ineffective
Allergy Response, Latex
Allergy Response, Risk for Latex
Anxiety
Anxiety, Death
Aspiration, Risk for
Attachment, Risk for Impaired
  Parent/Infant/Child
Autonomic Dysreflexia
Autonomic Dysreflexia, Risk for
Body Image, Disturbed
Body Temperature, Risk for Imbalanced
Bowel Incontinence
Breastfeeding, Effective
Breastfeeding, Ineffective
Breastfeeding, Interrupted
Breathing Pattern, Ineffective
Cardiac Output, Decreased
Caregiver Role Strain
Caregiver Role Strain, Risk for
Comfort, Impaired
Communication, Impaired Verbal
Conflict, Decisional
Conflict, Parental Role
Confusion, Acute
Confusion, Chronic
Constipation
Constipation, Perceived
Constipation, Risk for
Coping, Ineffective
Coping, Ineffective Community
Coping, Readiness for Enhanced
  Community
Coping, Defensive
Coping, Compromised Family
Coping, Disabled Family
Coping, Readiness for Enhanced Family
Denial, Ineffective
Dentition, Impaired
Development, Risk for Delayed

Diarrhea
Disuse Syndrome, Risk for
Diversional Activity, Deficient
Energy Field, Disturbed
Environmental Interpretation Syndrome,
  Impaired
Failure to Thrive, Adult
*Falls, Risk for*
Family Processes: Alcoholism,
  Dysfunctional
Family Processes: Interrupted
Fatigue
Fear
Fluid Volume, Deficient
Fluid Volume, Excess
Fluid Volume, Risk for Deficient
Fluid Volume, Risk for Imbalanced
Gas Exchange, Impaired
Grieving
Grieving, Anticipatory
Grieving, Dysfunctional
Growth and Development, Delayed
Growth, Risk for Disproportionate
Health Maintenance, Risk for Ineffective
Health-Seeking Behaviors
Home Maintenance, Impaired
Hopelessness
Hyperthermia
Hypothermia
Identity, Disturbed Personal
Incontinence, Functional Urinary
Incontinence, Reflex Urinary
Incontinence, Risk for Urge Urinary
Incontinence, Stress Urinary
Incontinence, Total Urinary
Incontinence, Urge Urinary
Infant Behavior, Disorganized
Infant Behavior, Readiness for
  Enhanced Organized
Infant Behavior, Risk for Disorganized
Infant Feeding Pattern, Ineffective
Infection, Risk for
Injury, Risk for

Injury, Risk for Perioperative-Positioning

Intracranial, Adaptive Capacity, Decreased

Knowledge, Deficient

Loneliness, Risk for

Memory, Impaired

Mobility, Impaired Bed

Mobility, Impaired Physical

Mobility, Impaired Wheelchair

Nausea

Neglect, Unilateral

Noncompliance

Nutrition: Less Than Body Requirements, Imbalanced

Nutrition: More Than Body Requirements, Imbalanced

Oral Mucous Membrane, Impaired

Pain, Acute

Pain, Chronic

Parenting, Impaired

Parenting, Risk for Imparied

Peripheral Neurovascular Dysfunction, Risk for

Poisoning, Risk for

Post-Trauma Syndrome

Post-Trauma Syndrome, Risk for

Powerlessness

*Powerlessness, Risk for*

Protection, Ineffective

Rape-Trauma Syndrome

Rape-Trauma Syndrome: Compound Reaction

Rape-Trauma Syndrome, Silent Reaction

Relocation Stress Syndrome

*Relocation Stress Syndrome, Risk for*

Role Performance, Ineffective

Self-Care Deficit

Self-Care Deficit, Bathing/Hygiene

Self-Care Deficit, Feeding

Self-Care Deficit, Toileting

Self-Esteem, Chronic Low

Self-Esteem, Situational Low

*Self-Esteem, Risk for Situational Low*

*Self-Mutilation*

Self-Mutilation, Risk for

Sensory Perception, Disturbed

Sexual Dysfunction

Sexuality Patterns, Ineffective

Skin Integrity, Impaired

Skin Integrity, Risk for Impaired

Sleep Deprivation

Sleep Pattern, Disturbed

Social Interaction, Impaired

Social Isolation

Sorrow, Chronic

Spiritual Distress

Spiritual Distress, Risk for

Spiritual Well-Being, Readiness for Enhanced

Suffocation, Risk for

*Suicide, Risk for*

Surgical Recovery, Delayed

Swallowing, Impaired

Therapeutic Regimen Management, Effective

Therapeutic Regimen Management, Ineffective

Therapeutic Regimen Management, Ineffective Community

Therapeutic Regimen Management, Ineffective Family

Thermoregulation, Ineffective

Thought Processes, Disturbed

Tissue Perfusion, Ineffective

Transfer Ability, Impaired

Trauma, Risk for

Urinary Elimination, Impaired

Urinary Retention

Ventilation, Impaired Spontaneous

Ventilatory Weaning Response, Dysfunctional (DVWR)

Violence, Risk for Other-Directed

Violence, Risk for Self-Directed

Walking, Impaired

*Wandering*

---

*Italicized diagnoses* are the most recent additions.

Copyright © 2001 by the North American Nursing Diagnosis Association.

# Index

Note: Page numbers followed by d indicate displays; those followed by f indicate figures; those followed by t indicate tables.

## A

AACN (American Association of Critical Care Nurses), standards of practice established by, 143
Abstract conceptualization, 12d
Accommodation, for conflict resolution, 51, 275–276
Accountability, 306–308, 307d
  in delegation, 269d, 269–270
  as responsibility of RNs, 293
Acquired immunodeficiency syndrome (AIDS), nursing profession and, 96
Active experimentation, 12d
Active learning, 107–108, 110–111
Active listening, 212
Administrative law, 305
ADN(s). *See* ADN education; Associate degree nurses (ADNs)
ADN education, 93, 103–108
  curricular content and learning domains for, 104–105
  curricular framework for, 104, 104d
  learning achievement levels for, 105, 106d
  learning process and, 106–108
  nursing process and nursing diagnosis and, 106, 107t
  philosophy and conceptual model for, 103–104
Adolescents, communication with, 221
Adult learner characteristics, assessment of, 125
Adult learning theory, 101–103, 102d

Advance directives, 311–312
Advice giving, 217
Affective domain, 104
  stimulating thinking and, 111
African Americans, in nursing, 84
Age. *See also specific age groups*
  as barrier to re-entry, 5
  learning and, 108–109, 110, 110d
Aging of population, nursing profession and, 95–96
AIDS (acquired immunodeficiency syndrome), nursing profession and, 96
Alarm reaction, 63
Ambivalence, about change, 64–65
American Academy of Nursing, 86–87
American Association of Critical Care Nurses (AACN), standards of practice established by, 143
*American Journal of Nursing,* 86
  founding of, 84
American Nurses Association (ANA), 85–87
  *Code for Nurses* of, 90, 91d, 287, 298t, 299, 318
  criteria for measurable outcomes of, 198, 198d
  *Nursing: A Social Policy Statement* of, 143, 295
  *The Nursing Practice Act: Suggested State Legislation* of, 144
  *Scope and Standards of Practice for Nursing Professional Development* of, 4–5
  *Social Policy Statement* of, 90

## M